Essential
Dermatopathology

Essential Dermatopathology

Sara Edward, MBBS, FRCPath, Dip Dermpath

Consultant Dermatopathologist
St James's University Hospital
Leeds, United Kingdom

Anthony Yung, MB, ChB, FRACP

Consultant Dermatologist
Waikato Hospital
Hamilton, New Zealand

Wolters Kluwer | Lippincott Williams & Wilkins
Health

Philadelphia • Baltimore • New York • London
Buenos Aires • Hong Kong • Sydney • Tokyo

Senior Executive Editor: Jonathan W. Pine, Jr.
Product Manager: Marian Bellus
Vendor Manager: Alicia Jackson
Senior Manufacturing Manager: Benjamin Rivera
Senior Marketing Manager: Angela Panetta
Designer: Teresa Mallon
Production Service: Aptara, Inc.

Printed in the People's Republic of China.

Library of Congress Cataloging-in-Publication Data

Edward, Sara.
  Essential dermatopathology / Sara Edward, Anthony Yung.
       p. ; cm.
  Includes bibliographical references and index.
   ISBN 978-1-60831-276-4 (alk. paper)
  1. Skin–Diseases–Handbooks, manuals, etc.   I. Yung, Anthony.   II. Title.
   [DNLM: 1. Skin Diseases–Handbooks. 2. Skin Physiological Phenomena–Handbooks.   WR 39]
   RL96.E295 2011
   616.5–dc22

                              2011008578

Care has been taken to confirm the accuracy of the information presented and to describe generally accepted practices. However, the authors, editors, and publisher are not responsible for errors or omissions or for any consequences from application of the information in this book and make no warranty, expressed or implied, with respect to the currency, completeness, or accuracy of the contents of the publication. Application of this information in a particular situation remains the professional responsibility of the practitioner; the clinical treatments described and recommended may not be considered absolute and universal recommendations.

The authors, editors, and publisher have exerted every effort to ensure that drug selection and dosage set forth in this text are in accordance with the current recommendations and practice at the time of publication. However, in view of ongoing research, changes in government regulations, and the constant flow of information relating to drug therapy and drug reactions, the reader is urged to check the package insert for each drug for any change in indications and dosage and for added warnings and precautions. This is particularly important when the recommended agent is a new or infrequently employed drug.

Some drugs and medical devices presented in this publication have Food and Drug Administration (FDA) clearance for limited use in restricted research settings. It is the responsibility of the health care provider to ascertain the FDA status of each drug or device planned for use in his or her clinical practice.

Visit Lippincott Williams & Wilkins on the Internet at: LWW.COM. Lippincott Williams & Wilkins customer service representatives are available from 8:30 am to 6 pm, EST.

9 8 7 6 5 4 3 2 1

To my parents for giving me everything in life.

To my husband, Sathish, for all things and everything, but especially for those flashes of inspiration that helped me on many occasions while writing this book.

To my daughters Diana and Sherin, for whom I am now free to cook dinners when they come back home from university.

SARA EDWARD

This book is dedicated to my wife Angela and my children Deborah and Olivia, whose patience and understanding allowed this book to become a reality.

ANTHONY YUNG

Foreword

Dermatology is a very difficult subject to teach. There are many different rashes and numerous types of lumps and bumps, and their recognition requires refined pattern recognition skills, aptitude, and experience. It is a clinical art. Dr. Yung is truly a dermatological "artist," having encyclopedic knowledge and a unique ability to combine that knowledge with clinical experience. My experience of him is that he is a unique clinician. Being a unique clinician does not necessarily translate into being a good teacher, but in the case of Dr. Yung, it does. In this book he has made a very special contribution to dermatology.

The dermatopathologist is also a specialized clinician and, in some ways, dermatopathologists and dermatologists require similar skills related to the ability to put together subtle differences in patterns in the skin. Dr. Edward shares with Dr. Yung a passion for dermatology and a talent for teaching. Putting them together in developing this book is inspired! I think *Essential Dermatopathology* will prove to be an essential book for all dermatologists and dermatopathologists.

Prof. Julia Newton-Bishop
Professor of Dermatology
St. James's University Hospital,
Leeds, United Kingdom

As new therapies have emerged in dermatology, the complications of many of these drugs have led to various complicated cutaneous eruptions. Furthermore, as more and more biopsies are being performed for lesions of all sorts, there has arisen a need for very clear dermatopathologic descriptions of various lymphomas, soft tissue tumors, and infections in the skin. As the specialty of dermatopathology evolves, the need for a clear text that describes the histopathology of the skin is critical. The content of *Essential Dermatopathology* forms a guide to very carefully described information that is of use and will be of interest to dermatologists, dermatopathologists, pathologist, students, and residents.

Dr. Edward has utilized her vast experience in dermatopathology to present very clearly from chapter to chapter, the variety of diseases one encounters and describes not only how they are diagnosed but also their important differential diagnoses. The need for such a book is great in the community. It will serve as a *vade mecum* for the medical profession involved in skin disease. I congratulate Dr. Edward on her efforts in presenting this wonderful new addition to the armamentarium of books describing dermatopathology and its fascinating, multiple presentations in the skin.

Prof. Martin Mihm Jr.
Professor of Dermatology and
Dermatopathology
Harvard Medical School
Boston, USA

There are many people at St James's University Hospital to whom I owe much and without whose help this book would have been nearly impossible:

All the staff in the histopathology laboratory who prepared the excellent tissue sections used in this book.

Martin Waterhouse and Michael Hale who have been unsparing in their time and commitment in the preparation of the digital images.

Silke Weischede, Mike Parsons, Paul Bennett, and Thomas Heaton for contributing to sections of the manuscript.

Steve Toms and Michael Todd who have always been obliging at short notice when I needed help with the images.

Finally to Jonathan Pine, Marian Bellus, and the team at Lippincott Williams & Wilkins without whose support and guidance this book would have remained just a dream.

Sara Edward

I am indebted to all the many dermatologists and dermatopathologists who have inspired and taught me in New Zealand and in the United Kingdom.

Thanks to all those who gave me the chance to work at the Leeds General Infirmary and St James's University Hospital in Leeds, United Kingdom.

A special thanks to Sara who has been the cornerstone for this project throughout. Thanks for convincing me that this project should become a book and working so hard to make it a reality. Without you this project would not have come to fruition.

A special mention also goes to the contribution of Jonathan Pine, Marian Bellus, and the whole production team at Lippincott Williams & Wilkins, whose patience and hard work have made this book possible.

Anthony Yung

Dermatopathology can be a daunting field to learn and understand. The innumerable disease processes and descriptive terminologies can make pursuit of knowledge in dermatopathology an arduous task. In *Essential Dermatopathology*, we have endeavored to break down the vast expanse of this subject into logical, smaller, and more manageable pieces, starting from the very basic level and building in level upon level of information to make the subject easier to grasp.

Dermatopathology is a very visually specialized field, so we felt it only right that we provide high quality images to help in the learning process—after all "a picture is worth a thousand words." This book in no way replaces the knowledge and information obtained by learning and being taught at the microscope or by viewing the many thousands of microscopic skin specimens that one needs to see in order to become proficient at reading dermatopathology specimens. We hope this book will serve as a helpful quick reference and an *aide-memoire* in facilitating the understanding of dermatopathology.

Sara Edward
United Kingdom

Anthony Yung
New Zealand

Contents

Structure of Skin and Regional Differences

INTRODUCTION

Skin is the largest organ in the body. It is unique not only in its size but also in various structures within it. The myriad of clinical and pathological features that a dermatologist and dermatopathologist faces on a day-to-day basis is again a reflection of the variability of its structure and the complexity of the immune system within the skin. Inter-racial variation of the skin and regional variations in the structure and physiology of the skin contribute significantly to the clinical presentation and histopathological appearance of skin conditions. Many skin conditions evolve in the clinical appearances with time (and with treatment). As as result there can be marked differences in the histological appearances of skin disease clinically and histologically, depending on the time at which a condition is seen and biopsied.

It is of paramount importance to understand the basic structure of skin in addition to knowing the site-specific variations seen in different parts of the body.

NORMAL SKIN

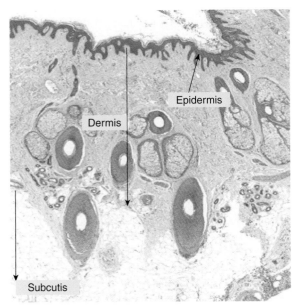

FIGURE 1.1   Normal Skin

Normal skin is composed of
- the epidermis (an epithelial layer),
- the dermis, consists mainly of thick bundles of collagen fibers running parallel to the epidermis, and
- the subcutis (or subcutaneous fat).

Deep layers: fascia, muscle, and bone lie below the subcutis.

EPIDERMIS

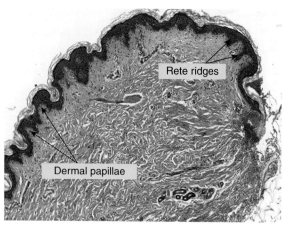

FIGURE 1.2   Epidermis

The epidermis undulates to form projections (rete ridges) into the superficial dermal layer (or papillary dermis). The "fingers" of dermis between the rete ridges are called "dermal papilla." They contain blood vessels and papillary dermal collagen. The thin layer of epidermis overlying the dermal papilla is called the "supra papillary plate." The prominence of the rete ridge pattern varies from region to region of the body.

LAYERS OF EPIDERMIS

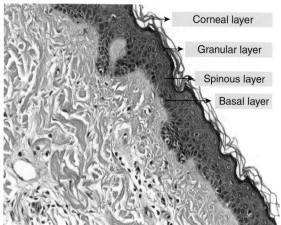

FIGURE 1.3   Layers of Epidermis

The epidermis consists of four layers:

1. Stratum corneum (or horny layer)—the most superficial layer
2. Stratum granulosum (or granular layer)
3. Stratum spinulosum (or spinous layer)
4. Stratum basale (or basal layer)—deepest layer that sits on basement membrane.

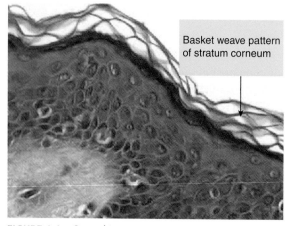

FIGURE 1.4   Corneal Layer

Corneal Layer

The keratinocytes of the stratum corneum (or cornified layer) are dark, compact, and lack nuclei. The cells form a "basket weave" arrangement. These cells are the most differentiated of the keratinizing system. They are eventually shed from the skin surface.

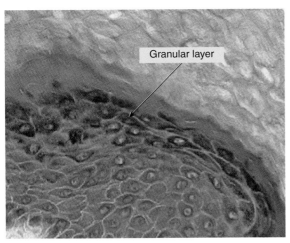

FIGURE 1.5   Granular Layer

Granular Layer

The keratinocytes of the granular cell layer are filled with basophilic (bluish coloured with haematoxylin & eosin staining) granules called "keratohyaline" granules.

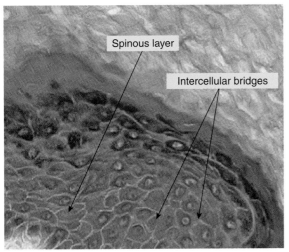

FIGURE 1.6   Spinous Layer

Spinous Layer

The keratinocytes of the spinous layer are large polygonal-shaped cells with a pinkish (eosinophilic) cytoplasm when stained with haematoxylin & eosin. The cytoplasm contains abundant keratin. The cells have characteristic "spines" that are intercellular bridges between the keratinocytes. Hence, this layer is also called the "prickle-cell layer." The intercellular bridges are the result of retraction of plasma membrane during processing while the desmosomes in between the cells remain intact.

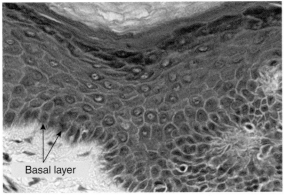

FIGURE 1.7   Basal Layer

Basal Layer

Basal cell keratinocytes consist of a single layer of cuboidal cells which sit along the basement membrane. These cells have large nuclei and a slightly bluish (basophilic) cytoplasm when stained with haematoxylin & eosin. They are mitotically active and contain melanin pigment transferred from adjacent melanocytes.

BASEMENT MEMBRANE OF THE SKIN

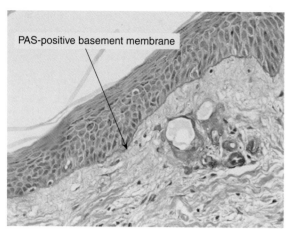

PAS-positive basement membrane

FIGURE 1.8   Basement Membrane of the Skin

The basement membrane is the thin extracellular matrix which separates the epidermis from the underlying dermis. It is composed of three layers: the lamina lucida, the lamina densa, and the sub-lamina densa (these layers can be identified only on electron microscopy).

The basal cells adhere to the basement membrane and the basement adheres to the dermis via a complex series of interactions between large molecules found on the basal cell membrane of the basal keratinocytes (called "hemidesmosomes"), basement membrane proteins, anchoring filaments, laminins, uncein, fibronectin, type IV collagen, and the anchoring fibrils (composed of type VII collagen) which arise in the dermis and traverse into the lower regions of the basement membrane.

MELANOCYTES

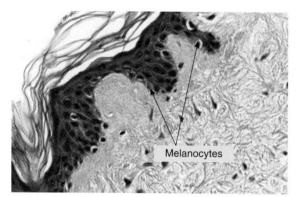

Melanocytes

FIGURE 1.9   Melanocytes

Melanocytes are derived from the neural crest and are seen as cells with a perinuclear halo along the basal layer of the epidermis. There are approximately 1:4-1:9 melanocytes per basal keratinocyte. The synthesis of melanin takes place within melanosomes that are transferred from the neural crest. Melanosomes transform to melanocytes when they reach the basal layer of the epidermis. The melanin is ultimately transferred to the basal keratinocytes by a process of pigment donation. The melanocytes have the important role of protecting the skin from nonionizing ultraviolet radiation.

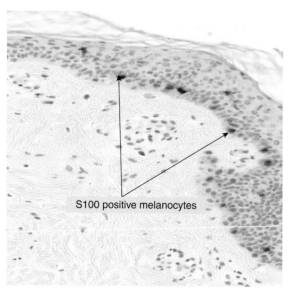

S100 positive melanocytes

FIGURE 1.10   Melanocyte Staining with S100

Melanocyte Staining with S100

Melanocytes located in the basal layer stain brown with S100 protein—an immunohistochemical stain that is highly sensitive but not specific for melanocytes.

MERKEL CELLS

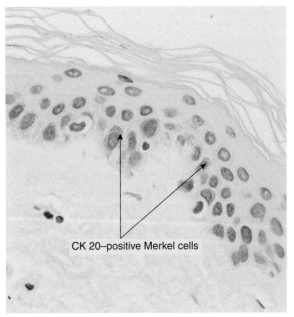

FIGURE 1.11   Merkel Cells Located in the Basal Layer

Merkel Cells Located in the Basal Layer

Merkel cells are difficult to visualize with haematoxylin & eosin staining in normal skin and are demonstrated more easily in Merkel cell carcinoma arising in the skin. Merkel cells can be visualized if the specimen is stained with immunohistochemical stains for cytokeratin 20 and Cam 5.2 (paranuclear dot-like staining is seen). The Merkel cell is a neuroendocrine cell whose function in the skin is unknown but is postulated to mediate tactile function.

LANGERHANS CELLS

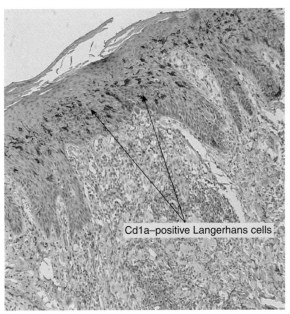

FIGURE 1.12   Langerhans Cells

Langerhans cells belong to the dendritic cell lineage but can appear anywhere in the epidermis. Langerhans cells are better visualized with immunohistochemical stains which stain for S100 and CD1a antibodies (seen as the brown staining cells in the image). Under the electron microscope they contain the characteristic Birbeck granules. Birbeck granules are rod-shaped organelles having a centrally striated density and an occasional bulb at one end.

DERMIS

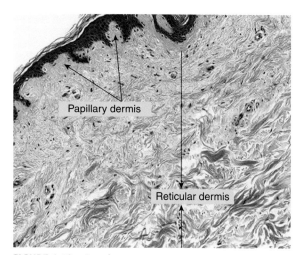

FIGURE 1.13   Dermis

The dermis is the layer immediately below the epidermis and basement membrane. It contains the components, which give the skin its mechanical properties such as strength (collagen fibers) and elasticity (elastin fibers). The superficial dermis is called the "papillary dermis" and the deeper dermal layer is called the "reticular dermis."

Papillary dermis and the reticular dermis differ in the thickness of the collagen fibers present. The relative proportion of the papillary dermis and reticular dermis varies from site to site.

The major components of the dermis are

- collagen fibers (Collagen I and small amounts of Collagen III),
- elastic fibers,
- ground substance (glycosaminoglycans or acid mucopolysaccharides), and
- other substances: hyaluronic acid, chondroitin-4-sulphate, and dermatan sulphate.

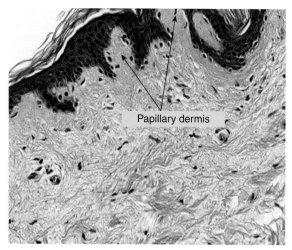

FIGURE 1.14   Papillary Dermis

Papillary Dermis

The collagen fibers of the papillary dermis consist of fine bundles of mainly Type I collagen fibers mixed with some Type III collagen fibers. They tend to be vertically orientated and contain the capillaries of the superficial plexus and fibroblasts.

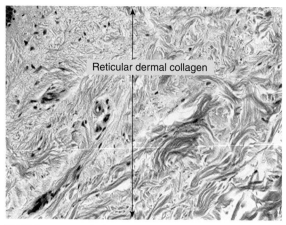

FIGURE 1.15   Reticular Dermis

Reticular Dermis

The collagen of reticular dermis is thicker and arranged parallel to the overlying epidermis. It is predominantly Type I collagen.

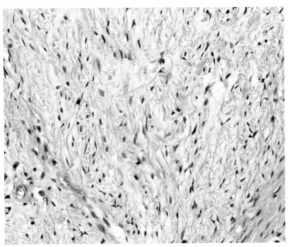

FIGURE 1.16   Fibroblasts

Fibroblasts

- Fibroblasts are cells with spindle-shaped nuclei haphazardly arranged in the dermis. Fibroblasts produce collagen which is the major constituent of extracellular matrix. There are 2 genetically distinct type of antibodies recognized, which are Type I and Type III.

- Type I and Type III collagens are the main constituents of the dermis. Type IV collagen is a major component of the basement membrane.

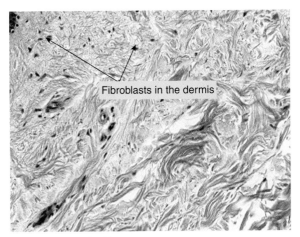

FIGURE 1.17   Fibroblasts

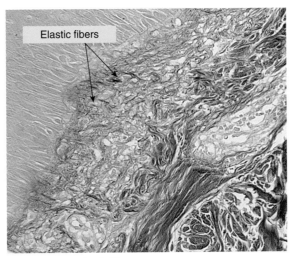

FIGURE 1.18   Elastic Fibers

Elastic Fibers

- Elastic fibers are a minor constituent of dermis. Elastic fibers are composed of elastin which are produced by fibroblasts.

- Elastic fibers consist of fine fibers in the papillary dermis, coarser fibers in the reticular dermis.

- Elastic fibers are best demonstrated by the use of Verhoeff's elastic van Gieson stain.

- On H&E sections they appear bluish in color.

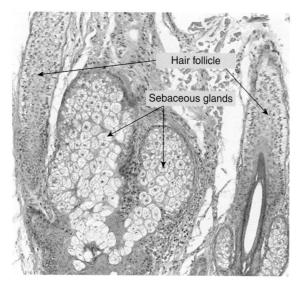

FIGURE 1.19   Sebaceous Glands

Sebaceous Glands

- Oil-producing glands associated with hair follicles.
- Most numerous on face, nose, scalp, midline of back, areola, and buccal and lip mucosa.
- Fordyce's spots in labial mucosa, Tyson glands in prepuce and Meibomian glands in eyelids are examples. They are absent in palms and soles.
- The cells of sebaceous glands are called sebocytes. The sebocytes are arranged in lobular or multilobulated aggregations and open into the hair follicle at the infundibulum region of the hair follicle.

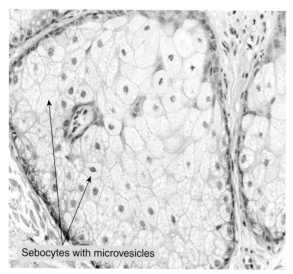

FIGURE 1.20   Sebaceous Glands

Sebaceous Glands

Sebocytes vary in size and are permanently linked to interlobular duct. The peripheral cells are flattened and have compressed nuclei whereas the central cells have rounded central nuclei and abundant vacuolated cytoplasm. The cytoplasm is rich in lipids and may be stained on frozen sections with Sudan 111 and 1V or Oil Red O.

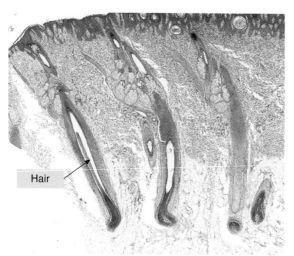

FIGURE 1.21   Hair Follicle

Hair Follicle

- The hair follicle has four parts.
  - The ostium which opens to the surface of the epidermis.
  - The infundibulum which extends from the ostium to the opening of the sebaceous glands.
  - The isthmus which extends from the opening of the sebaceous glands to the attachment of the arrector pili muscle.
  - The hair bulb which is normally located in the subcutaneous fat.
- Hair bulb is formed of the dermal papilla and collection of actively growing cells of the matrix.

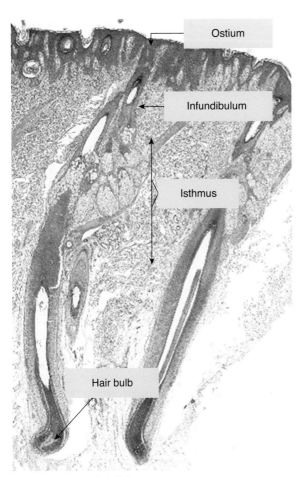

FIGURE 1.22 Hair Follicle

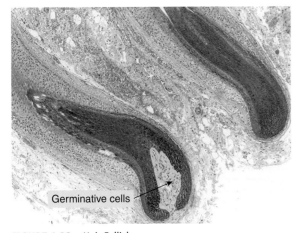

FIGURE 1.23 Hair Follicle

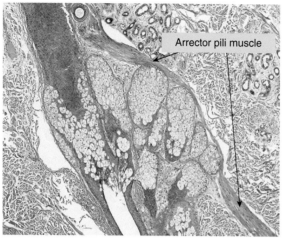

FIGURE 1.24   Arrector Pili Muscle

Arrector Pili Muscle

This is smooth muscle and is responsible for movement of hair and response to changes in temperature.

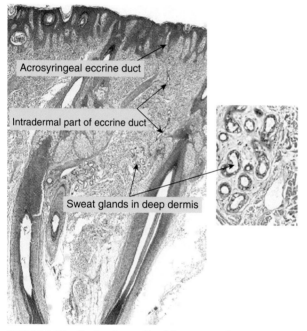

FIGURE 1.25   Eccrine Sweat Gland Secretory Coil

Eccrine Sweat Gland Secretory Coil

Eccrine sweat glands and are responsible for thermoregulation. They have secretory (coiled section) and excretory (ductal section) function. The transition between the secretory and excretory regions is very abrupt.

Eccrine sweat glands are seen in high concentration in the palms and soles, forehead and axillae.

- Eccrine sweat glands consist of three sections:
  - Coiled secretory gland found at the interface of reticular dermis and subcutis. The coiled secretory gland and intradermal ducts are surrounded by myoepithelial cells which are contractile cells involved with the secretion and transport of the sweat to the surface of the epithelium.
  - Intradermal duct coils which spiral toward the surface.
  - Intraepidermal component (also called the "acrosyringium").

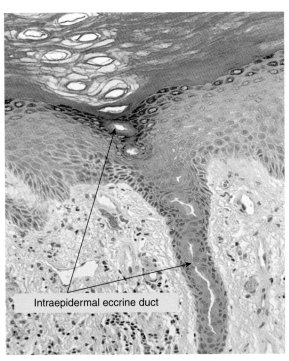

Intraepidermal eccrine duct

FIGURE 1.26   Eccrine Gland Intraepidermal Part

The intra epidermal part of the eccrine duct is called the Acrosyringium. The duct is lined by keratinocytes which are smaller than the keratinocytes of the epidermis. Eccrine poroma arises from the intra epidermal part of the eccrine duct.

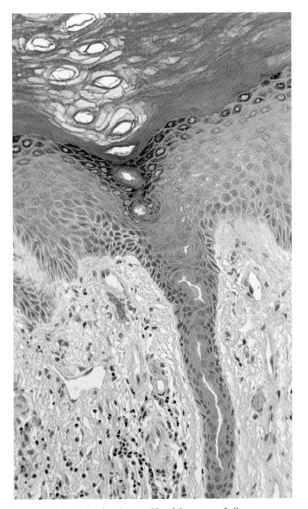

FIGURE 1.27   Eccrine Sweat Gland Secretory Coil

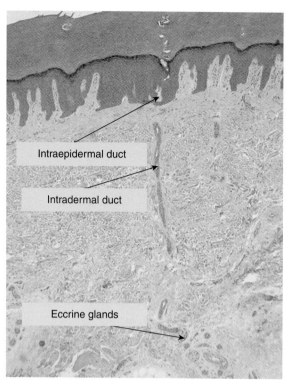

FIGURE 1.28   Eccrine Sweat Gland Secretory Coil

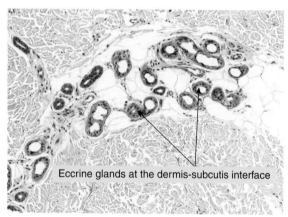

FIGURE 1.29   Eccrine Sweat Gland Secretory Coil

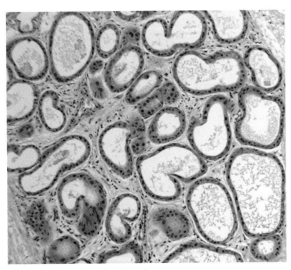

FIGURE 1.30   Apocrine Glands

Apocrine Glands

- Apocine glands occur most numerously in the axillae, groin, and anogenital region.

- Apocrine glands consist of a secretory component (coiled) and an intradermal duct (excretory) which opens into an orifice just above the sebaceous duct orifice in the hair follicle.

- The secretory coils are located in the subcutaneous fat and are lined by a layer of cuboidal cells and an outer myoepithelial layer. In addition, there is a luminal layer of cells which has abundant eosinophilic cytoplasm and a large nucleus located at the base.

- Apocrine cells exhibit characteristic apocrine "snouts" which are the decapitated secretions. The excretory components of apocirne glands do not have myoepithelial cells.

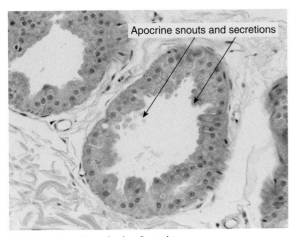

FIGURE 1.31   Decapitation Secretion

Decapitation Secretion

Apocrine cells secrete by "decapitation" secretion (small buds of the surface of apocrine cells pinch off into the lumen). The cells have abundant eosinophilic cytoplasm on staining with haematoxylin & eosin and basally located nuclei.

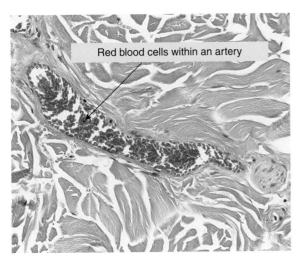

FIGURE 1.32   Arteries and Arterioles

Arteries and Arterioles

Arteries and arterioles are characterized by

- thick-walled vessels containing smooth muscle and an internal flattended endothelial cells lining the lumen of the vessel. Arteries and arterioles have small luminal diameter. Larger arterial and arteriolar vessels having internal elastic lamina with elastic fibres presnt in the vessel wall which can be demonstrated with Verhoeff's elastic van Gieson (EVG) stain.

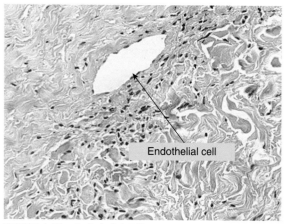

FIGURE 1.33   Endothelial Cells

Endothelial Cells

Endothelial cells are flattened cuboidal cells lining arteries.

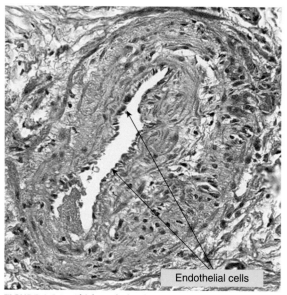

FIGURE 1.34   Thickened Blood Vessel

Thickened Blood Vessel

Thick walled blood vessel:

- Lined by endothelial cells internally.
- Larger vessels have smooth muscle in their wall. An internal elastic lamina may be present in the arterial wall.

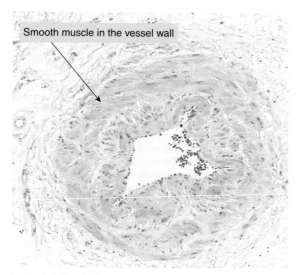

FIGURE 1.35   Vein

Vein

Veins are characterized by large luminal diameter and thin wall with a smooth muscle media. They do not have an elastic lamina.

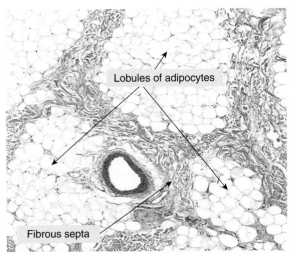

FIGURE 1.36   Subcutaneous Tissue

Subcutaneous Tissue

- The subcutis is the deepest layer of the skin and consists mainly of adipose or fat tissue.
- The components of the subcutis are
  - deepest portions of the appendageal structures in some sites (e.g., hair follicles),
  - fat cells arranged in aggregations called "lobules," and
  - fibrous "septa" which contain the
    - stroma
    - blood vessels (veins and arteries) and nerves

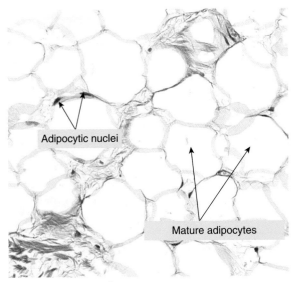

FIGURE 1.37   Fat Cells

Adipocytes (or fat cells)

Adipocytes are "signet ring"–shaped cells with eccentric nucleus, and cytoplasm filled with fat which is dissolved on normal haematoxylin & eosin staining/processing, leaving an empty appearance to the cells. Discrete collections of fat cells form a "lobule."

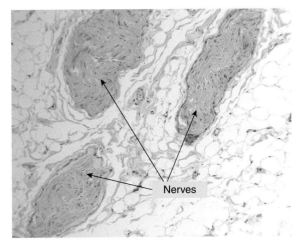

FIGURE 1.38   Nerve Cells

Nerve Fibers

Nerves consist of bundles of nerve fibers which are surrounded by fine collagen fibers (or endoneurium). The fibrous capsule surrounding the nerve bundle is called the "perineurium." Nerve fibers are positive for S100 and the perineurium is positive for EMA (epithelial membrane antigen), a glycoprotein found in normal epithelium, and also in the perineurial cells surrounding nerve fibers.

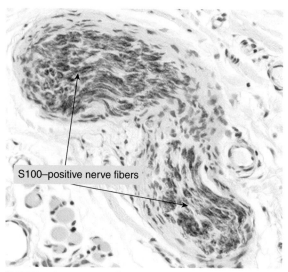

S100–positive nerve fibers

FIGURE 1.39   Nerve Cells

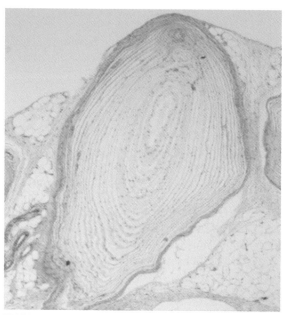

FIGURE 1.40   Pacinian Corpuscle

Pacinian Corpuscle

Pacinian corpuscles are neural structures which are responsible for the detection of pressure and vibrations sense. They lie deep in the deep dermis and subcutis, and most commonly seen on digits, and on the palms and soles. They have an "onion ring"–like appearances.

SCALP SKIN

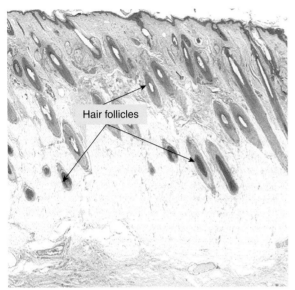

The characteristic feature of the scalp is the numerous hair follicles arising in the subcutis and exiting via follicular openings in the epidermis. Hair follicles consist of specialized invaginations of the epithelium.

FIGURE 1.41   Scalp Skin

SKIN OF LIP

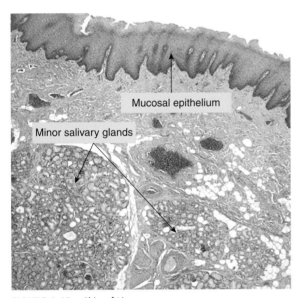

Skin from the lip is characterized by stratified squamous epithelium; however, unlike the epidermis, no keratin formation or granular layer is seen. The spinous layer of the epithelium of the lip may be vacuolated.

FIGURE 1.42   Skin of Lip

SKIN OF EYELID

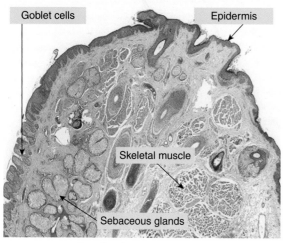

FIGURE 1.43   Skin of Eyelid

Eyelid skin is characterized by

- Two epithelial surfaces—conjunctival epithelium and cutaneous epidermis.
- The conjunctival epithelium is pseudostratified squamous epithelium type and contains vacuolated cells called "goblet cells."
- Prominent Meibomian glands (modified sebaceous glands) and orbicularis oculi muscle are seen in the dermis.

SKIN OF EAR

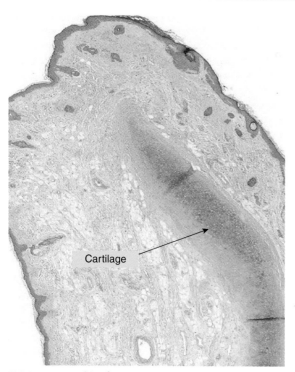

FIGURE 1.44   Skin of Ear

Skin from ear:

> The skin of the ear is characterized by a dual layer of normal epidermis and dermis with cartilage between the two layers of epidermis. Many vellous hairs may be found in the skin of ear.

SKIN OF NIPPLE

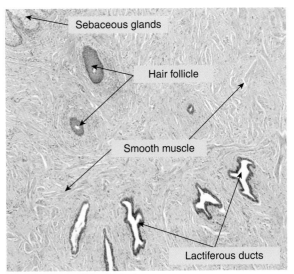

FIGURE 1.45   Skin of Nipple

Skin from the nipple is characterized by a papillomatous (warty, undulating) epidermis, lactiferous ducts, and abundant smooth muscle fibers in the dermis.

SKIN OF AXILLA

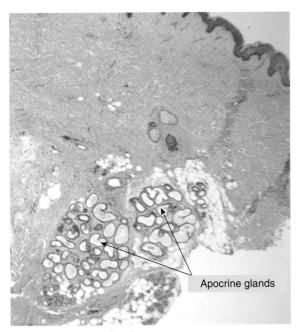

FIGURE 1.46   Skin of Axilla

Axillary skin is characterized by the presence of a papillomatous (thickened and undulating) epidermal layer, abundant hair follicles, and numerous apocrine glands present.

SKIN OF BACK

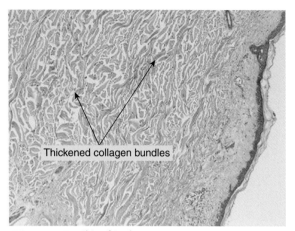

FIGURE 1.47   Skin of Back

Skin from the back is characterized by a normal thickness epidermal layer with a markedly thickened layer of collagen fibers in the dermis.

SKIN OF VULVA

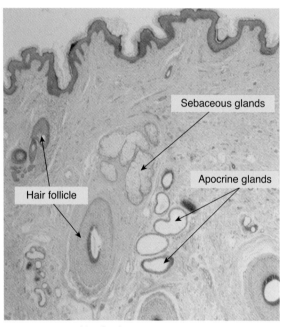

FIGURE 1.48   Skin of Vulva

The vulvar epithelium is stratified squamous epithelium. The superficial layers may be vacuolated. The sebaceous glands of the vulva open to the epidermal surface in some regions of the vulva. There is variable presence of granular layer in different regions of the vulva.

SKIN OF VULVA

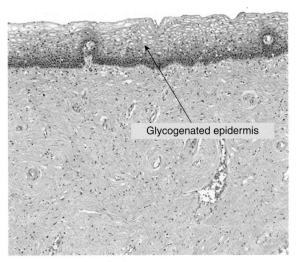

FIGURE 1.49   Skin of Vulva

LOWER LEG SKIN

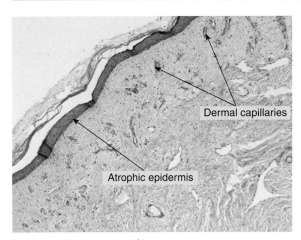

FIGURE 1.50   Lower Leg Skin

Lower leg skin is characterized by a thinner epidermis with less prominent rete ridge formation, multiple thin-walled small vessels in the dermis, often with red cell extravasation, and hemosiderin deposition.

ACRAL SKIN

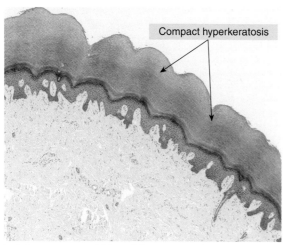

Compact hyperkeratosis

FIGURE 1.51   Acral (Skin of the Extremities) Skin

Acral site (e.g., sole and palms) skin is characterized by very thick stratum corneum (or "compact orthokeratosis"), prominent ridging pattern of epidermis, a dense dermis and the presence of numerous eccrine sweat glands at the junction of reticular dermis and subcutis.

BIBLIOGRAPHY

Mills SE, Carter D, Greenson JK, Reuter VE, Stoler MH, eds. Sternberg's Histology for Pathologists, 4th Ed. Philadelphia: Lippincott Williams & Wilkins, 2010.

Mooi W, Krausz T. Pathology of Melanocytic Disorders, 2nd Ed. New York: Oxford University Press, 2007.

Weedon D. Skin Pathology, 3rd Ed. New York: Churchill Livingstone, 2010.

The Cell Types and Other Structures

INTRODUCTION

This chapter aims to describe the different cells and structures which are encountered while assessing a skin biopsy. The cells are normal constituents of the epidermis and dermis or some of them may be found in blood vessels. Other structures and deposits which are not normal constituents of skin but encountered in different pathological processes are also described.

RED BLOOD CELLS

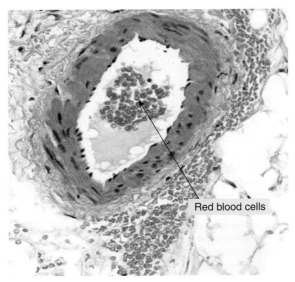

Red blood cells

FIGURE 2.1   Red Blood Cells

Red blood cells originate in the bone marrow from precursor cells called "erythroblasts." They are nonnucleated and appear pink-red in color on H&E staining. They are circular in shape and have an average diameter of 7.2 microns. Red blood cells contain hemoglobin which gives the red color to blood.

LYMPHOCYTES

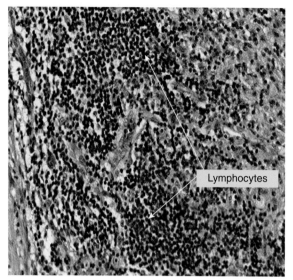

Lymphocytes originate from the hemopoietic stem cells in the bone marrow which differentiate toward the lymphoid stem cells. They are broadly classified into B and T lymphocytes which are generated from B cell and T cell progenitors. The maturation of the B and T lymphocytes happens within the microenvironment of the bone marrow. The mature B lymphocytes travel via the bloodstream into the B cell zone of the peripheral lymphoid tissue. The T cell precursors, however, migrate to the thymus via the bloodstream. The maturation occurs in the thymus and ultimately the mature T cells travel through the bloodstream to the T cell zone of the peripheral lymphoid organs. Lymphocytes are considered chronic inflammatory cells and have specific immunohistochemical staining properties (see Chapter 6).

FIGURE 2.2   Lymphocytes

EOSINOPHILS

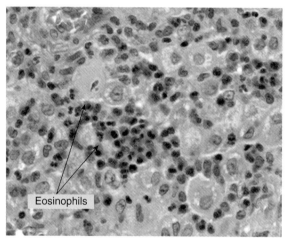

Eosinophils are derived from the stem cells of the bone marrow. They go through stages of maturation from the promyelocytes to the myelocytes and mature eosinophils. The mature eosinophils have bilobed nuclei and orange-red granules in their cytoplasm. The granules of eosinophils have cationic proteins and zinc-rich major basic protein. The eosinophils degranulate to release major basic proteins which contain histamine and histaminase which are involved with hypersensitivity reactions.

FIGURE 2.3   Eosinophils

FIBROBLASTS

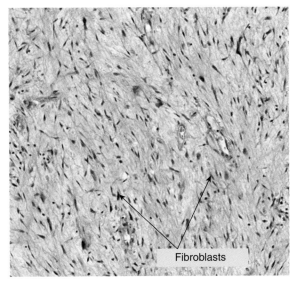

FIGURE 2.4   Fibroblasts

Fibroblasts are cells with spindle-shaped nuclei haphazardly arranged in the dermis. Fibroblasts produce collagen which is the major constituent of extracellular matrix. There are 2 types of collagen Type I and Type II.

- Type I and Type III collagen are the main constituents of the dermis. Type IV collagen is a major component of the basement membrane. (See Chapter 6 for immunohistochemical markers of fibroblasts.)

GHOST (SHADOW) CELLS

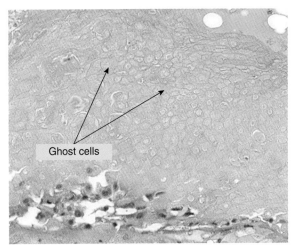

FIGURE 2.5   Ghost (Shadow) Cells

These cells are seen toward the central area of a pilomatrixoma. They have ample eosinophilic cytoplasm and distinct cell borders. The cells do not have a nucleus. These cells essentially originate from the basophilic cells seen toward the periphery of the lobule in a pilomatrixoma.

HISTIOCYTES

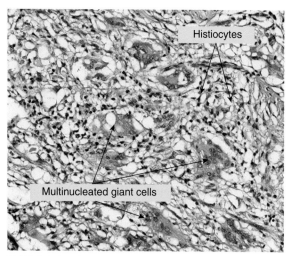

FIGURE 2.6   Histiocytes

Histiocytes belong to the monocyte family of cells in the bone marrow. They are also known as macrophages and belong to the mononuclear phagocyte system. The mature histiocyte is rounded or oval and has pale gray-blue cytoplasm. The nucleus may be eccentrically placed and may be oval, kidney-shaped, or lobulated. The chromatin may appear lacy. Histiocytes are chronic inflammatory cells. (See Chapter 6 for immunohistochemical markers of histiocytes.)

LANGERHANS CELLS

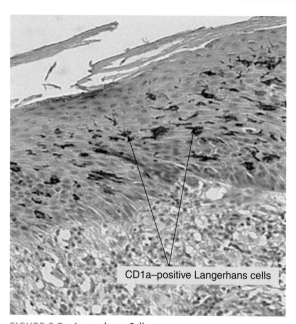

FIGURE 2.7   Langerhans Cells

Langerhans cells belong to the dendritic cell lineage but can appear anywhere in the epidermis. Langerhans cells are better visualized with immunohistochemistry stains which stain for S100 and CD1a antibodies (seen as the brown staining cells in the image). Under the electron microscope they contain the characteristic Birbeck granules. These are rod-shaped organelles having a centrally striated density and an occasional bulb at one end. (See Chapter 6 for immunohistochemical staining of Langerhans cells.)

MAST CELLS

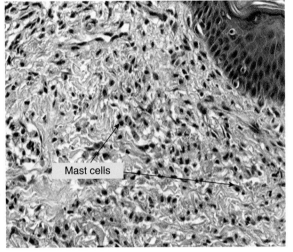

FIGURE 2.8   Mast Cells

In the skin mast cells are found in the dermis. They are derived from bone marrow stem cells. The density of mast cells varies in different parts of the body. The largest numbers are seen in the scrotum. Mast cells are round or oval and contain a central nucleus. The cytoplasm contains basophilic granules. The cells produce pharmacologically active agents such as histamine, leukotrienes, and prostaglandin D2. Mast cell degranulation with the release of these substances results in the symptoms such as pruritus, flushing, and syncope, which occur in mast cell disease with increase in their numbers. (See Chapters 5 and 6 for staining characteristics of mast cells.)

MELANOPHAGES

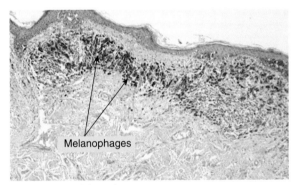

FIGURE 2.9   Melanophages

Melanophages are macrophages which have ingested melanin. The melanocytes at the dermoepidermal junction synthesize melanin. Melanophages in increased numbers are seen in disorders of abnormal pigmentation.

NEURAL CELL

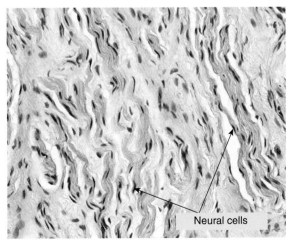

FIGURE 2.10   Neural Cell

Neural cells are derived from the neural crest. They have scanty cytoplasm and spindle-shaped nuclei with tapering ends. They are generally seen encased within the nerve sheath or perineurium. The nerves are normally located within the subcutaneous fat. (See Chapter 6 for staining characteristics of nerve cells.)

NEUTROPHILS

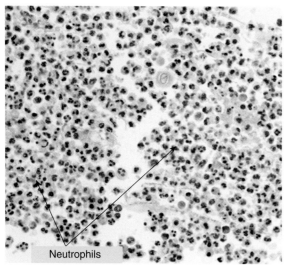

Neutrophils

FIGURE 2.11 Neutrophils

Majority of the neutrophils have two to five nuclear segments joined together by strands. The cytoplasm contains fine pink or bluish granules. Neutrophils are considered acute inflammatory cells. They are the major constituents of an abscess.

PLASMA CELLS

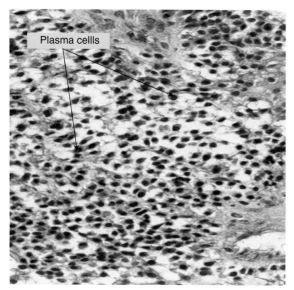

Plasma cellls

FIGURE 2.12 Plasma Cells

Plasma cells are not normally found in circulation or in the skin. They are chronic inflammatory cells and are seen as a component of an inflammatory process. They are also seen in neoplastic proliferation of plasma cells in plasmacytoma or cutaneous deposit of myeloma. Plasma cells are derived from antigenically stimulated B cells. They have abundant basophilic cytoplasm and eccentrically placed nuclei. Very rarely accumulations of immunoglobulins are seen in the cytoplasm as rounded eosinophilic inclusions called "Russell bodies." These inclusions are PAS-positive and diastase-resistant. (See Chapter 6 for staining characteristics of plasma cells.)

SMOOTH MUSCLE CELLS

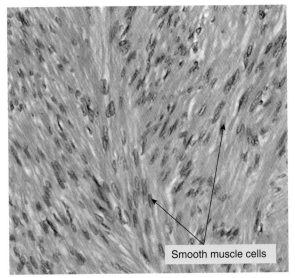

Smooth muscle cells in skin are seen in arrector pili muscle and around medium-sized and thick-walled blood vessels in the subcutaneous fat. The cells have abundant eosinophilic cytoplasm and spindle-shaped nuclei. The nuclei are characteristically blunt-ended or "cigar-shaped." Abnormal proliferation of smooth muscle cells gives rise to leiomyoma and leiomyosarcoma. (See Chapter 6 for staining characteristics of smooth muscle cells.)

FIGURE 2.13   Smooth Muscle Cells

SKELETAL MUSCLE CELLS

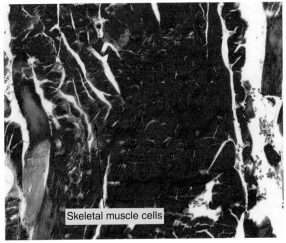

The normal adult myocyte is polygonal and contains multiple nuclei located at the periphery. The cytoplasm of the cells called the "sarcoplasm" has a textured appearance on H&E sections. The muscle groups are separated by connective tissue called "perimysium." The blood vessels and the nerves travel to the muscle through the perimysium.

FIGURE 2.14   Skeletal Muscle Cells

XANTHOMA CELLS

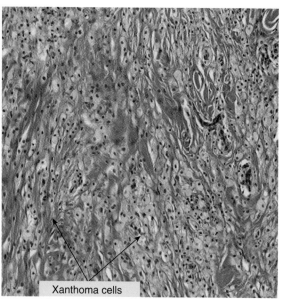

Xanthoma cells

FIGURE 2.15   Xanthoma Cells

Xanthoma cells contain lipid in their cytoplasm and so they appear foamy in H&E sections. They are basically histiocytes that have engulfed lipid in their cytoplasm. Xanthoma cells are associated with disorders of lipid metabolism. Proliferation of xanthoma cells results in xanthelasma and xanthoma in various anatomic locations of the body.

AMYLOID DEPOSITION

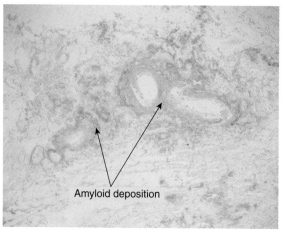

Amyloid deposition

FIGURE 2.16   Amyloid Deposition

Amyloid is deposited in an extracellular location as an eosinophilic hyaline material. Deposition of amyloid occurs in skin in localized cutaneous amyloidosis and systemic amyloidosis. There are several patterns of deposition of amyloid in the skin. The commonest patterns are nodular amyloidosis seen as large clumps of eosinophilic material in the dermis and around blood vessels and homogenous band-like infiltrate seen in the papillary dermis in lichen amyloidosis. Amyloid is protein in nature and is composed of straight nonbranching filaments ultrastructurally. Amyloid has very characteristic staining properties. (See Chapter 5 for special staining effects of amyloid.)

BONE

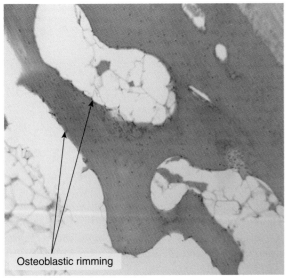

Osteoblastic rimming

FIGURE 2.17   Bone

There are two forms of cutaneous ossification. A primary type called "osteoma cutis" where there is an absence of a preexisting lesion and secondary type where the ossification develops secondary to trauma, inflammation, or neoplasia. There are several groups of primary cutaneous ossification and they are rare. The secondary form can be seen in association with basal cell carcinomas, trichoepitheliomas, hemangiomas, and lipomas. It can also be seen in association with trauma at injection sites and surgical scars.

CALCIUM DEPOSITION

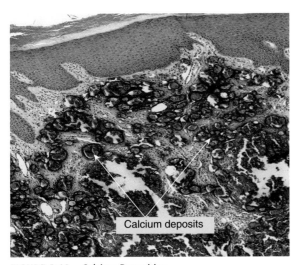

Calcium deposits

FIGURE 2.18   Calcium Deposition

Calcinosis cutis can be broadly divided into dystrophic and metastatic varieties. Dystrophic calcification is associated with damaged or degenerated tissue and metastatic calcification is associated with deranged metabolism of calcium and/or phosphorous. A rare idiopathic type has also been recognized which is best represented by tumoral calcinosis. In skin biopsies calcium is seen deposited in the dermis as intense uniformly basophilic substance. It may elicit a foreign body giant cell reaction in the dermis and sometimes pseudoepitheliomatous hyperplasia of the overlying epidermis.

CARTILAGE CELLS

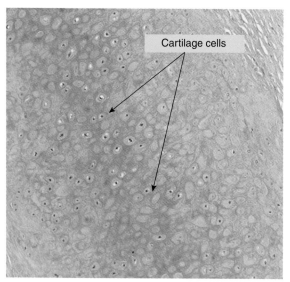

Cartilage cells

FIGURE 2.19   Cartilage Cells

Cutaneous deposition of cartilage is seen as primary cartilaginous tumors and as a metaplastic process. The cartilaginous tumors could be composed of pure cartilage or it could be cartilaginous metaplasia in a soft tissue tumor. On H&E sections, cartilage generally has a basophilic hue and the nuclei are seen within a clear space giving the appearance of lacunae.

CHOLESTEROL CLEFTS

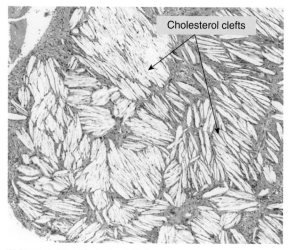

Cholesterol clefts

FIGURE 2.20   Cholesterol Clefts

These are needle-shaped structures with associated foreign body giant cell reaction. Cholesterol clefts are seen in a number of different conditions most notably in xanthogranulomatous reaction and more commonly in association with nonspecific inflammatory conditions.

HEMOSIDERIN DEPOSITION

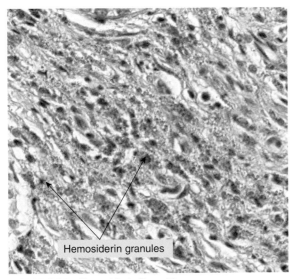

FIGURE 2.21   Hemosiderin Deposition

Hemosiderin is a breakdown product of hemoglobin. In the skin it is deposited in association with stasis dermatitis, pigmented purpuric dermatoses, hemochromatosis, and many other conditions. Any pathological process in which there has been previous bleeding results in hemosiderin deposition. (See Chapter 5 for staining characteristics of hemosiderin.)

MULTINUCLEATED GIANT CELLS

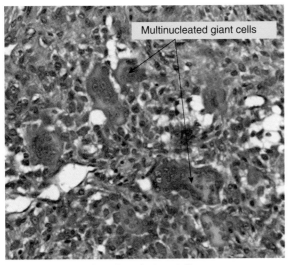

FIGURE 2.22   Multinucleated Giant Cells

Multinucleated giant cells are commonly formed by the coalescence of histiocytes. They are seen in connection with inflammatory conditions, infections, and neoplastic processes. There are several different types of multinucleated giant cells such as foreign body giant cells which are formed as result of an external foreign body or an internal foreign body such as keratin. Langhans giant cell is the type seen in tuberculosis. Tumor-type giant cells are seen classically in giant cell tumor of bone and soft tissues. They are also seen as a nondiagnostic feature in many benign and malignant melanocytic, epithelial, and soft tissue tumors.

OCHRONOSIS

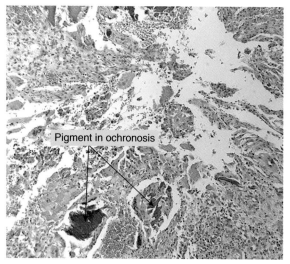

FIGURE 2.23   Ochronosis

Ochronosis is the result of deposition of yellow-brown ochre pigment in collagen-containing tissues in alkaptonuria. The pigment is homogentisic acid. This disorder is autosomal recessive and is the result of the absence of hepatic and renal enzyme called "homogentisic acid oxidase." Ochronosis is also used as a term when similar substances are deposited following topical use of phenol in the treatment of leg ulcers. It may also result following oral administration or injection of antimalarial drugs.

TUTON TYPE OF GIANT CELLS

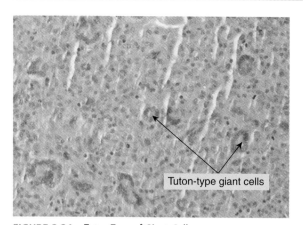

FIGURE 2.24   Tuton Type of Giant Cells

These are a special type of giant cells seen in juvenile xanthogranulomas and dermatofibromas. They characteristically have a wreath-like arrangement of nuclei at the periphery of the giant cell.

URIC ACID CRYSTALS

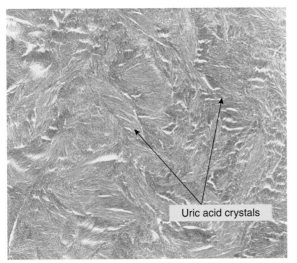

Uric acid crystals are seen in gout. If the material is fixed in alcohol, the crystals appear needle-shaped and brown in color. The crystals are doubly refractile. Usually, a foreign body giant cell reaction develops in the tissue surrounding the uric acid deposition.

FIGURE 2.25   Uric Acid Crystals

BIBLIOGRAPHY

David W. Skin Pathology, 3rd Ed. Churchill Livingstone, 2009.
Sharon WW, John RG. Enzinger & Weiss's Soft Tissue Tumors, 5th Ed. Mosby, Elseiver, 2007.
Stephen SS. Histology for Pathologists, 2nd Ed. Lippincott-Raven, 1997.

Techniques in Dermatology and Dermatopathology

INTRODUCTION

The primary aim in dermatology is to obtain an accurate diagnosis in order to select the most appropriate and effective treatment strategy for the patient. In some cases, the clinical appearance of a skin condition is sufficiently characteristic to start empiric treatment based on the presumptive clinical diagnosis. In many other cases, there is sufficient doubt or uncertainty clinically as to require a biopsy to confirm the diagnosis. In such cases, the clinical and histological diagnosis should be coherent (i.e., the histological appearances should be consistent with the clinical appearances and vice versa)—that is to say there should be clinicopathological correlation in all histological samples.

BIOPSY SPECIMENS IN DERMATOLOGY

Correct interpretation of dermatological biopsy specimens requires the following:
- Provision of an adequate
  - clinical history of the lesion or condition—an indication of duration/evolution of the lesion(s) or condition(s),
  - description (or more usefully, a printed image) of the lesion(s) or condition(s), and
  - working clinical diagnosis.
- Obtaining the correct biopsy specimen for the condition(s) or lesion(s).
- Correct handling and processing of the specimen.
- In selected cases, the dermatopathologist should be consulted to ascertain the best specimen to obtain and for suggestions about the following:
  - The priority of transporting the specimen to laboratory.
  - The best medium to transport the specimen in prior to it arriving in the laboratory.
  - Any special tests or specimens required, for example, microbiological examination and culture and T-cell gene rearrangement studies.
    - If in doubt, it's always wise to ask the dermatopathologist of the requirements well in advance of when the biopsy is actually being taken.
- Appropriate choice of histochemical and immunohistochemical stains and immunofluorescence study based on Bancroft and Gamble (1) and Sternberg (2).
- Clinicopathologic correlation. In selected cases, a multidisciplinary meeting of the dermatopathologist and clinicians and/or external expert review of the specimen may be required.

Biopsies may be taken for purely diagnostic purposes, but in some cases, these are used as a therapeutic measure (e.g., shave biopsies can be used to obtain a diagnosis and also as a treatment technique for a superficial lesion).

Clinicians use various methods to obtain a biopsy—each with its own advantages and disadvantages. The common methods used to obtain biopsy specimens in dermatology include the following.

METHODS USED TO OBTAIN A BIOPSY

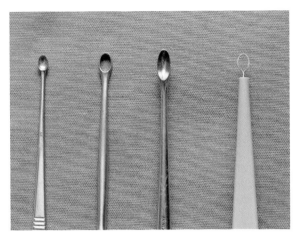

FIGURE 3.1   Types of Curettes

Curettes (from left to right): Three different styles of curettes-spoon-shaped curette, ovoid curette and ring curette

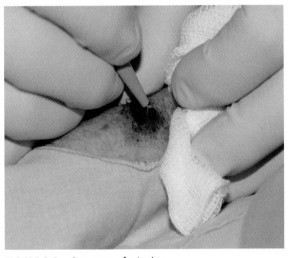

FIGURE 3.2   Curettage of a Lesion

Technique of curettage. Fragments of tissue obtained by scooping out the lesion by using relatively blunt ovoid "curettes" or alternatively sharper disposable "ring curettes"

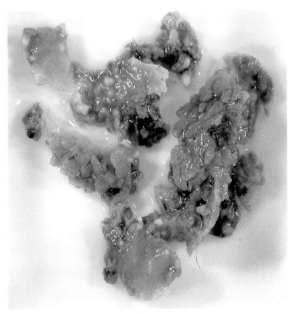

FIGURE 3.3   Macroscopy of Curettings

These are fragments of tissue with no specific orientation. Fragments of tissue obtained by scooping out the lesion using relatively blunt ovoid "curettes" or alternatively sharper disposable "ring curettes"

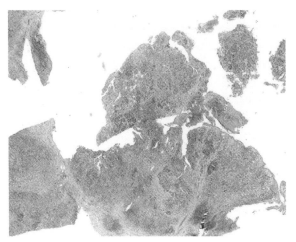

FIGURE 3.4   Microscopy of Curettings

H&E sections of curette showing melanoma (Fig. 3.4) and digital papillary adenocarcinoma (Fig. 3.5). It is prudent not to curette any lesion of indeterminate/non specific apperance or where the diagnosis is not clear. Lesions which may be treated with curative intent by curettage and cautrey include slected cases of basal cell cancers, squamous cell cancers and keratoacanthomas. If there is any clinical suspicion of a neoplasm it is best not to curette the lesion.

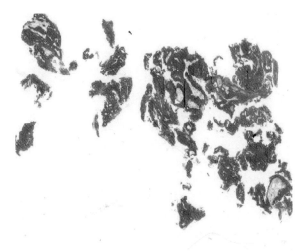

FIGURE 3.5   H&E Sections

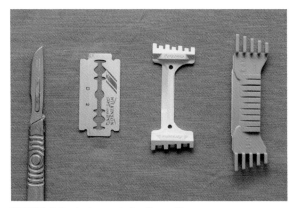

FIGURE 3.6   Instruments for Shave Biopsy

Instruments used to procure shave biopsy (from left to right): Number 10 Swann-Morton scalpel blade, Wilkinson's Sword™ **razor blade** Personna Dermablade®, Kai Biopsiblade®.

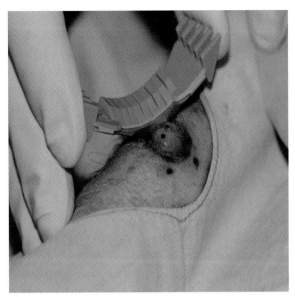

FIGURE 3.7   Performance of a Shave Biopsy

Performing of a Shave Biopsy

This is a technique for obtaining superficial tangential sampling of the skin with either Personna Derma blade®, Kai Biopsiblade® or Wilkinson Sword™ razor blade.

Shave biopsy of the skin lesion with a Kai Biopsi Blade® (similar technique is used with Wilkinson's Sword™ razor blade or Personna Dermablade®). The lesion is slightly elevated by infiltration of local anaesthetic (or alternatively, slightly elevated by pinching the surrounding skin) before shaving the lesion off at the underlying superficial to mid dermis level using simultaneous advancing and side to side movements using a blade held under fixed tension between the thumb and index finger. Broader lesions may need multiple overlapping shaves to remove the whole lesion.

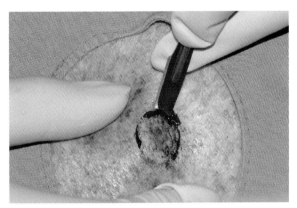

FIGURE 3.8   Saucerization

Saucerization

Shave biopsy using a Swann-Morton blade. The lesion is slightly elevated from the surrounding skin and shaved horizontally through the mid dermis by using broad strokes of a large scalpel (number 10 or larger). The resultant specimen is a round specimen with a saucer shaper-shaped profile (hence the term "saucerization"). Pedunculated (lesions arising from a narrow base) lesions can be shave excised by in a similar fashion by grasping the lesion with forceps, elevating the base and then shaving the lesion off at the superficial to mid dermal levels. Shave biopsy of a pedunculated (ie arising from a narrow base) lesion is achieved by grasping the lesion with fine toothed forceps, elevating the base and then shaving the lesion in a similar fashion.

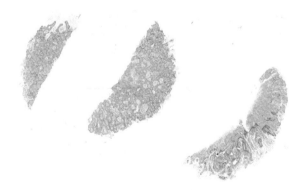

FIGURE 3.9   H&E Sections of a Shave of Seborrhoeic Keratosis

H&E Sections of a Shave of Seborrhoeic Keratosis

Shave biopsies are ideally performed as a diagnostic measure in benign superficial lesions.

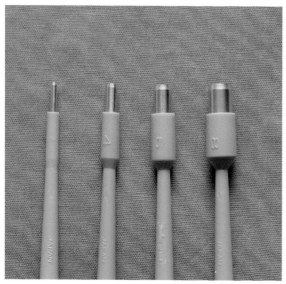

FIGURE 3.10   Punch Biopsy Various Sizes

Punch Biopsy

Punch biopsy various sizes.

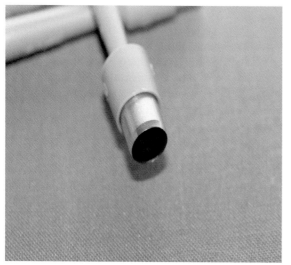

FIGURE 3.11   A Punch Biopsy Showing the Cutting Surface

A Punch Biopsy Showing the Cutting Surface.

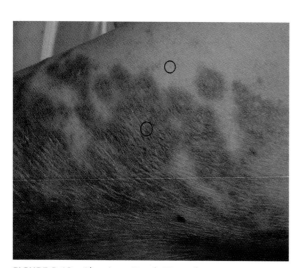

FIGURE 3.12   Planning a Punch Biopsy for Lupus Erythematosus and Perilesional Skin for DIF

The aim of punch biopsy is to obtain a representative sample of a lesion or alternatively a biopsy to encompass the entirety of a small lesion.

Samples for immunofluorescence are typically taken from surrounding normal skin in blistering conditions and connective tissues disease such as cutaneous lupus erythematosus.

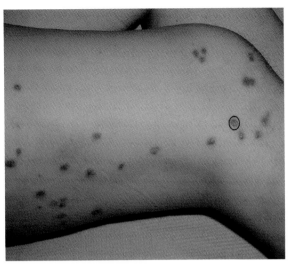

FIGURE 3.13   Planning a Punch Biopsy for Perforating Collagenosis

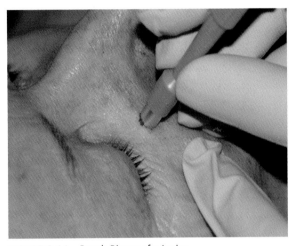

FIGURE 3.14   Punch Biopsy of a Lesion

Cylindrical sample of tissue obtained by using a disposable instrument called a "punch biopsy". Comes in various sizes from 1 mm–8 mm in diameter. Some punch biopsy instruments are elliptical in shape. Punch biopsies are analogous to a "core sample" or bone marrow Trephine.

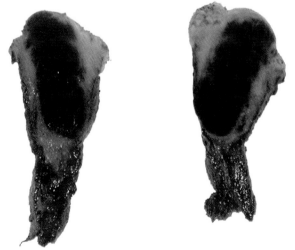

FIGURE 3.15   Longitudinal Slice of a Punch Biopsy

For routine histopathological examination, punch biopsies are sliced vertically from epidermis to the subcutaneous fat. It is ideal not to perform punch biopsies on pigmented lesions.

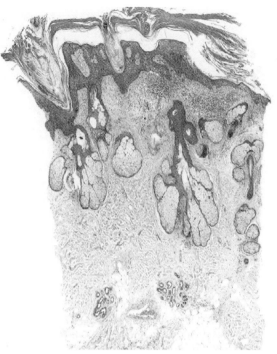

FIGURE 3.16   Microscopy of a Punch Biopsy

H&E microscopy of a punch biopsy showing moderate actinic keratosis.

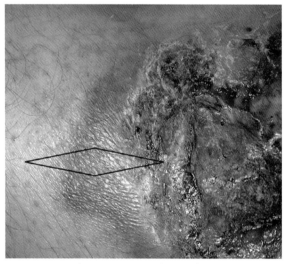

FIGURE 3.17   Planning an Incisional Biopsy for a Vasculitic Lesion

Incisional Biopsy

- Sample obtained by scalpel.
- Removal of an elliptical part of a lesion.
- Specimen is usually sectioned for histological evaluation vertically in the longitudinal axis of the specimen.
- Processing in this way gives a "panoramic" or "landscape" view of a skin condition/lesion and shows the transition from normal unaffected skin through to involved skin.

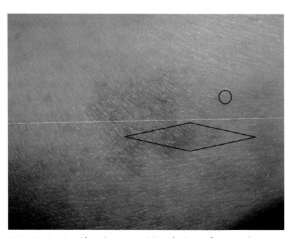

FIGURE 3.18   Planning an Incisional Biopsy for Pemphigus Foliaceus and Perilesional skin for DIF

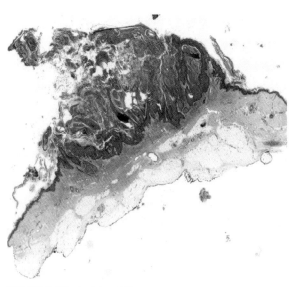

FIGURE 3.19   Incisional Biopsy

Incisional Biopsy

Incisional biopsy showing panoramic view of a keratoacanthoma.

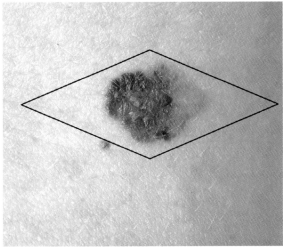

FIGURE 3.20   Planning an Excisional Biopsy for Melanoma

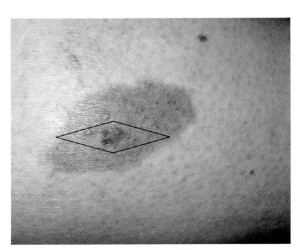

FIGURE 3.21   Planning an Excisional Biopsy for Congenital
Melanocytic Naevus

Excisional Biopsy

- Sample obtained by complete removal of a skin lesion using a scalpel.
- Small lesions can be removed by punch biopsies.
- Excision biopsies are performed as a curative procedure.
- There is usually a macroscopic wider margin for the lesion.

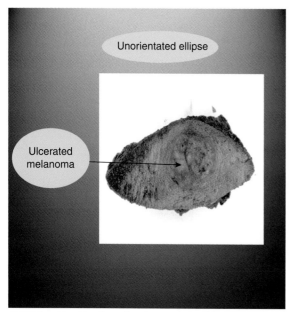

FIGURE 3.22   Unoriented Excision Biopsy of Skin

This specimen does not give an indication of the location of the lesion in relation to the anatomical position in the body. Marking the specimen with a suture or a small cut in the specimen (for example, at the superior aspect on the biopsy specimen) may be helpful to orientate the specimen to the anatomic position stated on the request form.

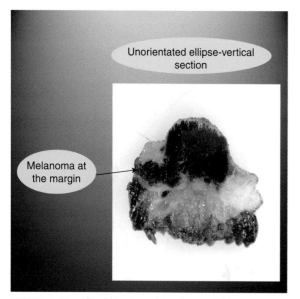

FIGURE 3.23   Sliced Unoriented Specimen of Skin

These specimens are painted with a single color at the resection margins and they are bread sliced. The image shows the middle slice of an excision of a malignant melanoma. The tumor is clearly seen at one of the peripheral margins of the biopsy.

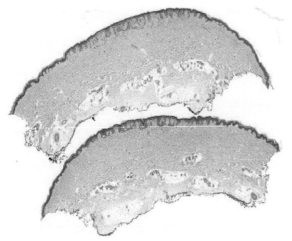

FIGURE 3.24   Excisional Biopsy-Unoriented

H&E section of an excision for a dysplastic naevus. The lesion appears well clear of the peripheral and deep margins of the biopsy.

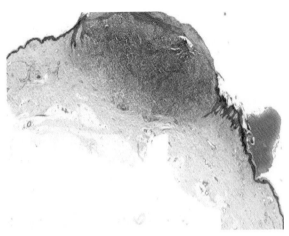

H&E section of an excision for a Nodular malignant melanoma. The tumor appears well clear of the peripheral and deep margins.

FIGURE 3.25   Excision Biopsy of a Nodular Melanoma

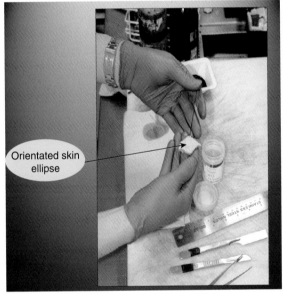

Orientated skin ellipse

FIGURE 3.26   Grossing Oriented Ellipse of Skin

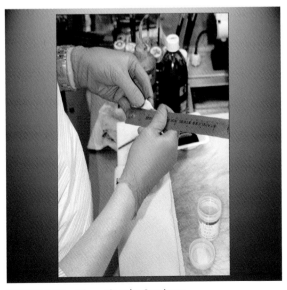

FIGURE 3.27   Measuring the Specimen

Orientated excision biopsies have a marker indicating the anatomical position in the body. While "grossing", this marker is designated a clock position for ease of orientation. Grossing is the process by which a specimen is described in terms of its macroscopic appearances and dimensions. It also involves identifying any markers on the specimen, and painting the resection margins appropriately. The presence or absence of a lesion described in the request form sent along with the specimen is particularly noted. There are standard protocols for dissection of the different types of biopsies as is being described in individual sections. Based on these protocols, slices of tissue are selected for processing.

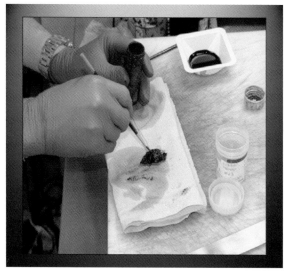

The marker suture is usually assumed to be at 12 o'clock position unless otherwise stated. The 3 o'clock and 6 o'clock positions are painted in two different colors.

FIGURE 3.28   Painting of the Specimen

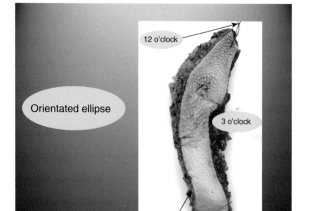

The image shows the painted orientated excision of skin with the marker at 12 o'clock and the 3 o'clock and 9 o'clock positions painted in two different colors.

FIGURE 3.29   Painted Oriented Ellipse of Skin

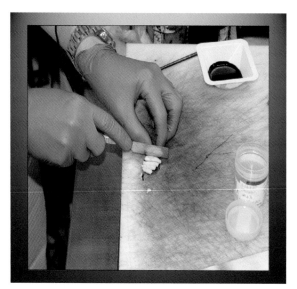

The specimen is bread sliced (that is, cut in a manner similar to loaf of bread) and appropriate block descriptions are made.

FIGURE 3.30   Slicing of Specimen

Table 3.1

Advantages and disadvantages of different biopsy techniques

Biopsy Specimen	Advantages	Disadvantages
Curettings from curettage and cautery	Quick and easy procedure to perform	Slow healing Possible slightly increased risk of infection Scar often becomes hypertrophic in nature; rarely, keloid scar formation Often leaves pigmentary changes, either hyperpigmentation or hypopigmentation Loss of orientation of lesions and normal anatomical structures Only fragments—cannot confidently assess completeness of removal of lesion or surgical margins Nondiagnostic if inadequate material submitted for histological assessment
Shave biopsy/excision	Quick and easy Suitable for removal of small (predominantly) epidermal-based lesions as a single specimen Maintains normal relationship of different skin structures	Slow healing Possible slightly increased risk of infection Possible anetoderma (loss of dermis) leading to herniation of underlying tissues Scar often becomes hypertrophic in nature; rarely, keloid scar formation Often leaves pigmentary disturbance (hyperpigmentation or hypopigmentation) Superficial—may not adequately characterize the whole lesion (e.g., may miss underlying dermal component of a desmoplastic melanoma underlying a lentigo maligna) May not result in adequate removal of a lesion requiring further surgical procedure
Punch biopsy	Quick and easy Small scar Heals rapidly with a small linear scar Small risk of infection and bleeding Multiple biopsies can be taken if there is heterogenous appearance to condition(s) or lesion(s) to give a better indication of evolution or progression of condition(s) or lesion(s) or alternatively if there are more than one pathological processes present Suitable to remove small lesion(s) in total without taking unnecessary tissue—a bit like a mini excision(al) biopsy Relatively quick and easy	Small risk of hypertrophic and keloid scar formation Smaller punch biopsies easier to malorientate during processing May not give a representative sample of a skin condition if the condition occupies a large area and has a degree of heterogeneity May not always adequately allow assessment of deeper structures in the subcutis (e.g., fat, hair bulbs, fascia), especially if too small a punch biopsy size is taken or if the sample only contains superficial layers of the skin Small risk of hypertrophic and keloid scar formation

(continued)

Table 3.1

Advantages and disadvantages of different biopsy techniques (*Continued*)

Biopsy Specimen	Advantages	Disadvantages
Incision(al) biopsy	Linear scar Usually quick healing Small risk of infection and bleeding Gives more representative sample of tissue—can encompass normal to abnormal tissue boundaries to allow comparison (e.g., annular lesions, blistering reactions) when sectioned vertically in the longitudinal axis of the sample Normal orientation to epidermis maintained More tissue available to do additional histo- and immunohistocyto-chemistry stains Full thickness of skin down to fascia and muscle can be sampled if needed	Diagnostic procedure—not used for treatment May not give a representative sample of the whole lesion (e.g., lentigo maligna) Larger biopsy, so larger scar
Excision(al) biopsy	Relatively quick and easy Linear scar Small risk of infection and bleeding Usually quick healing Whole lesion is contained in sample with normal orientation to epidermis Adequacy of excision can be assessed more accurately More tissue available to do additional histo- and immunohistocyto-chemistry stains Full thickness of skin down to fascia and muscle can be sampled if needed	Small risk of hypertrophic and keloid scar formation May be difficult to identify a small lesion(s) within the biopsy Larger biopsy, so larger scar

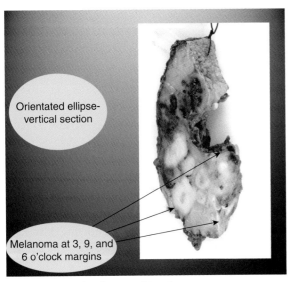

The middle slice of the specimen showing the tumor beneath the epidermis. The tumor is clearly seen reaching specific margins.

FIGURE 3.31   Sliced Oriented Specimen

PROCESSING OF SPECIMENS IN THE HISTOPATHOLOGY LABORATORY

All the aforementioned specimens are received in the pathology laboratory for routine histopathological examination in 10% formalin. All specimens are accompanied by a request form containing the demographic data of the patient and adequate detailed clinical history. If possible, a photograph of the lesion accompanying the request form would be ideal. The volume of formalin should be 10 times the size of the specimen.

Any specimen requiring fibroblast culture and tumor cytogenetics should be sent in the culture medium and not in Formalin. Specimens requiring electron microscopic examination should be transported in glutaraldehyde.

All specimens received in the histopathology laboratory are given a unique identifying number, which stays with the specimen ever after. The specimen is examined macroscopically as explained in the above section and undergoes processing as described below.

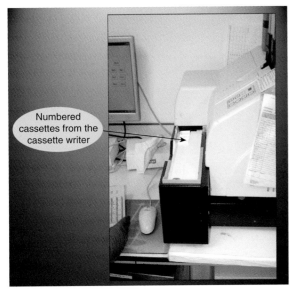

The cassette printer numbers the plastic cassettes which holds the tissue samples which are either small, as in a punch biopsy or slices of an excision biopsy.

FIGURE 3.32   Cassette Printed from the Cassette Writer

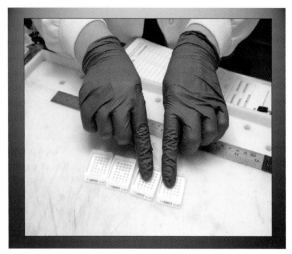

FIGURE 3.33   Numbered Cassettes

The cassettes and their lids have holes for thorough circulation of formalin and the processing fluids. The identifying histology number of the specimen is printed onto the cassette.

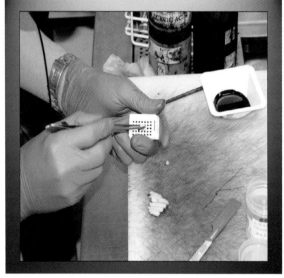

FIGURE 3.34   Sections Being Placed in Cassettes

The sliced specimens are placed inside individual cassettes and appropriate block descriptions are recorded on the report being prepared for the specimen.

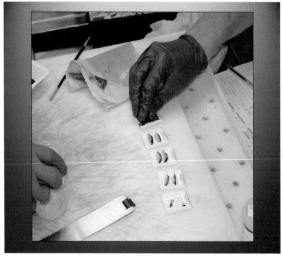

FIGURE 3.35   Complete Specimen in Cassettes

The entire specimen is thus placed in the numbered cassettes for the specimen and closed with a holed lid.

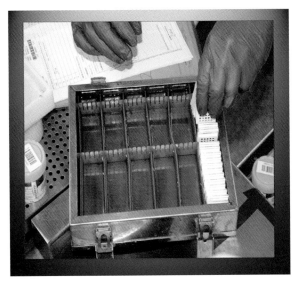

FIGURE 3.36   Cassettes in Trough Containing Formalin

The closed cassettes are immediately placed in a trough containing formalin so that the fixation of the specimen will still continue.

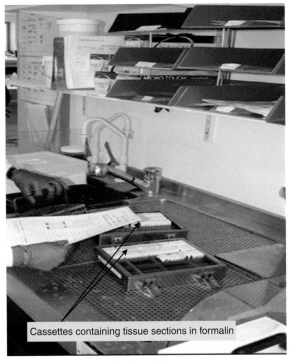

Cassettes containing tissue sections in formalin

FIGURE 3.37   Cross Checking of Cassettes

The blocks are cross-checked with the work sheet recorded at the time of blocking to make sure that there is no mismatch between the two entries.

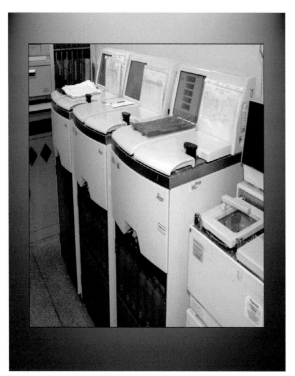

FIGURE 3.38   Processing Machines

Processing Machines

The processing of tissue involves mainly three different stages.

- *Dehydration*: This involves different concentrations of alcohol removing the fixatives and water from the tissues.
- *Clearing*: The dehydrating fluid is replaced with a another fluid which is compatible with the embedding medium. Commonly used clearing agents are Xylene and Chloroform. The tissue acquires a translucent appearance after it is treated with a clearing agent and hence the name "Clearing agent."
- *Impregnation*: Replacing the clearing fluid with the embedding medium.

The entire process is computerized and automated.

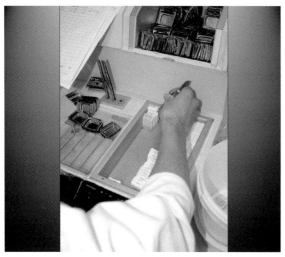

FIGURE 3.39   Cassettes Ready for Blocking

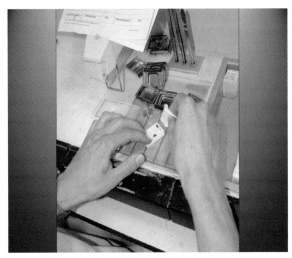

FIGURE 3.40   Cassettes with Tissue in Preblocking Stage

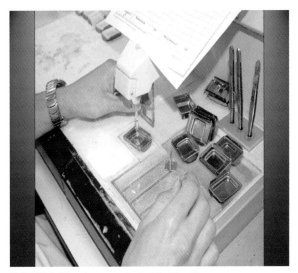

FIGURE 3.41   Cassettes in Preblocking Stage

Preparing the Blocks for Embedding

The processed tissue in cassettes are examined and prepared for embedding in paraffin wax.

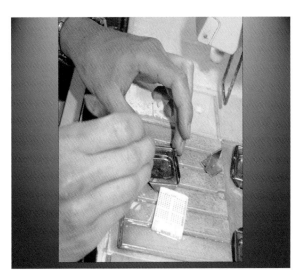

FIGURE 3.42   Tissue Being Embedded in Molten Wax

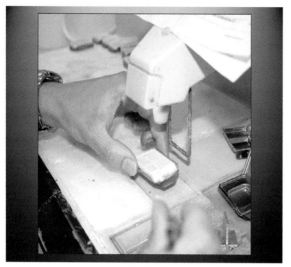

FIGURE 3.43   Adding More Molten Wax

Embedding in Paraffin Wax

Paraffin wax is the most popular embedding medium. It is cheap and has a wide range of melting points which makes it suitable in different climatic conditions. Embedding is a very important stage in the process of getting the optimum sections. This is particularly important with skin specimens which has a structural distinction and orientation of the specimen is crucial.

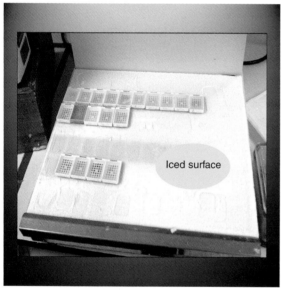

FIGURE 3.44   Solidifying the Paraffin Block

Solidifying the Paraffin Block

The molten paraffin wax is solidified on iced surface, so that the blocks are hard enough to be cut by the microtome.

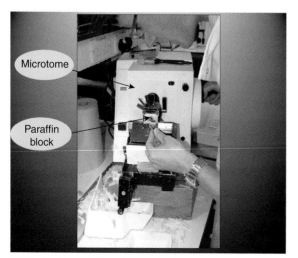

FIGURE 3.45   Blocks Being Cut by the Microtome

Blocks Being Cut by a Microtome

Sections of tissue which are 3–4 microns thick are produced by microtomes. The paraffin blocks are cut by very sharp and fine microtome knives in order to produce the sections. Microtomes are machines that will advance an object for a predetermined distance, then slide the object to the cutting tool, which is a steel knife or a blade and then the object through the knife to produce a section.

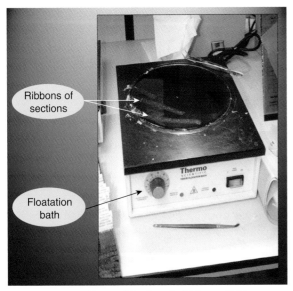

FIGURE 3.46   Ribbons of Sections 3–4 Microns Thick

Flotation Bath

Ribbons of sections 3–4 microns thick are transferred onto the water bath which is thermostatically controlled. The temperature of the water bath should be about 10 degree centigrade below the melting point of paraffin wax. A small quantity of alcohol or detergent will reduce the surface tension and allow the sections to flatten out with ease.

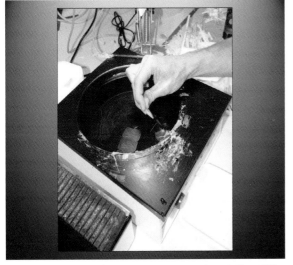

FIGURE 3.47   Transferring Sections to Numbered Glass Slides

Transferring Sections on to Glass Slides

Glass slides measuring 76 × 25 mm are routinely used. The slides are 1.00–1.2 mm thick. The unique histology number of the case is inscribed on the glass slide using lead pencil. The sections are carefully transferred on to the numbered glass slide.

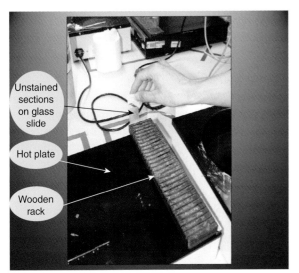

FIGURE 3.48   Racking of Unstained Sections

Sections on Slide Rack

The slides with unstained sections are arranged on the slide rack.

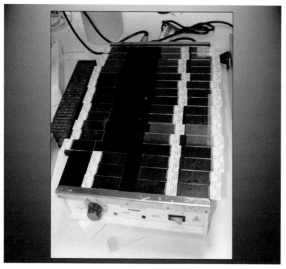

FIGURE 3.49   Unstained Sections on Hot Plate

Unstained Sections on Hot Plate

The slides holding the unstained sections are arranged on the hot plate. The temperature of the hot plate is set at the melting point of wax. The aim is to dry the sections and this is complete within 30 minutes.

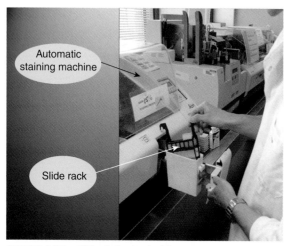

FIGURE 3.50   Slides Being Racked for Staining

Slides Being Racked for Staining

The slides are arranged in the rack to be fed into an automatic staining machine for routine haematoxylin and eosin staining.

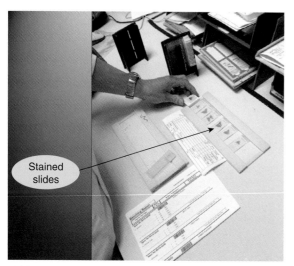

FIGURE 3.51   Sections Stained with Hematoxylin and Eosin

Sections Stained with Hematoxylin and Eosin

Haematoxylin and Eosin stain is the most commonly used stain in histopathology. Haematoxylin stains the cell nuclei blue/black and the eosin stains the cell cytoplasm from varying shades of pink to orange and red.

Haematoxylin is extracted from the heartwood of the tree *Haematoxylin campechianum* which originated in Campeche in Mexico. The different types of Haematoxylins commonly used in routine staining are Ehrlich's, Mayer's, and Harris's. Eosins are xanthene dyes and is the most suitable stain to combine with haematoxylin. It has a particular ability to distinguish between the cytoplasm of different types of cells staining them in different shades of pink and orange.

The staining procedure is fully automated and it usually takes half an hour for a batch of 30 slides to stain.

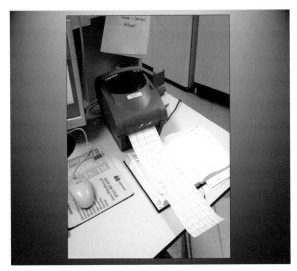

FIGURE 3.52   Labels Being Printed for Glass Slides

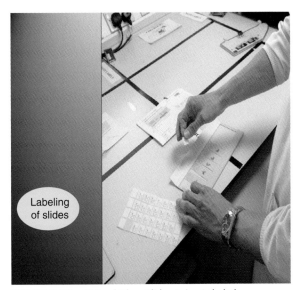

FIGURE 3.53   Stained Glass Slides Being Labeled

Labelling Stained Slides

The stained slides are labelled with the identifying number. This is the number which is allocated to the specimen at the time of booking in.

Before the slides are booked out to pathologists, the labelled slides are finally checked in the laboratory against the request form to identify any discrepancies in

- Identification of the specimen
- The nature and number of sections on the slide
- Quality of the sections
- Quality of staining

All the events from the time of reception of the specimen to authorisation of the report by the pathologist are recorded on the computer in the chronological order.

BIBLIOGRAPHY

Bancroft JD, Gamble M, eds. Theory and Practice of Histological Techniques, 6th ed. New York: Churchill Livingstone, 2007.
Mills SE, ed. Histology for Pathologists, 3rd ed. Philadelphia: Lippincott Williams & Wilkins, 2006.
Eady D, Brethnack S, Walker N. Surgical Dermatology. London: Blackwell Science, 1996.

Descriptive Terms in Dermatopathology

INTRODUCTION

Dermatopathology as a specialty is unique in its lexicon. Skin is the largest organ in the body with a very complex microenvironment. The three main subdivisions of skin namely the epidermis, the dermis, and the subcutaneous fat are functionally and morphologically complicated. The abnormalities or the disease processes which occur in these structures itself are numerous and intricate. The assessment of skin biopsy requires a thorough understanding of the different morphological changes in different parts of the skin. This chapter aims to explain the different descriptive terms used in dermatopathology to elucidate the pathological processes.

ABSCESS WITHIN A FOLLICLE

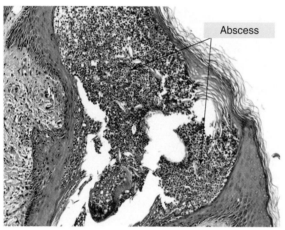

Abscess is a collection of neutrophils. Abscesses can form in any part of the skin such as epidermis, hair follicle, eccrine glands, dermis, or subcutaneous fat. This could be due to several reasons such as release of the contents of the cyst and secondary inflammation, bacterial or fungal infections, or secondary to an external injury. It may also be seen as part of a benign or malignant neoplastic process. Collection of neutrophils within a follicle is generally termed "acute folliculitis."

FIGURE 4.1   Abscess Within a Follicle

ACANTHOSIS OF EPIDERMIS

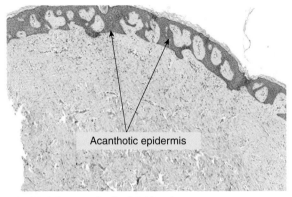

FIGURE 4.2   Acanthosis of Epidermis

Acanthosis of the epidermis is the term used to refer to the increased thickness of the epidermis. This is the result of an increase in the number or size of the spinous layer of the epidermis. The mechanism underlying acanthosis varies in different disease conditions. Acanthosis may be seen in inflammatory conditions such as psoriasis or neoplastic conditions such as Bowen disease and squamous cell carcinoma.

ACANTHOLYSIS

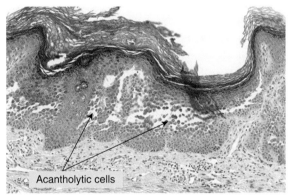

FIGURE 4.3   Acantholysis

Acantholysis is the result of loss of cohesion of the keratinocytes. This could happen in the corneal, granular and spinous layers of the epidermis and the lining of the adnexal structures. Acantholysis could be induced by external agents such as oil or it could be the effect of immunoglobulins and/or complement, which is the mechanism of acantholysis in pemphigus vulgaris or foliaceous. In the lower part of the epidermis it could be induced by toxins released by neutrophils as it happens in dermatitis herpetiformis. Acantholysis is also seen in malignancies such as squamous cell carcinoma.

ANTONI A AND ANTONI B AREAS

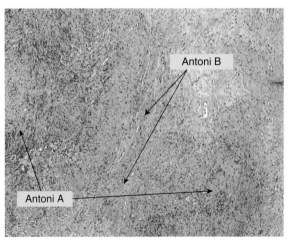

FIGURE 4.4   Antoni A and B Areas

Antoni A area refers to the cellular component of a schwannoma. Interlacing fascicles of spindle-shaped cells are seen with nuclear pallisading. The nuclei exhibit very minimal nuclear pleomorphism. Antoni B areas are less cellular and exhibit hyalinization, xanthomatous change, and pseudocystic areas. In a classical schwannoma alternating areas of Antoni A and Antoni B may be seen. In a cellular schwannoma Antoni A area predominates in comparison with Antoni B area which may be seen in less than 10% of the tumor area.

APOPTOSIS

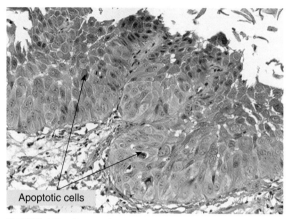

Apoptosis is individual cell necrosis (or cell death). The cells undergo fragmentation of the nuclei with subsequent phagocytosis. Apoptotic cells are seen in physiological and pathological conditions. The keratinocytes of the catagen follicle undergoing apoptosis and transforming to a telogen follicle is an example of apoptosis in physiological conditions. Pathologically it may be seen in inflammatory and neoplastic conditions. The classical example of apoptosis is Civatte bodies or colloid bodies seen in lichen planus. Apoptotic keratinocytes are also seen in drug-induced dermatitis.

FIGURE 4.5   Apoptosis

BORST-JADASSOHN PHENOMENON

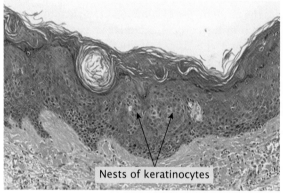

The presence of sharply defined areas of morphologically similar cells within the epidermis is termed "Borst-Jadassohn phenomenon." This is a variant of clonal proliferation of cells. This type of proliferation is seen in Bowen disease, seborrheic keratoses, and hidroacanthoma simplex.

FIGURE 4.6   Borst-Jadassohn Phenomenon

BULLA

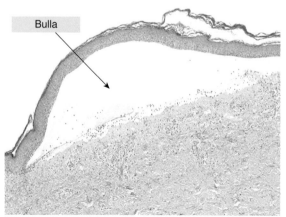

Bullae are blisters which are generally more than 1 cm in diameter. Smaller lesions are referred to as vesicles. Either of these occurs in the different layers of the epidermis or in a subepidermal location. The location and the content of the bulla are crucial in diagnosing the pathological entity.

FIGURE 4.7   Bulla

CIVATTE BODIES

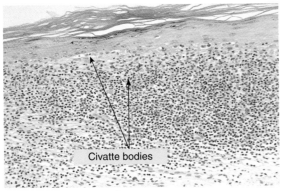

FIGURE 4.8   Civatte Bodies

Civatte bodies are seen as nonnucleated eosinophilic structures in the epidermis or the papillary dermis. These are considered to be keratinocytes that have undergone apoptosis. Civatte bodies are synonymous with colloid bodies.

CORNOID LAMELLA

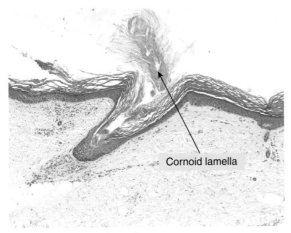

FIGURE 4.9   Cornoid Lamella

Cornoid lamella is a tissue reaction pattern seen in a range of inflammatory and neoplastic conditions. It is considered as a characteristic feature of porokeratosis and its many variants. On histological sections it is seen as a "tier" of parakeratotic cells (i.e., a multilayered column of nucleated epidermal cells through all layers of the epidermis) with absent or markedly decreased granular layer just beneath it. The keratinocytes of the spinous layer appear vacuolated. Pathogenetically cornoid lamellation is a result of abnormalities of keratinization.

CORPS RONDS

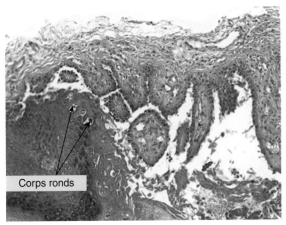

FIGURE 4.10   Corp Ronds

Corps ronds are dyskeratotic epidermal cells with rounded nuclei and slightly basophilic (bluish) cytoplasm when stained with haematoxyllin & eosin. In comparison, normal dyskeratotic epithelial cells normally have intensely eosinophilic (pink) cytoplasm in usual dyskeratotic cells. Corp ronds are seen in dyskeratotic conditions such as Darier disease.

CRUST

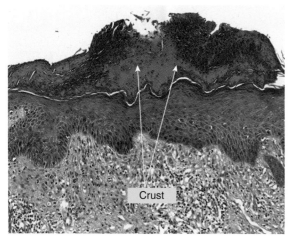

FIGURE 4.11   Crust

Crust is seen on the surface of the epidermis as a collection of plasma mixed with red blood cells, lymphocytes, and neutrophils. The term "scale crust" is used when parakeratotic cells are admixed with it. Scale crust is seen in conditions such as spongiotic and allergic dermatitis. The underlying mechanism is thought to be spongiosis or excoriation, following which the accumulation of the cells occurs.

DESMOPLASIA

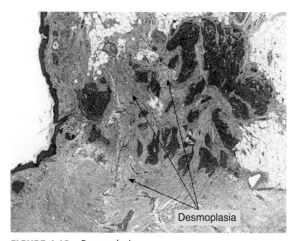

FIGURE 4.12   Desmoplasia

Desmoplasia refers to the dense accumulation of fibrous tissue as response to a benign or malignant neoplasm. The process is activated by the cytokines released by the fibroblasts.

DYSKERATOSIS

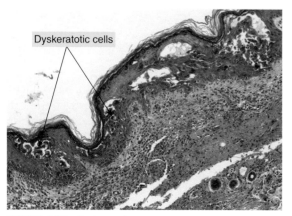

FIGURE 4.13   Dyskeratosis

Dyskeratosis is abnormal and premature cornification seen within the keratinocytes of the epidermis and the adnexal structures. Dyskeratosis is considered slow death of keratinocytes with eventual abnormal cornification. Dyskeratotic cells have intensely eosinophilic (pink) cytoplasm and pyknotic (dark and condensed) nuclei when stained with haematoxylin & eosin. These cells are seen in a variety of inflammatory conditions such as Darier's disease and Grover's disease and also neoplastic conditions such as Bowen's disease.

EPIDERMOTROPISM

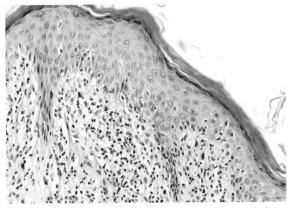

FIGURE 4.14   Epidermotropism

Epidermotropism is the term usually used to refer to the migration of atypical cells into the epidermis. The term is classically used to refer to the process in cutaneous T cell lymphoma (also known as mycosis fungoides) where atypical lymphocytes are seen within the lower half of the epidermis. These cells tend to have a surrounding halo.

EXOCYTOSIS

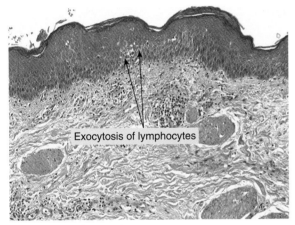

FIGURE 4.15   Exocytosis

Exocytosis refers to the migration of inflammatory cells on to the epidermis. They could be located in all levels of the epidermis and are very commonly associated with spongiosis, the inflammatory pattern associated wth eczematous conditions.

FIBRINOID NECROSIS

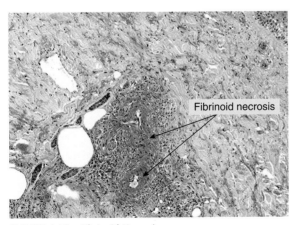

FIGURE 4.16   Fibrinoid Necrosis

Fibrinoid necrosis refers to the extravasation of fibrin outside the blood vessel secondary to injury to the vessel wall. Fibrinoid necrosis of the vessel wall is a common histological finding in vasculitis due to any cause.

LYMPHOID FOLLICLES

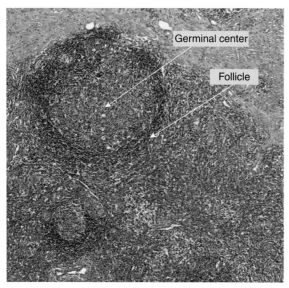

FIGURE 4.17   Follicles with Germinal Centers

Lymphoid follicles are seen in lymph nodes. However, in the skin they are encountered in cutaneous lymphoid hyperplasia and cutaneous lymphomas. A follicle is the active structure seen within the lymph node. A follicle that has acquired a germinal center is called a "secondary follicle." The germinal center is seen in the middle of the follicle and the surrounding cells form the mantle zone. The germinal center is formed of the dendritic reticulum cells, lymphoid cells, and the tingible body macrophages. The mantle zone is composed of mature lymphocytes.

FOLLICULOCENTRIC INFLAMMATION

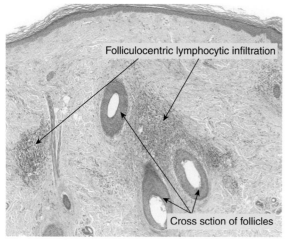

FIGURE 4.18   Folliculocentric Inflammation

This is an inflammatory reaction pattern seen characteristically in lupus erythematosus. The lymphocytes of the inflammatory infiltrate have a predilection for the hair follicles and other adnexal structures. In later stages of the disease there is infiltration and destruction of the follicular epithelium.

FOLLICULOSEBACEOUS INDUCTION

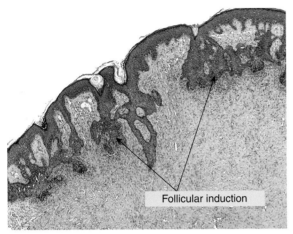

Follicular induction

FIGURE 4.19   Folliculosebceous Induction Overlying Dermatofibroma

This is a reaction pattern seen specifically overlying dermatofibroma. The basal epithelial cells are hyperplastic and they proliferate giving the appearance of a basaloid proliferation simulating a basal cell carcinoma. Occasionally sebaceous glands are also seen within the basaloid proliferation. It is important to recognize this pattern and not to overcall this as a basal cell carcinoma.

GRANULOMAS

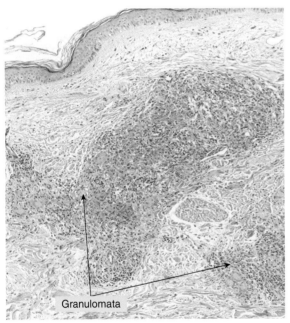

Granulomata

FIGURE 4.20   Granuloma

Granulomatous inflammation of the dermis is seen in various inflammatory and neoplastic conditions. They are defined as "a collection of epithelioid histiocytes (histiocytes which have an appearance resembling epithelial cells of the skin), lymphocytes, and multinucleated giant cells," which are formed by fusion of histiocytes. Three different types of giant cells have been described. (a) Langhans type in which the nuclei are arranged in a horseshoe pattern, (b) Tuton type of giant cell in which the nuclei are arranged as a wreath, and (c) multinucleated giant cell in which the nuclei are randomly arranged within a big cell.

There are different histological types of granulomas. They have been classified as tuberculoid, sarcoidal, foreign body, and suppurative. Different inflammatory mechanisms are involved in each type of granuloma. Granulomatous pattern is also seen in granuloma annulare, necrobiosis lipoidica, and malignant tumors.

GRENZ ZONE

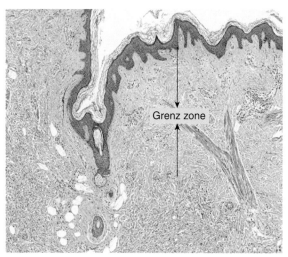

FIGURE 4.21   Grenz Zone

Grenz zone literally means "wall" or "an area of separation." This is an area of normal dermis separating the dermis from the epidermis and is commonly seen in dermatofibroma as a diagnostic clue.

HYPERGRANULOSIS

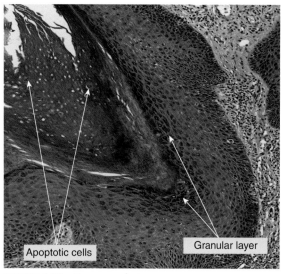

FIGURE 4.22   Hypergranulosis

Hypergranulosis is a term used to indicate the increased thickness and numbers of the granular layer of the epidermis. Wedge shaped hypergranulosis is seen in Lichen Planus and is a diagnostic clue. Hypergranulosis is commonly seen in viral warts.

HYPERKERATOSIS-BASKET WEAVE TYPE

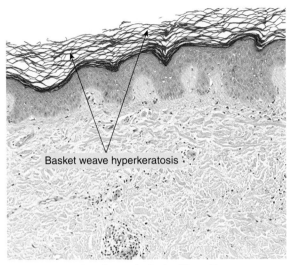

FIGURE 4.23   Hyperkeratosis, Basket Weave Type

It means thickening of the corneal layer of the epidermis in a basket weave pattern. The nuclei are absent in the epithelial cells of this layer. Basket weak hyperkeratosis is also referred to as "orthokeratosis" or "orthokeratotic hyperkeratosis."

HYPERKERATOSIS-COMPACT TYPE

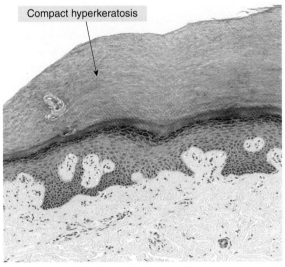

FIGURE 4.24   Hyperkeratosis, Compact Type

This type of hyperkeratosis is seen in acral skin. The corneal layer is markedly thickened and the basket weave is not retained as the layers appear to be compressed together.

HYPERKERATOSIS-FOLLICULAR TYPE

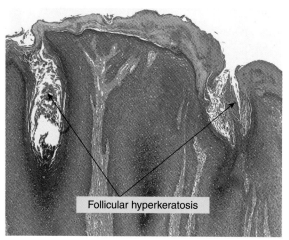

FIGURE 4.25   Hyperkeratosis of Follicles

It is also referred to as follicular plugging. The follicular ostium (opening in the epithelial layer) is plugged by excessive amounts of keratin. It is considered as one of the diagnostic features of discoid lupus erythematosus but can be seen in other conditions.

INTERFACE DERMATITIS

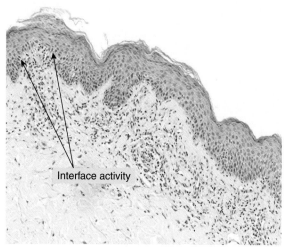

FIGURE 4.26   Interface Dermatitis

It is a very loosely used term in dermatopathology. It refers to inflammation at the dermoepidermal interface. The inflammatory cell involved is invariably a lymphocyte. The intensity of the inflammation and the degree of involvement of the basal layer vary to a considerable degree depending on the lesion. The lymphocytic infiltrate may be lichenoid or focal. The infiltrate may or may not obscure the dermoepidermal junction, in addition to causing basal cell vacuolation as seen in erythema multiforme and lichen planus or may just obscure the dermoepidermal interface as in lymphomatoid papulosis. Some authors use this term to specifically indicate the prescence of a "lichenoid" type inflammatory infiltrate (see below) which has a more diffuse, sparse lymhocytic infiltrate (as opposed a "band like" lymphocytic infiltrate) without obscuration of the basal layer.

KAMINO BODIES

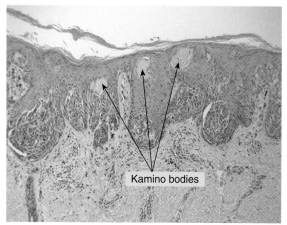

FIGURE 4.27   Kamino Bodies, H & E Stain

Kamino bodies are seen within the epidermis and are a characteristic feature of Spitz nevi. On H&E sections they appear as pink globules (Fig. 4.27) and they are PAS (periodic Acid Schiff stain) positive and diastase resistant (Fig. 4.28). Sometimes they coalesce to form large pink structures in the epidermis. Ultrastructurally they have been identified to contain Collagen IV and VII and laminin, thus identifying to be basement membrane substance. Many studies suggest that the presence of Kamino bodies is a feature of benign Spitz nevus. The bodies get smaller or disappear in malignant Spitz nevi.

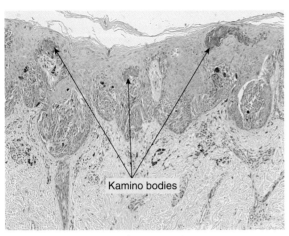

FIGURE 4.28   Kamino Bodies, PAS Stain

KERATINOUS CYSTS

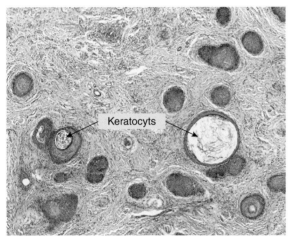

FIGURE 4.29   Keratocysts

These are cysts lined by squamous epithelium and containing keratinous material within them. They are a constant feature of trichoepithelioma.

LENTIGINOUS MELANOCYTES

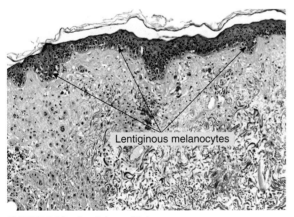

FIGURE 4.30   Lentiginous Melanocytes

This is the arrangement of melanocytes at the dermoepidermal junction in a picket fence pattern. Lentiginous pattern of melanocytes is seen in sun-damaged skin referred to as lentiginous melanocytic hyperplasia. In lentigo maligna, the cells are atypical and sometimes nested.

LICHENOID INFILTRATE

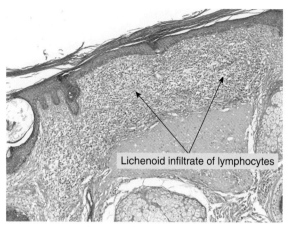

FIGURE 4.31   Lichenoid Infiltrate

This is band-like infiltrate seen in the papillary dermis. In majority of the cases the infiltrate is composed of lymphocytes with an admixture of histiocytes. In lichenoid tissue reaction basal cell damage may be seen in addition to Civatte bodies. Lichenoid infiltrate can be seen in conditions such as lichenoid actinic keratosis, lichen planus, squamous cell carcinoma, and melanoma.

LEUKOCYTOCLASIS

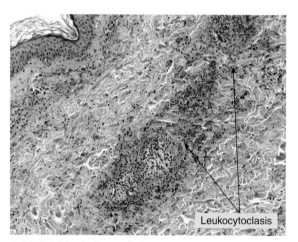

FIGURE 4.32   Leukocytoclasis

This is a process of disintegration of the neutrophils secondary to usually a hypersensitivity reaction. The neutrophil loose the lobulation of the nuclei and they appear pyknotic or dense. This results in the formation of nuclear dust. Leukocytoclasis is most commonly seen in leukocytoclastic vasculitis.

METAPLASIA IN A NEVUS

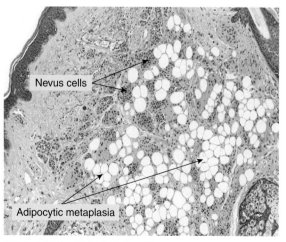

FIGURE 4.33   Metaplasia in a Nevus

Metaplasia is the presence of a cell type which is not normally present in that location where they occur (i.e., aberrant expression). Adipocytic metaplasia is seen in many benign and malignant neoplasms as seen in this nevus. Other types of metaplasia include cartilaginous and osseous.

MUNRO MICROABSCESS

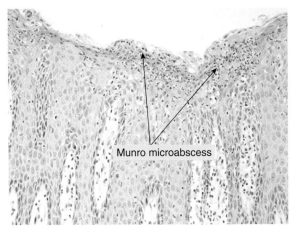

FIGURE 4.34   Munro Microabscess

Munro microabscess is the collection of neutrophils in an intra-corneal location. This is a feature seen in psoriasis. The adjacent skin shows areas of parakeratosis with intervening layers of orthokeratosis.

PAGETOID SPREAD

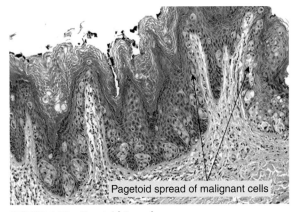

FIGURE 4.35   Pagetoid Spread

The upward migration of single or small groups of atypical melanocytes into the spinous and granular layer of the epidermis in melanoma is referred to as "Pagetoid spread." Characteristically these cells should be seen at the peripheral aspect of the dermal component in a melanoma. Pagetoid spread in melanoma is known to correlate with bRAF mutation. Spitz nevi, acral nevi, pigmented spindle cell nevi, and congenital nevi are known to manifest upward spread. In these benign lesions the upward spread is generally of single cells and they are confined to the epidermis above the dermal component. Spitz nevi are also known to manifest larger nests within the epidermis.

Other nonmelanocytic lesions are also known to have Pagetoid spread of cells within the epidermis. These include Paget's disease of the nipple, extramammary Paget's disease, Bowen disease, intraepidermal sebaceous carcinoma, and intraepidermal Merkel cell carcinoma. Less commonly Pagetoid reticulosis (a localized form of cutaneous T cell lymphoma occurring on the dorsa of the feet) and Langerhans cell histiocytosis also manifest pagetoid spread of cells.

Immunohistochemistry is of paramount importance in establishing a diagnosis in the above-mentioned conditions.

PAPILLOMATOSIS

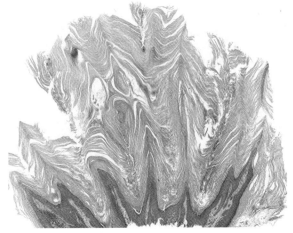

FIGURE 4.36   Papillomatosis

Papillomatosis refers to the projection of papillary dermis toward the surface resulting in an undulated and uneven epidermis. Usually papillomatosis is associated with marked hyperkeratosis. Squamous papilloma, viral wart, seborrheic keratosis, and verrucous carcinoma are some of the common conditions exhibiting papillomatosis.

PAPILLARY MESENCHYMAL BODIES

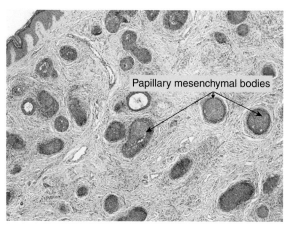

FIGURE 4.37   Papillary Mesenchymal Bodies

These are primitive hair structures seen in trichoepithelioma. This feature could be used as one of the diagnostic clues for distinguishing trichoepitheliomas from basal cell carcinomas.

PAPILLARY MICROABSCESSES

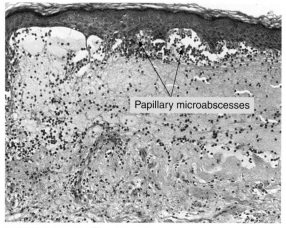

FIGURE 4.38   Papillary Microabscess

Papillary microabscesses are a collections of neutrophils in the dermal papillae. This is most commonly seen in dermatitis herpetiformis. It could also be seen in linear IgA disease and cicatricial pemphigoid.

Immunofluorescence studies should be helpful in establishing the diagnosis.

PARAKERATOSIS

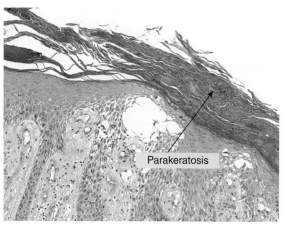

FIGURE 4.39   Parakeratosis

Parakeratosis refers to the retention of keratinocyte nuclei in the corneal layer. The nuclei appear flattened and parallel to the underlying epidermis. Parakeratosis is the result of too rapid elimination of keratinocytes due to varying pathological processes.

PERIVASCULAR LYMPHOCYTES

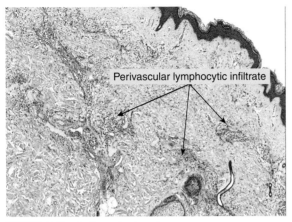

FIGURE 4.40 Perivascular Lymphocytes

This is one of the most common patterns of arrangement of lymphocytes in an inflammatory dermatoses where the inflammotry infiltrate of lymphocytes aggragates around blood lessels in the dermis. On its own it does not have any diagnostic significance.

PIGMENT INCONTINENCE

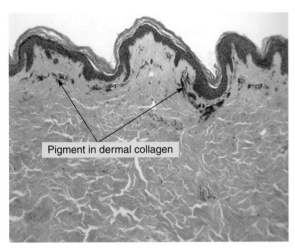

FIGURE 4.41 Pigment Incontinence

This is a term used to denote the presence of melanin pigment within the papillary dermis and within the macrophages. Pigment incontinence is seen in inflammatory dermatoses and melanocytic abnormalities.

PLEOMORPHISM

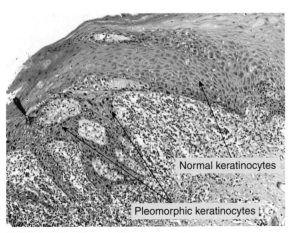

FIGURE 4.42 Pleomorphism

It refers to variation in size and shape of the nuclei and the cell as a whole. Pleomorphism is considered a hallmark of malignancy. The degree of pleomorphism varies in different tumors.

POIKILODERMA

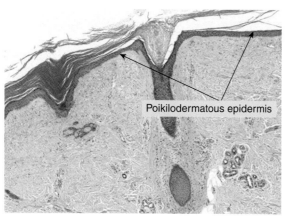

FIGURE 4.43   Poikilodermatous Epidermis

Poikilodermatous epidermis refers to the triad of epidermal atrophy, erythema (or telangiectasia) and mottled pigmentation. On H&E sections the epidermis appears very thinned out with possibly telangiectasia or dilation of blood vessels. Poikiloderma could be a manifestation of many inflammatory and neoplastic conditions, notably lichen planus and cutaneous T-cell lymphoma.

PSORIASIFORM HYPERPLASIA

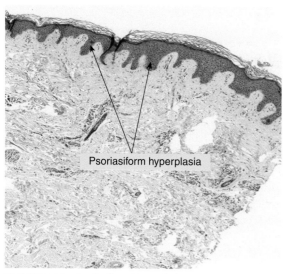

FIGURE 4.44   Psoriasiform Hyperplasia

This is a reaction pattern seen in a number of inflammatory diseases, the notable ones include psoriasis and its variants, Pityriasis rubra pilaris and lichen simplex chronicus. On H&E sections the epidermis shows regular elongation of rete ridges with occasional clubbing of the rete. There will be variable infiltration of inflammatory cells which includes neutrophils and lymphocytes in the papillary dermis and into the dermis. Psoriasis and its variants classically shows collections of neutrophils in the spinous and/or corneal layer and suprapapillary thinning of the epidermis.

SAW TOOTHING

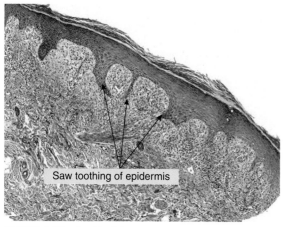

FIGURE 4.45   Saw Toothing

This is a pattern of epidermal reaction seen most commonly in lichen planus. The epidermis projects into the underlying dermis as thinned pointed structures giving the appearance of claws or the appearance of the cutting edge of a saw. The papillary dermis shows a lichenoid infiltrate.

SCAR WITH KELOID

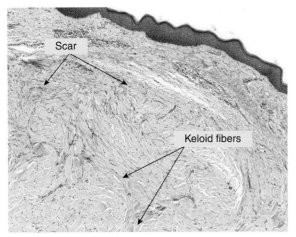

FIGURE 4.46   Scar with Keloid

Scar and keloid results following injury to the skin. On H&E, the scar shows parallel arrangement of collagen and fibroblasts with the overlying epidermal surface. Thin-walled vascular channels with mild infiltration of inflammatory cells are seen. Keloids within a scar are recognized by hypereosinophilic thick bundles of collagen.

SOLAR ELASTOSIS

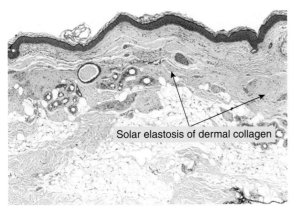

FIGURE 4.47   Solar Elastosis

Dermal solar elastosis is seen as pale blue structureless area in the superficial dermis. The overlying epidermis shows mild increase in the number of melanocytes termed "photo-activated melanocytes." The keratinocytes show varying degrees of atypia and are termed mild-moderate-to-severe actinic keratosis.

SPONGIOSIS

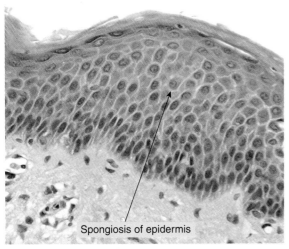

FIGURE 4.48   Spongiosis

Spongiosis refers to the separation of the keratinocytes due to intercellular edema. The intercellular bridges are prominent on H&E sections. The degree of spongiosis varies in with the etiological factor and in extreme cases can result in a spongiotic vesicle. Mild infiltration of lymphocytes, neutrophils, and eosinophils may be seen which may give a clue to the diagnosis. One of the major reaction patterns.

SPONGIOTIC VESICLE

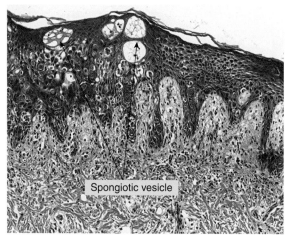

FIGURE 4.49 Spongiotic Vesicle

Extreme degrees of spongiosis results in "spongiotic vesicle" within the epidermis leading to blister formation clinically. There may be accumulation of lymphocytes, neutrophils or eosinophils within them.

SPONGIFORM PUSTULE OF KOGOJ

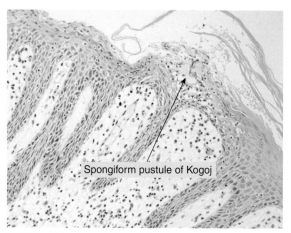

FIGURE 4.50 Spongiotic Vesicle

This is accumulation of neutrophils within the thin layer of corneal layer and/or degenerate cells of the spinous layer. This is a feature seen in psoriasis and its variants.

STORIFORM PATTERN

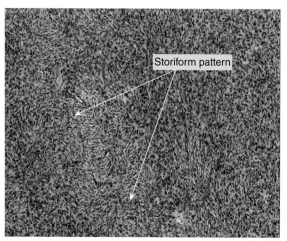

FIGURE 4.51 Storiform Pattern

This is a pattern of arrangement of cells characteristically seen in dermatofibrosarcoma protuberans and less commonly in dermatofibromas. The spindle and stellate cells are arranged around a central point in radial pattern. Storiform pattern may be seen less commonly in other soft tissue tumors.

SUBCORNEAL PUSTULE

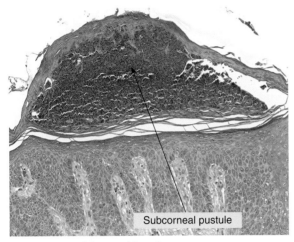

There is collection of neutrophils beneath the corneal layer. This is a feature seen in various conditions including subcorneal pustular dermatoses, impetigo, dermatophytosis, variants of pemphigus, and acute generalized exanthematous pustulosis.

FIGURE 4.52   Subcorneal Pustule

SUPRAPAPILLARY PLATE

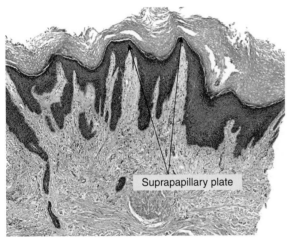

This is the area of the epidermis seen just above the dermal papillae. Thinning of the supra papillary plate is a feature considered diagnostic of Psoriasis.

FIGURE 4.53   Suprapapillary Plate

BIBLIOGRAPHY

Ackerman AB. Subtle clues to histopathologic findings from gross pathology (clinical lesions) Collarettes of scales as signs of spongiosis. Am J Dermatopathol 1979;1:267–272.

David W. Skin Pathology, 3rd Ed. Churchill Livingstone, 2009.

Jones RR. Spongiosis—a passive phenomenon? J Am Acad Dermatol 1982;6:547–549.

Leboit PE. Interface dermatitis. How specific are its histopathologic features? Arch Dermatol 1993;129: 1324–1328.

Nickoloff BJ. Light microscopic assessment of 100 patients with patch/plaque stage mycosis fungoides. Am J Dermatopathol 1988;10:469–477.

Oliver GF, Winkleman RK, Muller SA. Lichenoid dermatitis. A clinicopathological and immune pathologic review of sixty two cases. J Am Acad Dermatol 1989;21:284–292.

Sharon WW, John RG. Enzinger & Weiss's Soft Tissue Tumors, 5th Ed. Mosby, Elsevier, 2007.

Stephen SS. Histology for Pathologists, 2nd Ed. Lippincott-Raven, 1997.

Weedon D, Searle J, Kerr JFR. Apoptosis. Its nature and implications for dermatopathology. Am J Dermatopathol 1979;1(2):133–144.

Yancey KB. From bedside to bench and back. The diagnosis and biology of bullous diseases. Arch Dermatol 1994;130:983–987.

Histochemical Stains in Dermatopathology

INTRODUCTION

Histochemistry is that branch of histopathology that deals with the identification of chemical components of cells and tissues. In recent years there has been a greater understanding of the different chemical substances synthesized in different tissues of the body, particularly in disease conditions. The identification of the different chemical substances has gone a long way in establishing a particular diagnosis.

The tissues identified by the histochemical stains relevant to dermatopathology can be broadly classified under the following headings.

1. Carbohydrates: (a) mucins and (b) glycogen

2. Proteins: amyloid

3. Connective tissues: (a) elastic fibers and (b) collagen

4. Microorganisms: stains for carbohydrates

5. Pigments and minerals

ALCIAN BLUE STAINING MUCIN IN THE DERMIS

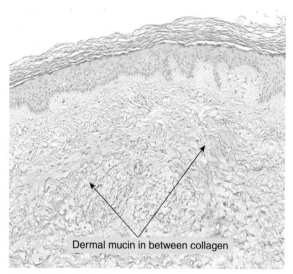

Dermal mucin in between collagen

FIGURE 5.1   Alcian Blue

Mucins are hexosamine-containing polysaccharides covalently bonded to various amounts of protein. Mucins are of different types and histochemically they can be identified as connective tissue and epithelial mucins. Both are sulphated acidic mucins. The different types of mucin may be present as a single type or in combination in different tissues. Hyaluronic acid is a sulphated sialomucin and is normally present in the dermis but in increased quantities in myxoedema.

Alcian blue is a dye used to demonstrate mucin. The connective tissue and epithelial mucins being acidic are periodic acid schiff (PAS) negative and are produced mainly by fibroblasts, mast cells, endothelial cells, chondrocytes, osteocytes, and certain tumors. Hyaluronic acid is a sulphated sialomucin and is normally present in the dermis but in increased quantities in myxoedema. Mucin deposition in the dermis in the different varieties of cutaneous mucinoses, granuloma annulare, lupus erythematosus, and scleredema can be demonstrated at pH2.5.

Alcian blue was one of the earliest Alcian dyes to be introduced and it shows intense staining. The staining technique can be varied using varying pH to identify the specific type of mucin. Mucin deposition in the dermis in the different varieties of cutaneous mucinoses including lupus erythematosus and scleredema can be demonstrated at pH2.5.

GLYCOGEN IN THE GOBLET CELLS OF THE CONJUNCTIVAL EPITHELIUM

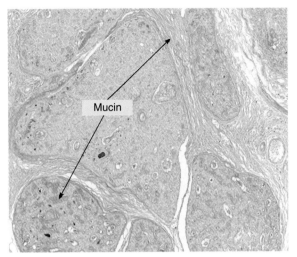

FIGURE 5.2   Alcian Blue Stain Adenoid Cystic Carcinoma

Adenoid Cystic Carcinoma produces abundant sulphated sialo-mucin called "hyaluronic acid." This is seen in between the lobules of tumour and in the smaller cysts.

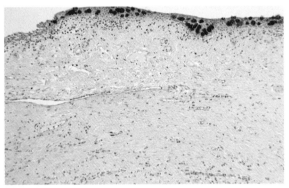

FIGURE 5.3   PAS Staining Glycogen in the Goblet Cells of Conjunctival Epithelium

Glycogen in normally present in the goblet cells of the conjunctiva, gastrointestinal and respiratory tracts, and the liver. The PAS stain produces the magenta color to glycogen. Normal glycogen present in tissues is not digested by diastase.

STAINS FOR PROTEINS

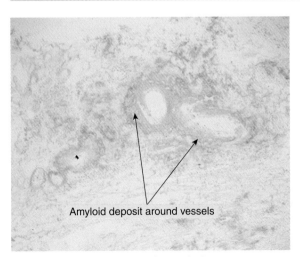

FIGURE 5.4   Congo Red Stain for Amyloid

Congo Red Staining Amyloid

Congo red is a dye which is used to stain amyloid. The reaction between Congo red and amyloid is through nonpolar hydrogen bonding.

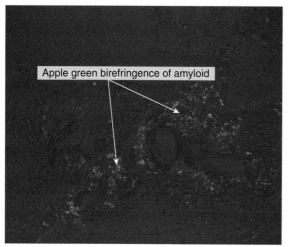

FIGURE 5.5   Congo Red Stain Demonstrating Apple Green Birefringence

Congo Red Demonstrating Apple Green Birefringence

Amyloid stained with Congo red exhibits apple green birefringence when viewed under polarized light. Birefringence is the property of a crystalline substance which has asymmetrical or laminated molecular structure. Two rays of light vibrating in perpendicular planes will travel in different velocities through the substance producing a fast ray and a slow ray. Such a substance will have two refractive indices and is said to show positive birefringence if the plane of vibration of the slow ray is parallel to the length of the fiber or crystal. A negative birefringence is produced when the plane of vibration of the slow ray is perpendicular to the length of the fiber. The bright apple green birefringence of amyloid following staining with Congo red or Sirius red is highly sensitive and is an intrinsic property of amyloid fibril-Congo-red complex.

Amyloid also has the ability to fluoresce following treatment with fluorochromic dyes. One of the most popular dyes used has been thioflavin T. However, this is a sensitive but not a specific stain. Keratin, arteriolar hyaline, and fibrin are known to stain with thioflavin T in addition to amyloid.

Immunohistochemical methods have also been used to detect the various types of amyloid.

Under the electron microscope amyloid exhibits a beta-pleated appearance of the fibrils. This is used as a reliable technique for the detection of amyloid.

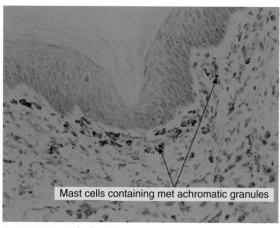

FIGURE 5.6   Toluidine Blue

Toluidine Blue Staining Mast Cells

The purple granules seen within mast cells are a demonstration of metachromasia of the dye toluidine blue. Metachromasia is a phenomenon by which a dye exhibits different colors depending on the wavelength of light it absorbs and the concentration of the surroundings. Toluidine blue transmits in the blue at low concentrations and in the purple at higher concentrations.

CONNECTIVE TISSUE STAINS

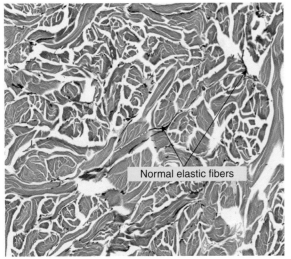

FIGURE 5.7   Elastic Van Gieson Stain for Normal Elastic Fibers

Elastic Fibers Stained with Verhoeff's Stain

Elastic fibers are seen in skin, respiratory system, and circulatory system. They are seen as fine single fibers in the skin. The elastic tissue is stained black.

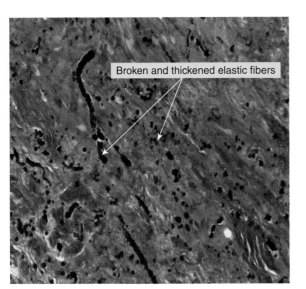

FIGURE 5.8   Elastic Van Gieson in Elastofibroma

Abnormal Elastic Fibers Stained with Verhoeff's Stain

The elastic fibers are thickened, corded, and broken in elastofibroma. The fibers are stained black.

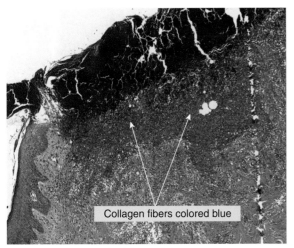

FIGURE 5.9   Masson's Trichrome LP

Masson's Trichrome Staining Collagen

Collagen fibers are found in abundance as an intercellular substance in most sites of the body. They may be seen as individual fibers or as clumped fibers as in a tendon. Collagen is synthesized by the fibroblasts. The synthesis of collagen is controlled genetically and four major types and several minor types of collagen have been recognized. All of them have the characteristic amino acid content. Collagen types I and III are major constituents of skin and collagen type IV is an important component of the lamina densa of the basement membrane of skin. Collagen type VII is seen in the sublamina densa region of the basement membrane. There are several disorders associated with the abnormal production and deposition of collagen in the skin. These include scleroderma, perforating collagenoses, and atrophic collagenoses to name a few.

Masson's trichrome stains the collagen blue green in color and elastin pale red.

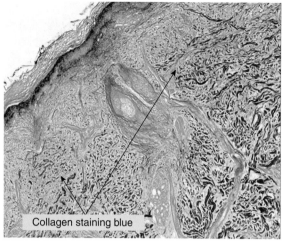

FIGURE 5.10   Masson's Trichrome Stain Morphea

Masson's Trichrome Staining Abnormal Collagen Deposition in Morphea

The excess amount of collagen deposited in the papillary dermis is stained blue by Masson's trichrome.

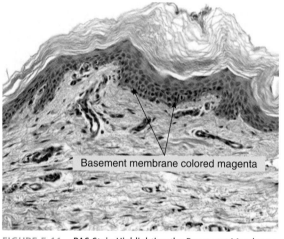

FIGURE 5.11   PAS Stain Highlighting the Basement Membrane

PAS Stain Highlighting the Basement Membrane

The basement membrane of skin is made of predominantly collagens IV and VII. The association of collagen IV with significant amounts of carbohydrates explains the strong reaction of basement membrane with periodic acid-Schiff reagent, which is an indicator of the presence of carbohydrates.

STAINS FOR MICROORGANISMS

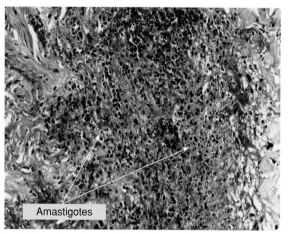

FIGURE 5.12   Giemsa Stain Positive for the Amastigotes of Leishmania Tropica

Leishman Donovan Bodies Stain with Giemsa

Cutaneous Leishmaniasis or oriental sore is transmitted by sand fly bite. Leismania Tropica is the organism most commonly involved. They are seen within swollen histiocytes and can be highlighted with Giemsa stain as haematoxyphilic bodies.

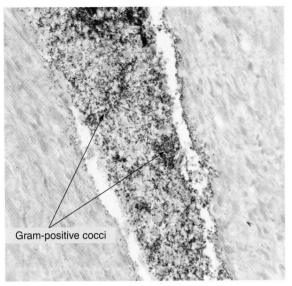

FIGURE 5.13   Gram Stain

Gram Stain Demonstrating Bacteria

The stain demonstrates the bacteria that appear blue in color. The common gram-positive cocci are *Streptococcus* sp. and *Staphylococcus* sp. The gram-positive bacilli are *Clostridium* and *Corynebacterium*.

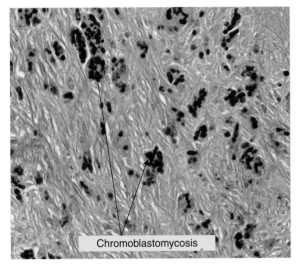

FIGURE 5.14   Grocott's Methenamine Silver

Grocott's Methenamine Silver Stain

Fungal spores of chromoblastomycosis are stained black with the silver stain.

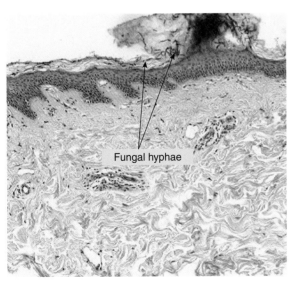

FIGURE 5.15   PAS Stain Highlighting the Fungal Hyphae

PAS Stain Highlighting Fungal Hyphae

Fungal hyphae are highlighted with the PAS stain which stain the cuticle of the hyphae magenta in color. Hematoxylin and eosin sections of the biopsy show three characteristic features in suspected fungal infections. These are the presence of neutrophils within the corneal layer, compact orthokeratosis, and the presence of the sandwich sign. Sandwich sign refers to the hyphae being sandwiched between the upper normal basket weave hyperkeratosis and the lower abnormal compact or parakeratotic hyperkeratosis. These three features were first described by Ackerman.

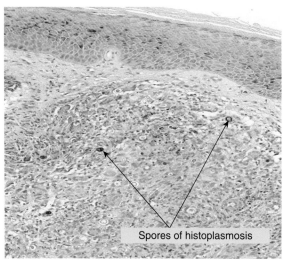

FIGURE 5.16   PAS Stain Highlighting Spores of Histoplasmosis

PAS Stain Highlighting Histoplasmosis

The capsule of *Histoplasma capsulatum* is highlighted by the PAS stain.

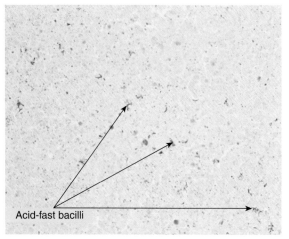

FIGURE 5.17   Zeihl-Neelsen Stain Demonstrating Acid-Fast Bacilli

Ziehl-Neelsen Stain Demonstrating Mycobacteria

Mycobacteria are rod-shaped or bacilli and they possess a capsule containing a long-chain fatty acid called "mycolic acid," which makes them hydrophobic. This fatty capsule influences the penetration and removal of the stain by acid and alcohol. This is referred to as being acid and alcohol fast. Mycobacteria possess carbohydrates in their wall and hence they could be demonstrated using the PAS stain. But this is possible only when the concentration of the organism is quite high.

STAINS FOR PIGMENTS

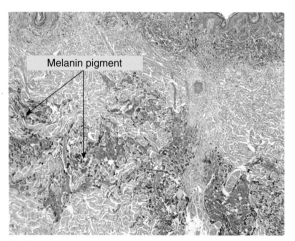

FIGURE 5.18   Masson Fontana Staining Melanin

Masson Fontana Staining Melanin Pigment

Melanin is a brownish-black pigment found in the skin, eye, and substantia nigra of the brain. Melanin is synthesized within melanosomes contained in the cytoplasm of the melanocytes. Melanin is produced from tyrosine by the action of an enzyme tyrosinase. Dihydroxyphenylalanine is an intermediary product in the sequence of events prior to the synthesis of melanin. The melanin thus produced is transferred to the keratinocytes through the melanocyte dendritic processes. The melanocytes and the keratinocytes that receive the melanin together form the epidermal melanin unit.

The Masson Fontana stains the melanin pigment black.

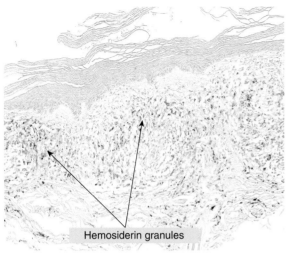

FIGURE 5.19   Perl's Prussian Blue Staining Hemosiderin
Pigment

Perl's Prussian Blue

Perl's Prussian blue stain is considered to be the first histochemical reaction. Hemosiderin is stained blue in color. Hemosiderin is a breakdown product of hemoglobin and is seen as golden-yellow intracellular granules. It contains iron in the form of ferric hydroxide.

BIBLIOGRAPHY

Bancroft JD, Gamble M. Theory and Practice of Histological Techniques, 5th Ed. Churchill Livingstone, 2002.
Mooi WJ, Krausz T. Pathology of Melanocytic Disorders, 2nd Ed. Hodder Arnold, 2007.
Weedon D. Skin Pathology, 3rd Ed. Churchill Livingstone, 2009.

Immunohistochemical Stains in Dermatopathology

INTRODUCTION

Immunohistochemistry is a specialized technique by which the antigen-antibody interaction is utilized to detect a specific antigen in the cell. The analysis of the interaction is done at a light microscopic level. An antibody is a molecule that has the property of combining specifically with a second molecule termed the "antigen." Antibodies are immunoglobulin molecules consisting of light chains and a pair of heavy chains. Immunoglobulin molecules can be both antibodies, binding specifically to tissue antigens, and antigens providing antigenic determinants to which secondary antibodies may be attached. An antigen is a complex three-dimensional structure capable of inducing antibody formation. Some of the commercially available antibodies are designated by CD, which refers to cluster of differentiation or cluster of designation. This is a system intended for the classification of monoclonal antibodies generated by different laboratories around the world against epitopes on the surface molecules of white blood cells. Since then the use of CD designation has expanded to a wide variety of cell types and currently more than 320 CD numbers have been identified in different cells.

The antibody used in immunohistochemistry is evaluated purely on the basis of the sensitivity and specificity of the antigen-antibody reaction. The immunohistochemical staining of any tissue section is performed with a simultaneous control tissue section. The controls are tissue sections that are known to be positive for that antibody. The use of controls ensures that the antibody has worked. Some of the specimens may have internal controls, for example there is positive staining of the epidermis and the adnexal structures with cytokeratins and epithelial membrane antigen (EMA). When assessing immunohistochemical stains it is always useful to check the control. If there is absence of staining in the controls and the specimen sections, the reason is bound to be a technical problem. In this instance it is wise to ask for repeat staining of the antibody.

The following sections give an account of the different immunohistochemical stains of diagnostic significance in dermatopathology.

CYTOKERATINS

Ultrastructurally, the cell cytoplasm contains intermediate filament proteins together with microfilaments and microtubules. In epithelial cells that are rich in high-molecular-weight keratins, the intermediate filaments are arranged in a parallel pattern. Keratins have a high degree of specificity and sensitivity in the diagnosis of epithelial neoplasms. Keratins are broadly divided into Type I (acidic) and Type II (basic) keratins. There are 12 type 1 keratins and 8 type 2 keratins.

Cytokeratins are present in the epidermis and the adnexal structures of the skin. Hence, the usefulness of cytokeratins in dermatopathology is for the confirmation of tumors primarily arising from the epidermis and the adnexa. Additionally, cytokeratins are also used to confirm metastatic epithelial tumors of the skin.

The commonest tumors of keratinocyte origin are squamous cell carcinomas and basal cell carcinomas. There are many microscopic subtypes of both these tumors described. Most often there is no diagnostic difficulty with the classical morphological appearances in squamous cell carcinomas. Immunohistochemical stains are of use when diagnostic difficulty is encountered with unusual or hybrid morphological appearances as in spindle cell or epithelioid cell tumors or when there is a combination of cell types.

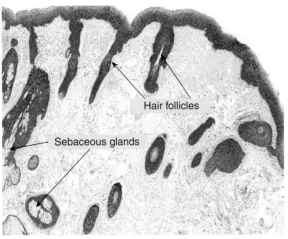

FIGURE 6.1   EMA Staining the Epidermis and Adnexal Structures

EMA Staining Epidermis and Adnexal Structures

The normal epidermis and its adnexal structures contain the cytokeratin tonofilaments and they stain with high molecular cytokeratin antibodies such as EMA, AE1/AE3, MNF116, CK 14, and CK5/6. All these antibodies demonstrate the same staining patterns.

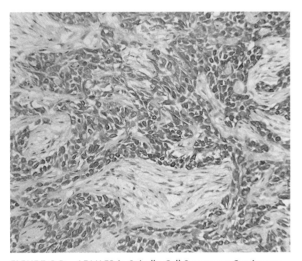

FIGURE 6.2   AE1/AE3 in Spindle-Cell Squamous Carcinoma

AE1/AE3 and CK14 Staining the Spindle-Cell Squamous Carcinoma

Squamous carcinomas with spindle cell, small cell, or pleomorphic cell morphology can be diagnostically challenging. Spindle-cell melanomas, sarcomas, and atypical fibroxanthomas enter the differential diagnosis. Immunohistochemical staining with cytokeratins is crucial in establishing the diagnosis of a spindle-cell squamous carcinoma also known as "sarcomatoid carcinoma." Spindle-cell carcinomas stain with AE1/AE3, MNF 116, CK14, and EMA in a diffuse and strong pattern. The diagnosis is also established by demonstrating the negative staining with S100, Melan A (melanocytic markers), SMA, desmin, h-caldesmon (mesenchymal markers), CD68, and CD163 (histiocytic markers).

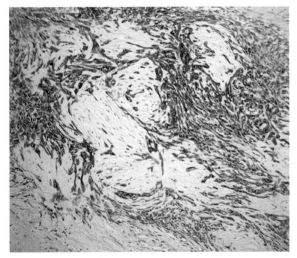

FIGURE 6.3   CK 14 in Spindle-Cell Carcinoma

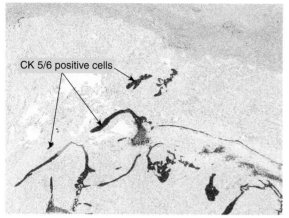

FIGURE 6.4   CK5/6 in Spindle-Cell Carcinoma

CK5/6 Staining Spindle-Cell Squamous Carcinoma

CK5/6 is a selective high-molecular-weight cytokeratin and decorates the spindle cells in poorly differentiated sarcomatoid carcinomas.

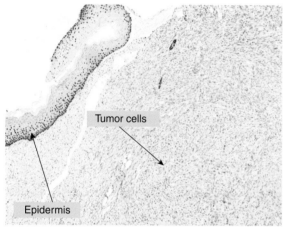

FIGURE 6.5   p63 in Spindle-Cell Carcinoma

p63 in Squamous Carcinoma

Squamous carcinomas which are poorly differentiated stain with p63 in a nuclear pattern. It is well known as a basal cell marker and can be used to differentiate poorly differentiated squamous cell carcinoma from poorly differentiated adenocarcinoma. It is expressed in nonneoplastic and neoplastic squamous epithelium.

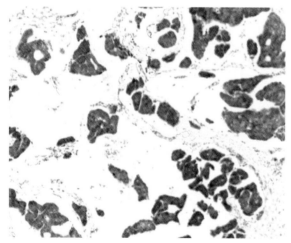

FIGURE 6.6   MNF 116 in Mucinous Carcinoma

MNF116

MNF 116 is a cocktail of high- and low-molecular-weight cytokeratins. Hence, it is broad spectrum and stains epidermal and adnexal tumors. Mucinous and adenoid cystic carcinomas are either primary or metastatic to skin. The distinction can be made only on clinical grounds as in finding a primary at a different site. Mucinous carcinomas are known to show in situ changes in some cases which helps to differentiate primary from metastatic tumors.

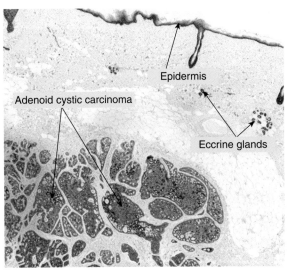

FIGURE 6.7   MNF Staining Adenoid Cystic Carcinoma and Epidermis

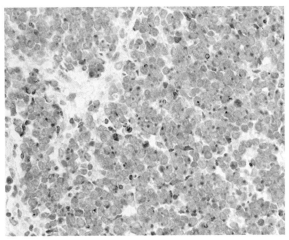

FIGURE 6.8   AE1/AE3 Staining Merkel Cells

AE1/AE3 Staining Merkel Cell Carcinoma

AE1/AE3 is a cocktail of high- and low-molecular-weight cytokeratins. Merkel cell carcinomas stain for the cytokeratins in a membranous pattern.

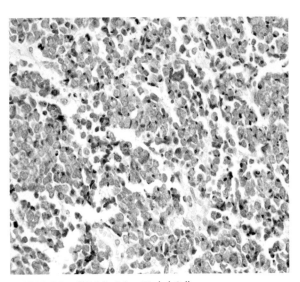

FIGURE 6.9   CK20 Staining Merkel Cells

CK20 Staining Merkel Cells

CK 20 is a selective cytokeratin known to demonstrate a para nuclear dot positivity in Merkel cell carcinoma. CK 20 is also useful in confirming the primary origin of a metastatic cutaneous carcinoma. The primary sites stained by CK20 are those of colorectal and urothelial origin.

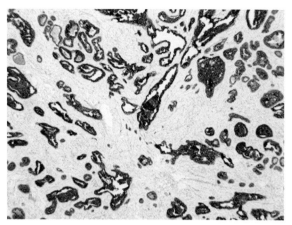

FIGURE 6.10   CK7 in Apocrine Tubular Adenoma

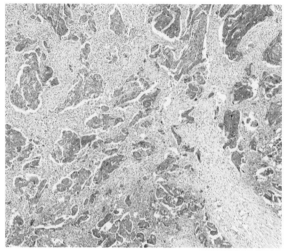

FIGURE 6.11   CK7-Positive Tumor Cells in St. Mary Joseph's Nodule

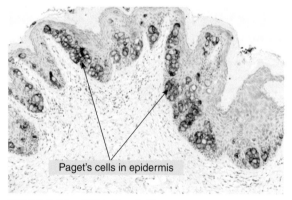

FIGURE 6.12   CK7 in Paget's Disease

CK 7 Staining Apocrine Tubular Adenoma

CK7 is a selective cytokeratin and stains the adnexal tumors of the skin, particularly of the head and neck area. It is also useful in differentiating primary and metastatic cutaneous tumors. Tumors originating from breast, right-sided colon and stomach, gynecological tract, urological tract, and respiratory tract are positive for CK7.

CK 7 Staining Metastatic Tumor of Ovarian Origin

Sister Mary Joseph's nodule is metastatic adenocarcinoma arising in the umbilical area. The primary sites are usually from the gynecological or gastrointestinal tract. The adenocarcinoma cells stain positively for CK7.

CK7 in Extra Mammary Paget's Disease

The vacuolated cells present within the epidermis in primary extramammary Paget's disease are considered to be of intraepidermal apocrine origin. Hence, these cells show positive stain with CK7, EMA, and carcinoembryonic antigen. However, secondary extramammary Paget's disease could have the primary carcinoma arising in the breast, gynecological tract, gastrointestinal tract, urological tract, or prostate. Paget's cell secondary to breast carcinomas is positive for CK7 and GCDFP-15 (gross cystic disease protein fluid-15). Primary tumors of the gynecological tract are positive for CK7 and CK20 in selected tumors of the endocervix. Primary ovarian tumors in addition stain for CA125 and WT1. Left-sided colonic tumors are positive for CK20 in 100% of cases. Fifteen percent of left-sided colonic tumors also stain for CK7. Right-sided colonic, esophageal, and gastric tumors are CK7 positive. CDx2 stains positive for primary mucinous tumors of colonic origin and not of ovarian origin. Tumors of the urological tract, the commonest being transitional cell carcinomas stain positive for CK20, CK5/6, thrombomodulin, and uroplakin 111. Villin is useful in distinguishing a CK20-positive tumor as colonic or urothelial in origin. Villin is positive in 90% of the tumors of colonic origin. Prostate specific antigen and prostate specific acid phosphatase confirm a primary of prostatic origin. The final diagnosis rests on clinicopathological correlation.

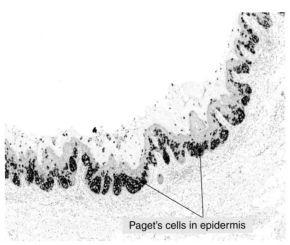

FIGURE 6.13   Cam 5.2 Staining Cells of Extramammary Paget's Disease

Cam 5.2 Staining Extramammary Paget's Cells

Cam 5.2 is a cocktail of low-molecular-weight cytokeratins and stains the adenocarcinoma cells in primary and secondary extramammary Paget's disease.

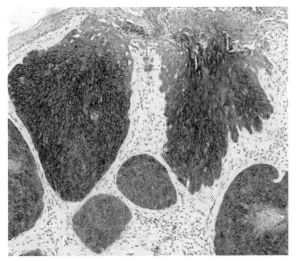

FIGURE 6.14   BerEP4 Staining Basal Cell Carcinoma

BerEp4 Staining Basal Cell Carcinoma

BerEp4 stains basal cell carcinoma and adenocarcinoma cells. In dermatopathology BerEp4 is particularly useful in distinguishing morpheic basal cell carcinoma from poorly differentiated squamous cell carcinoma, which is negative.

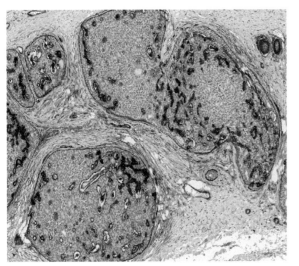

FIGURE 6.15   Collagen IV Stain in Adenoid Cystic Carcinoma

Collagen Staining of the Basement Membrane

Collagen and laminin are the principal components of the basement membrane in any tissue. Laminin is an active component of the lamina lucida. Type IV collagen is found in lamina densa and type VII collagen in the anchoring filaments. In discoid lupus erythematosus, there is exaggerated thickening of the basement membrane with collagen IV (Fig. 6.16) and thickening with fronds into the dermis with collagen VII (Fig. 6.17).

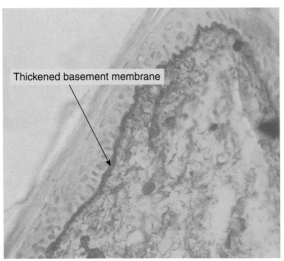

FIGURE 6.16 Collagen IV in DLE. By Courtesy of Dr. K Al-Refu, University of Jordan

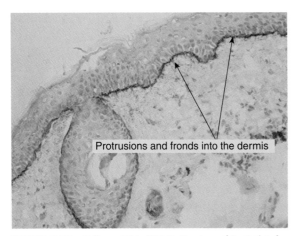

FIGURE 6.17 Collagen VII in DLE. By Courtesy of Dr. K Al-Refu, University of Jordan

MARKERS FOR CELLS OF MELANOCYTIC AND NEURAL ORIGIN

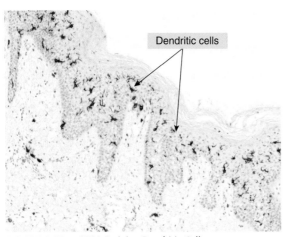

FIGURE 6.18 S100 Staining Dendritic Cells

S100 Staining Dendritic Cells

S100 protein has acquired its name from the fact that it is completely soluble in 100% ammonium sulphate. Three isoforms of S100 have been identified. They are S100ao (alpha dimer), S100a (alpha-beta isoform), and S100b (beta dimer). S100 protein is identified in a wide range of tissues. These include Schwann cells, neurons, melanocytes, chondrocytes, and various epithelial cells. The dendritic cells are Langerhans cells distributed within the epidermis.

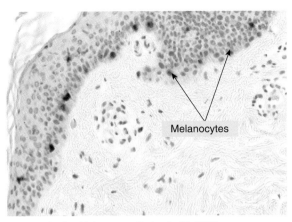

FIGURE 6.19   Melanocytes Stained with S100

S100 Staining Melanocytes

S100 protein stains melanocytes in the normal epidermis. Melanocytes are located in the basal layer of the epidermis in a ratio of 1 for 4–10 keratinocytes.

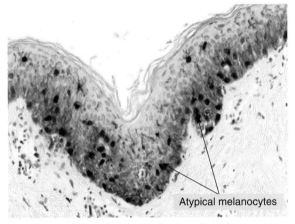

FIGURE 6.20   S100 Staining Melanocytes in Melanoma In Situ

S100 Staining Melanocytes in Melanoma In Situ

The melanocytes in melanoma in situ are pleomorphic and markedly increased in number.

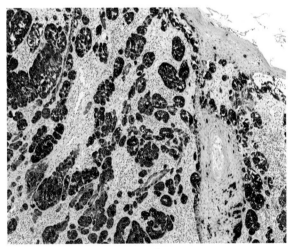

FIGURE 6.21   S100 Staining Melanoma

S100 Staining Melanocytes in Melanoma

The atypical melanocytes are found in the epidermis and the dermis.

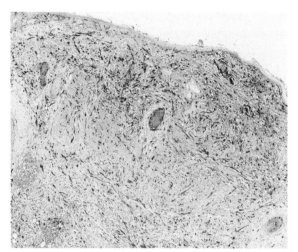

FIGURE 6.22 S100 in Desmoplastic Melanoma

S100 Staining Melanoma Cells in Desmoplastic Melanoma

Desmoplastic melanoma is a variant of melanoma showing slender spindle-shaped cells in the dermis. The cells stain with S100 and not with Melan A or HMB45 because the cells do retain part of its myofibroblastic characteristics.

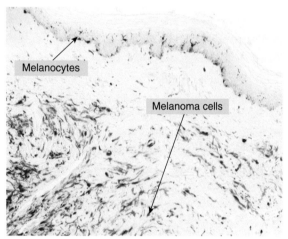

Melanocytes

Melanoma cells

FIGURE 6.23 S100 with Blue Chromogen

S100 with Blue Chromogen

In heavily pigmented lesions such as blue nevus, the presence of melanocytes can be demonstrated using a different color to the antibody. The usual brown color of immunohistochemical stains is masked by the blue color which highlights the melanocytes. This is particularly useful in assessing dermal invasion in an early radial growth phase melanoma, when the scattered atypical cells are obscured by inflammatory cells.

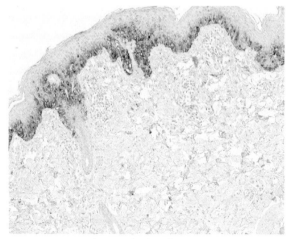

FIGURE 6.24 Melan A with Blue Chromagen in Melanoma In Situ

Melan A with Blue Chromogen

Melan A also known as Mart-1 (melanoma antigen recognized by T-cells-1) is a monoclonal antibody raised against a glycoproteinaceous antigen restricted to cells of melanocytic lineage. The protein is localized to the inner membranes of Types 1, 2, and 3 premelanosomes. Melan A is considered specific in the range of 60–80%.

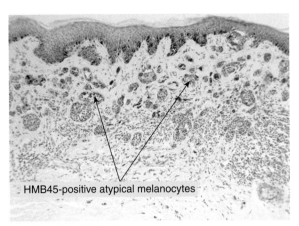

FIGURE 6.25   HMB 45

Human Melanoma Black (HMB45)

HMB45 is a monoclonal antibody that recognizes gp-100, a melanosomal glycoprotein. HMB45 denotes active melanogenesis. It is present in junctional melanocytes of junctional and compound nevi. It is present in many melanomas, but desmoplastic melanomas are generally negative.

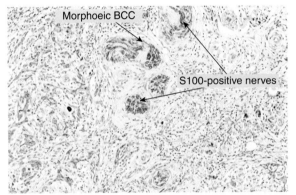

FIGURE 6.26   S100 Demonstrating Perineural Infiltration

S100 Staining the Nerves

S100 protein has been identified in the nerve cells. Nerve cells are of neural crest in origin.

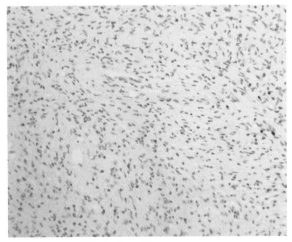

FIGURE 6.27   S100 in Neurofibroma

S100 in Neurofibroma

A subset of cells of neurofibroma stains with S100 protein, confirming the fact that neurofibroma contains a mixture of cells.

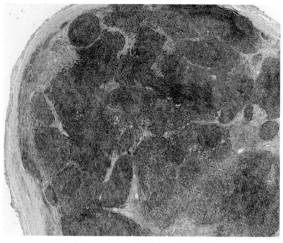

FIGURE 6.28   Schwannoma Stained with S100

S100 Staining Schwannian Cells

S100 stains the spindle cells of Schwannoma diffusely and strongly.

VASCULAR MARKERS AND LYMPHATIC MARKERS

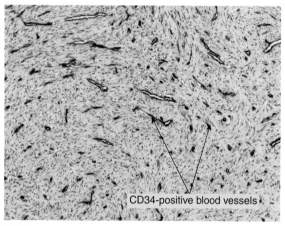

CD34-positive blood vessels

FIGURE 6.29   CD34 Staining Vessels

CD34 Staining Blood Vessels

CD34 is expressed by the embryonic progenitor cells and endothelial cells. It is a very sensitive indicator of vascular differentiation.

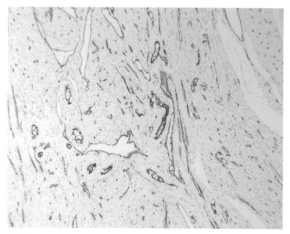

FIGURE 6.30   CD31 Staining Blood Vessels

CD31 Staining Blood Vessels

CD 31 is vascular endothelial marker staining the endothelial cells of normal blood vessels.

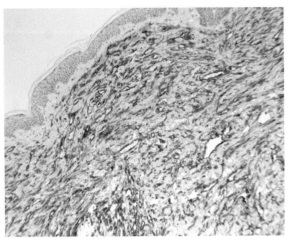

FIGURE 6.31   CD31 in Angiosarcoma

CD31 in Angiosarcoma

CD31 being a marker highly sensitive for endothelial differentiation, stains the cells of Angiosarcoma, regardless of the grade of the tumour.

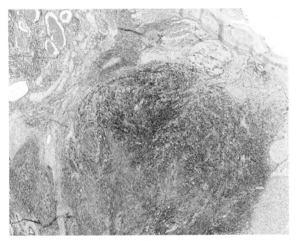

FIGURE 6.32   CD34 in Kaposi's Sarcoma

CD34 in Kaposi's Sarcoma

The vascular proliferation seen in Kaposi's sarcoma is stained strongly and diffusely by CD34.

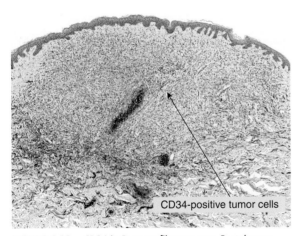

FIGURE 6.33   CD34 in Dermatofibrosarcoma Protuberans (DFSP)

CD34 Staining in Dermatofibrosarcoma Protuberans

Dermatofibrosarcoma protuberans is a fibrohistiocytic tumor of intermediate malignancy. The CD34 stains the dendritic cell population of cells that proliferate in the dermis. The CD34 staining is seen strong and diffuse in the dermis.

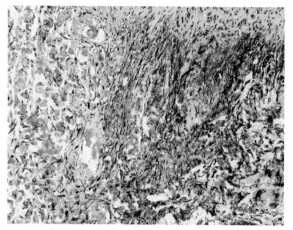

FIGURE 6.34   Staining Tumor in Dermatofibroma (DF)

CD34 Staining in Dermatofibroma

The fibrohistiocytic cells of dermatofibroma stain in a peripheral edge pattern in dermatofibromas.

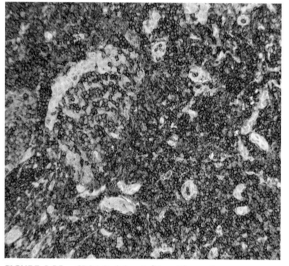

FIGURE 6.35   CD34 Staining Solitary Fibrous Tumor

CD34 Staining in Solitary Fibrous Tumor

CD34 is used as reliable marker for the diagnosis of solitary fibrous tumor. The sensitivity and specificity are in the range of 80–90%.

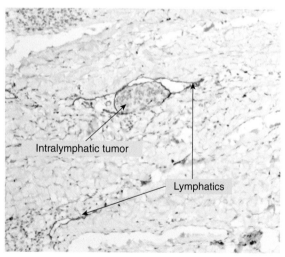

FIGURE 6.36   D2-40 Tumor in Lymphatics

D2-40 Tumor in Lymphatics

D2-40 is also known as podoplanin and is a highly sensitive marker to detect lymphatic channels.

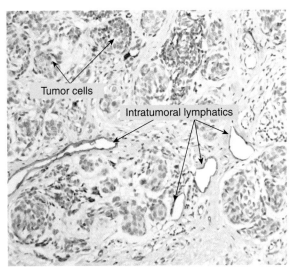

FIGURE 6.37   D2-40 Calponin Staining the Smooth Muscle Cells

D2-40 Stains the Intratumoral Lymphatics

The density of lymphatics within the tumor is a good indicator of the probability of lymph node metastasis, particularly in malignant melanoma as is demonstrated by this example.

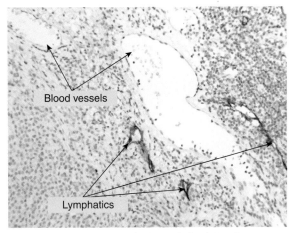

FIGURE 6.38   D2-40, Lymphatics and Blood Vessels

D2-40 Selectively Staining Lymphatics

D2-40 stains the lymphatic endothelium as opposed to the vascular endothelium.

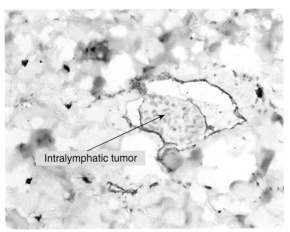

FIGURE 6.39   Lyve 1, Tumor in Lymphatics

LYVE-1 (Lymphatic Vessel Endothelial Hyaluronan Receptor) Staining Lymphatics

Lyve-1 is a lymphatic-specific gene. The antibody is a sensitive marker of lymphatic endothelium.

MARKERS FOR CELLS OF MESENCHYMAL ORIGIN

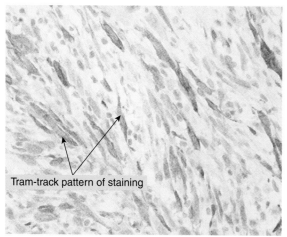

FIGURE 6.40   Calponin Staining the Smooth Muscle Cells

Calponin Staining Smooth Muscle Cells

Calponin stains the smooth muscle cells with partial smooth muscle differentiation in a tram-track pattern. Calponin is unique to smooth muscle and is known to activate the actomyosin adenosine triphosphatase activity in the smooth muscle contractile apparatus. Calponin is used as a reliable marker to identify the myofibroblasts which also demonstrates partial muscle differentiation.

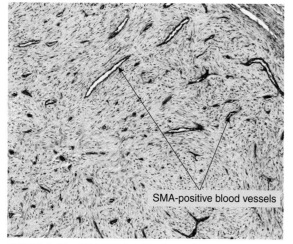

FIGURE 6.41   SMA Staining Blood Vessels

Smooth Muscle Actin Staining Blood Vessels

Smooth muscle cells present in the wall of blood vessels are stained with smooth muscle actin. Here the staining is uniformly cytoplasmic and nuclear unlike myofibroblasts which stain in a tram-track pattern.

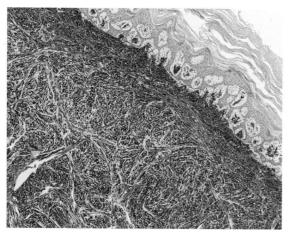

FIGURE 6.42   SMA Staining Leiomyoma

Smooth Muscle Actin Staining Leiomyoma

Cutaneous leiomyomas arise from the arrector pili muscles, which are true smooth muscles. The staining is uniformly cytoplasmic and nuclear.

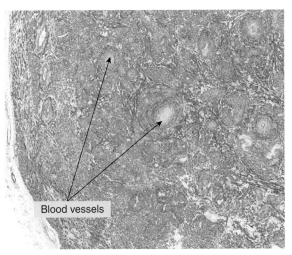

FIGURE 6.43   Smooth Muscle Actin Staining the Smooth Muscle Around Vessels—Angioleiomyoma

SMA Staining Smooth Muscles in Angioleiomyoma

Angioleiomyoma shows proliferation of smooth muscles around the blood vessels. This is true smooth muscle differentiation and stains strongly and diffusely with smooth muscle actin.

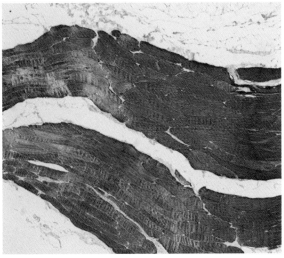

FIGURE 6.44   Desmin Staining Normal Skeletal Muscle

Desmin Staining Normal Skeletal Muscle

Desmin stains smooth muscle and skeletal muscle and is an intermediate filament protein. It is a highly sensitive marker of muscle differentiation.

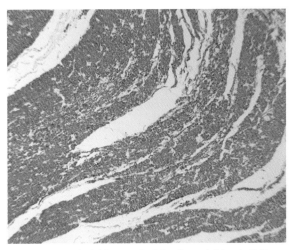

FIGURE 6.45   h-Caldesmon Staining Smooth Muscle Cells

h-Caldesmon Staining Smooth Muscle Cells

Heavy Caldesmon is a cytoplasmic protein specific for smooth muscles and myoepithelial cells.

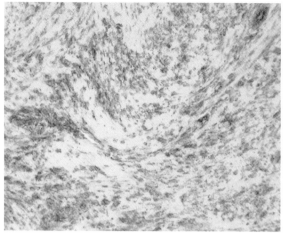

FIGURE 6.46   Beta-Catenin

Beta-Catenin in Fibromatosis

Nuclear expression of beta-catenin is seen in 90% of cases of fibromatosis as a result of mutation of beta-catenin. Beta-catenin is involved in intracellular signaling as part of the Wnt signaling pathway.

MARKERS FOR HEMOPOIETIC CELLS

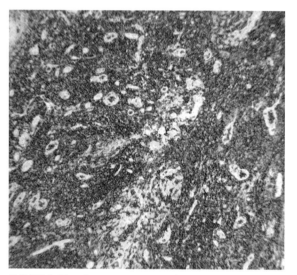

FIGURE 6.47   CD45 Staining Normal Lymphocytes

CD45 Staining Normal Lymphocytes

CD45 is found on all white blood cells as a membrane protein tyrosine phosphatase. It is a useful as pan lymphocytic marker.

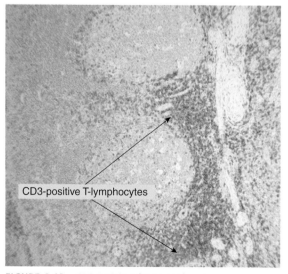

FIGURE 6.48   CD3 Staining the T-Lymphocytes

CD3 Staining the T-lymphocytes

CD3 is very specific for cells of T-cell derivation. The CD3 protein complex is located in the cell membrane.

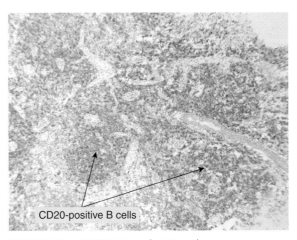

FIGURE 6.49   CD20 Staining the B-Lymphocytes

CD20 Staining the B-lymphocytes

CD 20 is a membrane protein acquired late in the stage of pre-B cell maturation. CD79a has very similar staining pattern for B-lymphocytes and it also stains plasma cells.

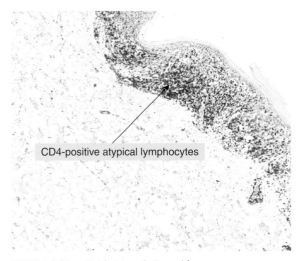

FIGURE 6.50   CD4 in Mycosis Fungoides

CD4 in Mycosis Fungoides

CD4 identifies the helper subset of T-lymphocytes. It interacts with HLA class 11 antigen during antigen recognition. The helper lymphocytes are best identified by flow cytometry or in frozen tissue.

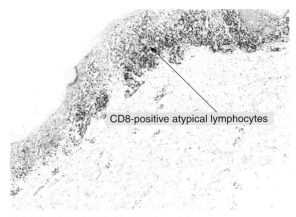

FIGURE 6.51   CD8 in Mycosis Fungoides

CD8 in Mycosis Fungoides

CD8 identifies the suppressor/cytotoxic T-lymphocytes. Normally CD4:CD8 ratio is 2:1. It can be altered in conditions such as mycosis fungoides, infections, and other inflammatory conditions.

FIGURE 6.52   CD30

CD30

CD30 belongs to the tumor necrosis factor receptor super family. It is a diagnostic marker for anaplastic large cell lymphomas, lymphomatoid papulosis, Hodgkin's disease, and CD30+ lymphoproliferative disorders. Alk-1 is the protein product of anaplastic lymphoma kinase gene. Cutaneous anaplastic large cell lymphomas can be positive for ALK-1, and it indicates cutaneous involvement from a nodal primary and subsequent bad prognosis.

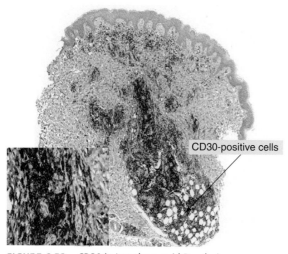

FIGURE 6.53   CD30 in Lymphomatoid Papulosis

CD30 in Lymphomatoid Papulosis

Lymphomatoid papulosis is considered a latent lymphoma and is a CD30-positive lymphoproliferative disorder. It shows a wedge-shaped proliferation of CD30-positive cells.

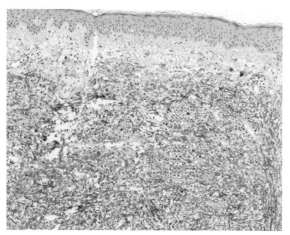

FIGURE 6.54   Myeloperoxidase Staining the Leukemic Deposit

Myeloperoxidase Staining Leukemic Deposit

Myeloperoxidase is a monocyte/granulocyte–related marker and is useful in the confirmation of myeloid tumor of skin.

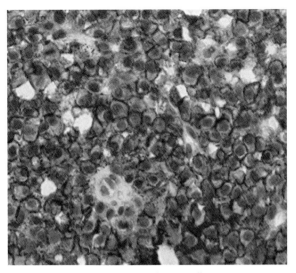

FIGURE 6.55   CD138 Staining Plasma Cells

CD138 Staining Plasma Cells

CD138 is a sensitive and specific marker for plasma cells. It shows the characteristic membrane staining.

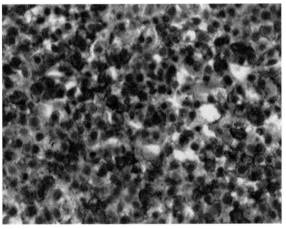

FIGURE 6.56   Epithelial Membrane Antigen Staining Plasma Cells

EMA Staining Plasma Cells

Epithelial membrane antigen is one of the human milk fat globules derived from the mammary epithelium. It is positive in tumors of different derivations and plasma cells. It shows the characteristic membrane staining.

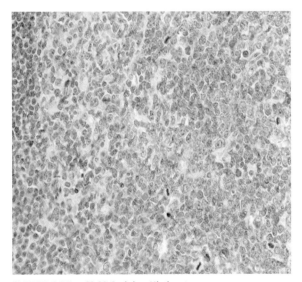

FIGURE 6.57   CD68 Staining Histiocytes

CD68 Staining Histiocytes

CD68 is a sensitive marker for histiocytes or macrophages and it shows characteristic membrane staining pattern.

FIGURE 6.58 CD163 Staining Histiocytes

CD163 Staining Histiocytes

CD163 is another reliable marker of histiocytes. It is much more specific and sensitive marker for histiocytes and shows membrane staining and cytoplasmic staining.

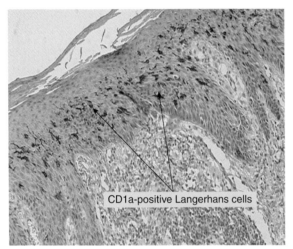

CD1a-positive Langerhans cells

FIGURE 6.59 CD1a Staining Normal Langerhans Cells

CD1a Staining Normal Langerhans Cells

Langerhans cells make up 3-8% of the cells of the epidermis and they are seen in different layers of the epidermis normally. They are also located in other organs, lung, and lymph nodes. Langerhans cells contain the characteristic granules called Langerhans cell granules or Birbeck granules and they stain with CD1a, S100, and a small percentage of them with CD68. Normal Langerhans cells have long dendritic processes and they process and present antigen to the T-lymphocytes.

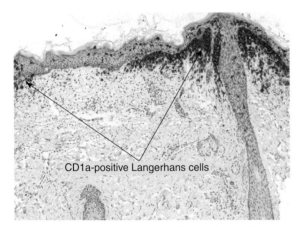

CD1a-positive Langerhans cells

FIGURE 6.60 CD1a Staining Cells of Langerhans Cell Histiocytosis

CD1a Staining Langerhans Cell Histiocytosis

Langerhans cell histiocytosis is a neoplastic condition in which the proliferating cells are seen in the dermis in addition to the epidermis.

IMMUNOHISTOCHEMICAL STAINS USED IN CUTANEOUS METASTATIC TUMORS

Skin is a very common site for metastasis, scalp being the commonest site due to its rich vascularity. Carcinomas with primary sites in breast, colon, kidney, endometrium, ovary, and thyroid frequently metastasize to the skin. Melanomas are well known for cutaneous metastasis. Cutaneous deposits are well documented from leukemias and lymphomas. Sarcomas although rare also target skin as a site for metastasis.

When a cutaneous metastasis is encountered, the use of immunohistochemical stains are crucial in arriving at the correct diagnosis. Considering the morphological appearances, a judicious use of relevant immunohistochemical stains will help in identifying the primary site. It goes without saying that clinicopathological correlation is very important in the diagnostic process.

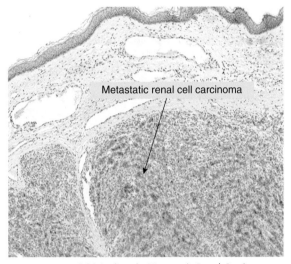

FIGURE 6.61   RCC Antigen in Metastatic Renal Carcinoma

Renal Cell Carcinoma Antigen

Renal cell carcinoma antigen is positive in about 67% of metastatic renal cell carcinomas. Two percent of metastatic nonrenal cell carcinomas are positive, particularly from the breast.

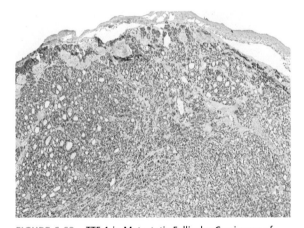

FIGURE 6.62   TTF-1 in Metastatic Follicular Carcinoma of Thyroid

Thyroid Transcription Factor (TTF-1) in Metastatic Thyroid Carcinoma

TTF-1 is a nuclear tissue-specific protein transcription factor found in all histologic types of thyroid tumors, lung carcinomas (small and large cell carcinomas), and small cell carcinomas of other sites. It is a useful marker for confirming a primary from these sites in the event of a metastasis.

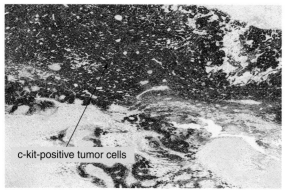

FIGURE 6.63 c-kit Staining in Metastatic Gastrointestinal Stromal Tumor

c-kit (CD117) in Gastrointestinal Stromal Tumors

CD117 is a transmembrane tyrosine kinase receptor and plays a significant role in the development and function of interstitial cells of Cajal. CD117 has been localized in several tumors, the notable one being gastrointestinal stromal tumor. About 4% of GISTs are c-Kit-negative. GISTs metastasizing to the skin are rare but have been documented. In dermatopathology, CD117 is also used as a reliable marker in the detection of mast cells.

NEUROENDOCRINE MARKERS

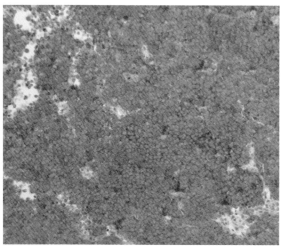

FIGURE 6.64 Synaptophysin

Synaptophysin

Synaptophysin is a very sensitive but less specific marker that recognizes the glycoprotein which is an integral part of the neurosecretory granule membrane. It has a membranous pattern of staining. Other neuroendocrine markers are chromogranin, Leu7, and neuron-specific enolase. Neuroendocrine markers are generally used in dermatopathology to confirm neuroendocrine carcinomas of the skin, the most common being Merkel cell carcinoma.

OTHER USEFUL IMMUNOHISTOCHEMICAL MARKERS

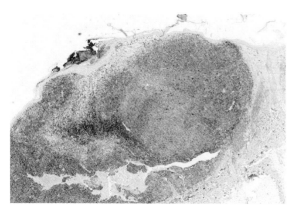

FIGURE 6.65 CD10 in Atypical Fibroxanthoma

CD10

CD10 is more commonly used as a lymphoid marker to identify lymphoblastic leukemias and lymphomas. It is also positive in atypical fibroxanthoma and thus is useful in confirming the diagnosis as the only consistently positive marker for atypical fibroxanthoma.

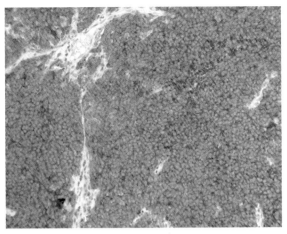

FIGURE 6.66   CD99 Staining Ewing's Sarcoma

CD99 in Ewing's Sarcoma

CD99 is an intercellular adhesion molecule. This is also a marker of lymphomas and leukemias and also stains solid tumors. CD99 is a confirmatory marker for Ewing's sarcoma and also stains solitary fibrous tumor.

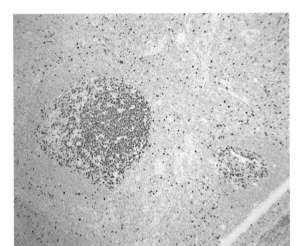

FIGURE 6.67   Ki 67

Ki 67 (MIB 1)

Ki 67 is a nuclear protein and recognizes the proliferative portion of the cell cycle. The proliferation index can be estimated by dividing the number of positive cells by all the cells present. Ki67 index correlates well with tumor grade.

MARKERS FOR VIRAL INCLUSIONS

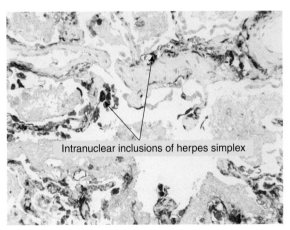

Intranuclear inclusions of herpes simplex

FIGURE 6.68   Intranuclear Inclusions in Herpes Simplex Infection

Herpes Simplex Virus Antibody

Antibodies against herpes simplex virus (HSV) are useful for the detection of intranuclear inclusions. Monoclonal and polyclonal antibodies are available for the detection of HSV. They are very sensitive but not specific as they can also stain other viral antigens such as varicella-zoster. Moreover they are not useful to differentiate HSV1 and HSV2.

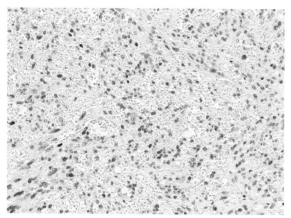

FIGURE 6.69   HHV-8 in Kaposi's Sarcoma

Human Herpes Virus-8 Antibody

The antibody against human herpes virus-8 (HHV-8) is useful in the confirmation of Kaposi's sarcoma. The diagnosis of Kaposi's sarcoma can sometimes be problematic particularly in the early patch stage and when it occurs in an unusual location. The antibody demonstrates a nuclear pattern staining the latent associated nuclear antigen-1 (LANA-1).

BIBLIOGRAPHY

Al-Refu K, Edward S, Ingham E, Goodfield M. Alterations in the basement membrane zone in cutaneous lupus erythematosus as demonstrated by immunohistochemistry. Poster presented at: 2nd International conference on Cutaneous Lupus Erythematosus (ICCLE 2008); May 2008; Kyoto, Japan.

Al-Refu K, Goodfield M. Immunohistochemistry of ultrastructural changes in scarring lupus erythematosus. Clin Exp Dermatol 2010;36(1):63–68.

Bancroft JD, Gamble M. Theory and Practice of Histological Techniques, 5th Ed.

Dabbs DJ. Diagnostic Immunohistochemistry, 2nd Ed.

Mooi WJ, Krausz T. Pathology of Melanocytic Disorders, 2nd Ed. Hodder Arnold, 2007.

Weedon D. Skin Pathology, 3rd Ed. Churchill Livingstone, 2009.

Immunofluorescence Study in Dermatopathology

INTRODUCTION

Immunofluorescence is a method of identifying particular antigen(s) within a tissue by utilizing the specific unique binding properties of antibodies to a corresponding antigen.

In "direct immunofluorescence," a fluorescent dye is conjugated or coupled to an antibody. When the conjugated dye-antibody is mixed/incubated with tissue, the antibody binds to the target antigen in the tissues forming a conjugated fluorescent dye-antibody-antigen complex (Table 7.1). After washing away excess conjugated dye-antibody, the remaining tissue-bound conjugated dye-antibody-target antigen complex is detectable by the presence of fluorescence within the tissue. The fluorescent dyes commonly used are fluorescein and rhodamine. They have the property of absorbing ultraviolet or visible light, which causes the molecule to redistribute the electrons and emit radiation of a different wavelength. Fluorescein is the popular fluorochrome and has the absorption spectrum over ultraviolet and blue light range with a characteristic apple-green emission. Rhodamine, Texas Red, and phycoerythrin are other dyes with orange-red emissions. This property is best exploited in the fluorescence-activated cell sorter system which allows two different emission colors to be measured simultaneously. In this process two different antibodies are conjugated, one with fluorescein and the other with phycoerythrin, and they are excited with a single blue laser beam. The green and red emissions can be measured at the same time.

The immunofluorescence staining is performed on thin (3–4 microns) sections of unfixed tissue. The tissue is transported in Michel's medium. Michel's medium is 10% ammonium sulphate with buffer (potassium citrate, magnesium sulphate, ethyl maleimide, distilled water, and potassium hydroxide to pH 7). The other transport medium used is phosphate buffered saline (0.1 M sodium phosphate, 0.15 M sodium chloride with pH 7.3). The specimens should be kept in the transport medium for less than 24 hours so that the immunopathological findings are comparable with those obtained from fresh tissue.

"Indirect immunofluorescence" is the method used to detect autoantibodies in patients' sera. This method is used to detect one or more autoantibodies in a single dilution of the patient's serum. The antibodies include antinuclear antibodies, antimitochondrial, and smooth muscle antibodies to name a few.

The optimal site for taking a biopsy for direct immunofluorescence is uninvolved or normal perilesional skin for autoimmune bullous diseases. In cases of suspected leukocytoclastic vasculitis and Henoch-Schönlein purpura, lesional skin is preferred as it appears to detect a greater number of immune deposits compared with perilesional uninvolved skin. Involved sun-exposed skin is positive in 100% of cases of lupus erythematosus. Uninvolved sun-exposed skin is positive in 90% of cases. Uninvolved sun-protected skin is positive only in 30% of cases. The positive staining for IgG, IgM, and C3c is popularly known as the lupus band test. The site of the biopsy is important in interpreting the results of the lupus band test. The Lupus band test may be negative in early lesions, remissions and some cases of drug induced Lupus erythematosus.

IgG, IgA, IgM, fibrin, and C3c are the antibodies used in dermatopathology. The selective staining of the different antibodies together with the location of the fluorescent antigen-antibody complex decides the final diagnosis. The immunofluorescence findings are always correlated with the histological appearances and also with the clinical features before a final diagnosis is arrived at.

Table 7.1

Intraepidermal staining of C3c

Skin Diseases	Antibody	Location
Pemphigus vulgaris	IgG +/− C3c	Sieve-like pattern within the epidermis
Bullous pemphigoid	IgG +/− C3c (linear)	Basement membrane zone
Dermatitis herpetiformis	IgA (granular)	Dermal papillae
Lupus erythematosus	IgG, IgM, C3c	Basement membrane zone (systemic lupus erythematosus-lesional and nonlesional), discoid lupus erythematosus (lesional only)
Alopecia areata	C3c	Around the hair bulb
Vasculitis	Fibrin, C3c	Around dermal blood vessels
Linear IgA disease	IgA	Basement membrane zone

Sometimes the direct immunofluorescence findings can be negative or nonspecific in nature (e.g., connective tissue disorders other than lupus erythematosus). Despite well-described patterns of fluorescence in autoimmune blistering conditions, the pattern in any given patient may show variations in the type of antibody deposited.

IMMUNOFLUORESCENCE STUDIES WITH SALT-SPLIT SKIN

Indirect and direct immunofluorescence studies of perilesional skin is done using the salt-split technique. This technique is based on the principle that incubation of the patient's skin in 1 mol/L sodium chloride (saline) artificially splits the basement membrane at the level of lamina lucida. The incubation is done for 48 hours at 4-degree centigrade. The site of the dermo-epidermal separation is determined with indirect immunofluorescence mapping. More commonly direct immunofluorescence of the NACL-split skin biopsy is performed. The technique is useful in distinguishing bullous pemphigoid from epidermolysis bullosa acquisita. IgG and or C3c is located on the roof (epidermal side) or roof and floor (dermal side) of the blister in bullous pemphigoid. Epidermolysis bullosa acquisita is characterized by deposition of IgG along the floor of the blister since the split actually occurs at the level of lamina densa.

The immunoglobulin deposition is found along the roof of the blister in cicatricial pemphigoid and pemphigus gestationis. In bullous dermatosis of lupus erythematosus and cicatricial pemphigoid, the immunoglobulin deposition is seen on the floor of the blister.

Immunoperoxidase antigen mapping also known as blister mapping is another technique by which the site of dermoepidermal split can be mapped. Paraffin-embedded sections of lesional skin can be stained for the immunoglobulin, complement and antibodies such as laminin and collagen IV. The localization of the antibody determines the level of split.

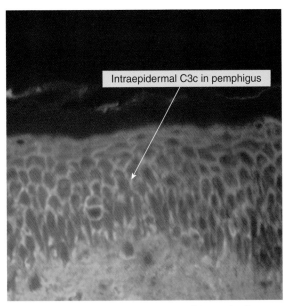

FIGURE 7.1   Intraepidermal C3c in Pemphigus Vulgaris

Intraepidermal Staining of C3c

Intraepidermal staining of C3c in a sieve-like pattern is seen in pemphigus vulgaris.

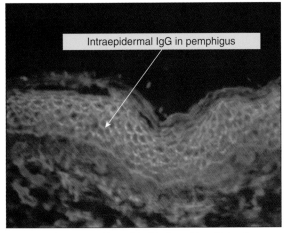

FIGURE 7.2   Intraepidermal IgG in Pemphigus Vulgaris

Intraepidermal Staining of IgG

This pattern of staining of IgG which is similar to that of C3c is diagnostic of different variants of pemphigus.

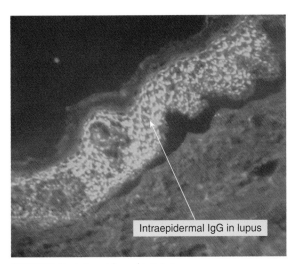

FIGURE 7.3   Intraepidermal IgG in Lupus

Nuclear staining of the keratinocytes by IgG is a pattern well recognized in cutaneous lupus erythematosus. Although it is seen only in a small percentage of cases, it is known to correlate with oral involvement. A similar pattern of IgA deposition is seen in IgA pemphigus.

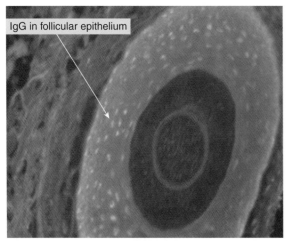

FIGURE 7.4   IgG in Follicular Epithelium

IgG in the Follicular Epithelium

IgG is deposited in the follicular epithelium in a nuclear pattern in lupus erythematosus.

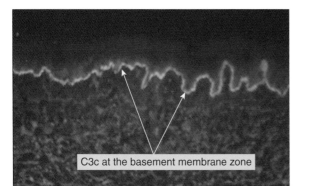

FIGURE 7.5   C3c at the Basement Membrane Zone

C3c at the Basement Membrane Zone

A homogenous pattern of staining of C3c is seen at the basement membrane zone in bullous pemphigoid. C3c may be the only antigen present in the early stages. IgG shows a similar staining pattern. The salt-split skin shows the antibodies on the epidermal side (roof) of the blister in majority of cases. It may also be seen on the floor of the blister in a small number of cases. It is seen on the dermal side (floor) of the blister in epidermolysis bullosa acquisita.

C3c at the basement membrane zone is a confirmatory feature of cutaneous lupus erythematosus.

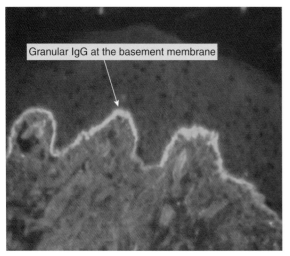

FIGURE 7.6   IgG at the Basement Membrane Zone

IgG at the Basement Membrane Zone

Similar to C3c, IgG is a component of lupus band test in the confirmation of lupus erythematosus. IgG is usually seen in a granular pattern in lupus and a homogenous pattern in bullous pemphigoid. In the salt-split skin for a bullous disorder, IgG is seen on the epidermal side (roof) of the blister in bullous pemphigoid and on the dermal side(floor) of the blister in epidermolysis bullosa acquisita.

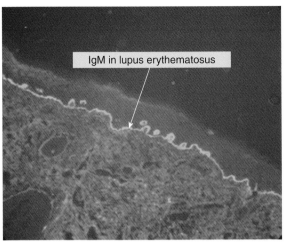

FIGURE 7.7   IgM in Lupus Erythematosus

IgM at the Basement Membrane Zone

IgM is deposited at the basement membrane zone in 50–90% of discoid lupus erythematosus, along with IgG.

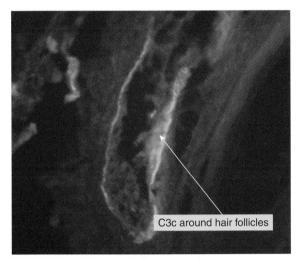

FIGURE 7.8   C3c Around Follicles

C3c Around Hair Follicles and Bulb

C3c along with IgG and sometimes IgM is seen in alopecia areata and is considered a diagnostic finding.

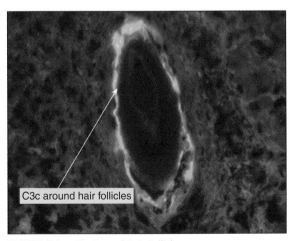

FIGURE 7.9   C3c Around Hair Follicles

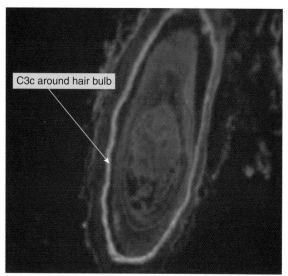

FIGURE 7.10   C3c Around Hair Bulb

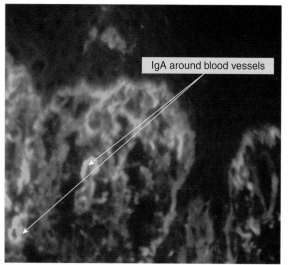

FIGURE 7.11   IgA Around Blood Vessels

IgA Around Blood Vessels

IgA is seen around blood vessels in early cases of Henoch-Schönlein purpura. It may be seen in involved and uninvolved skin.

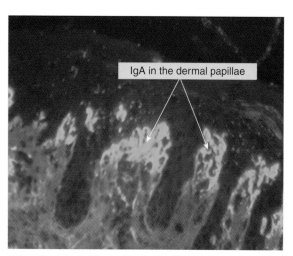

FIGURE 7.12   IgA in the Dermal Papillae

IgA in the Dermal Papillae

Granular deposition of IgA is a consistent finding in dermatitis herpetiformis. It is seen in the dermal papillae of perilesional and uninvolved skin. Dermatitis herpetiformis is associated with celiac disease, a gluten sensitive enteropathy in 90% of cases. Dermal IgA is not demonstrated in cases of celiac disease in which there are no skin lesions. IgA antiendomysial antibodies are identified in 100% of cases.

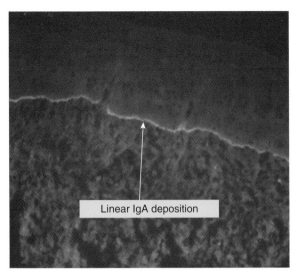

FIGURE 7.13   Linear IgA Deposition

Linear IgA Deposition

Linear IgA deposition at the basement membrane zone is seen in a number of cutaneous diseases. It is a useful feature to differentiate from dermatitis herpetiformis. It is seen in linear IgA disease of nonlesional skin in 80% of the cases.

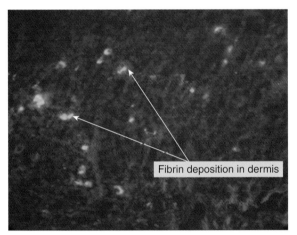

FIGURE 7.14   Fibrin Deposition in Dermal Vessels

Fibrin Deposition Around Vessels

Fibrin is deposited around blood vessels in leukocytoclastic vasculitis. They are also seen as pericapillary fibrin cuffs in venous leg ulcers and adjacent to any ulcer.

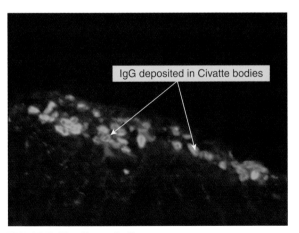

FIGURE 7.15   Civatte Bodies

Civatte Bodies

Civatte bodies are basement membrane substance globules seen in the papillary dermis in a number of different conditions, the most common being lichen planus. Occasionally, Civatte bodies are seen to stain with antibody for fibrin.

BIBLIOGRAPHY

Megahead M. Histopathology of Blistering Diseases. Springer, 2004.
Weedon D. Skin Pathology, 5th ed. Churchill Livingstone, 2009.

Epidermis—Inflammatory and Neoplastic Diseases

INTRODUCTION

The epidermis is the outermost layer of the skin. It is embryologically derived from the ectoderm and is composed of keratinocytes. In addition, there are melanocytes, Langerhans cells, and Merkel cells within the epidermis. The keratinocytes contain tonofilaments that are composed of keratin intermediate filaments. Keratin consists of a group of more than 30 antigenically different subtypes. There are two main subtypes of epidermal keratins.

1. Small acidic keratins (K10-K20)

2. Larger neutral-basic keratins (K1-K19)

Keratins exist in pairs in vivo, one being contributed from each group. The suprabasal keratins are keratin types 1 and 10, and the basal keratins are keratin types 5 and 14. Mutations of keratin genes result in several pathological processes, for example, epidermolysis bullosa simplex variants result from mutations of keratin types 1 and 10.

The epidermis undergoes a process of maturation, which is poorly understood. Maturation is expressed in the form of keratinization where the basal cells transforms into the cells of stratum corneum, which is formed of keratin only and are devoid of nuclei.

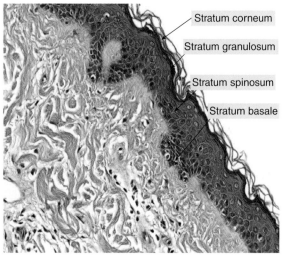

Stratum corneum

Stratum granulosum

Stratum spinosum

Stratum basale

FIGURE 8.1 Epidermis

Layers of the Epidermis

The epidermis consists of four layers:

1. Stratum corneum (or horny layer)—the most superficial layer.

2. Stratum granulosum (or granular layer).

3. Stratum spinosum (or spinous layer).

4. Stratum basale (or basal layer)—deepest layer that sits on basement membrane.

PATHOLOGY

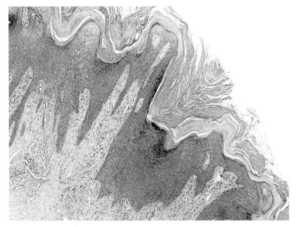

FIGURE 8.2   Acanthosis

Acanthosis

Acanthosis is the term used to refer to the increased thickness of the epidermis. This is the result of an increase in the number or size of the spinous layer of the epidermis. Acanthosis may be seen in inflammatory conditions such as psoriasis or neoplastic conditions such as Bowen's disease and squamous cell carcinoma.

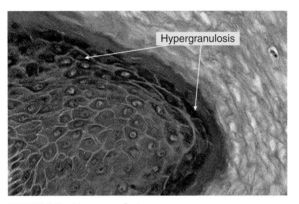

FIGURE 8.3   Hypergranulosis

Hypergranulosis

Hypergranulosis is a term used to indicate the increased thickness and number of the granular layer of the epidermis. Hypergranulosis is commonly seen in viral warts. Wedge-shaped hypergranulosis is seen in Lichen planus as a diagnostic clue.

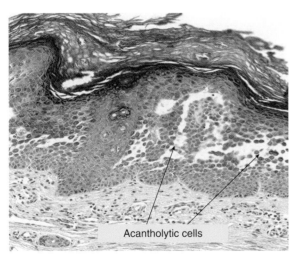

FIGURE 8.4   Acantholysis

Acantholysis

Acantholysis is the result of loss of cohesion of the keratinocytes. This could happen in the corneal, granular, or spinous layers of the epidermis and the lining of the adnexal structures. Acantholysis could be induced by external agents such as oil, or it could be the effect of immunoglobulins and or complement, which is the mechanism of acantholysis in pemphigus vulgaris or foliaceus. Acantholysis may be seen in other conditions such as squamous cell carcinoma.

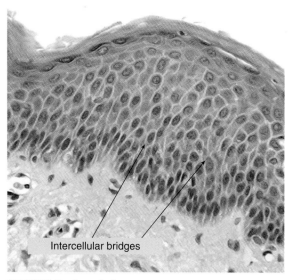

FIGURE 8.5   Spongiosis

Spongiosis

Spongiosis refers to the separation of the keratinocytes due to intercellular edema. The intercellular bridges are prominent on H&E sections. Eosinophilic spongiosis is the signature finding in eczematous conditions (e.g., atopic and allergic contact dermatitis) but may also be seen in the pre-bullous phase of blistering conditions (pemphigus and bullous pemphigoid), drug reactions, insect bites, incontinentia pigmenti, and in id reactions (hypersensitivity reactions) to fungi. The degree of spongiosis varies with the etiological factor and in extreme cases can result in a spongiotic vesicle (= intraepidermal blister). Spongiosis may be localized to the acrosyringium (miliarial spongiosis) or hair follicles (follicular spongiosis). Spongiosis may be less obvious in chronic eczematous conditions such as lichen simplex chronicus. Mild infiltration of lymphocytes, neutrophils, and eosinophils may be seen, which may give a clue to the diagnosis.

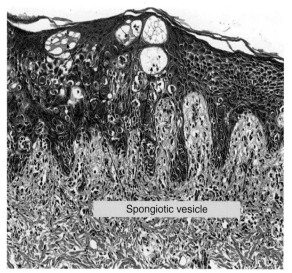

FIGURE 8.6   Spongiotic Vesicle

Spongiotic Vesicle

Extreme degrees of spongiosis result in spongiotic vesicle within the epidermis. There may be accumulation of lymphocytes, neutrophils, or eosinophils within the vesicles.

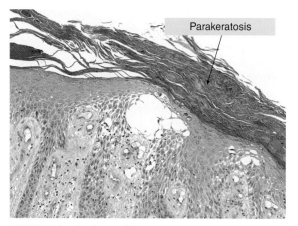

FIGURE 8.7   Parakeratosis

Parakeratosis

Parakeratosis refers to the retention of keratinocyte nuclei in the corneal layer. The nuclei appear flattened and parallel to the underlying epidermis. Parakeratosis is the result of too rapid elimination of keratinocytes due to varying pathological processes. Parakeratosis often reflects that previous injury or damage to the epidermis has occurred.

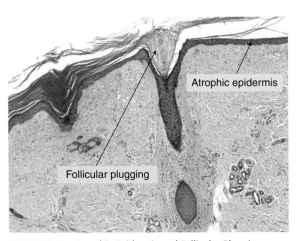

FIGURE 8.8   Atrophic Epidermis and Follicular Plugging

Atrophic Epidermis and Follicular Plugging

Atrophy or thinning of the epidermis occurs in many inflammatory and neoplastic disorders. The striking histological feature is the decreased numbers of the keratinocytes and the loss of rete ridges. There may be associated loss of the dermal collagen with telangiectasia. Atrophy of the epidermis is an important histological finding in poikilodermatous conditions such as cutaneous T-cell lymphoma, following cutaneous lupus, dermatomyositis, and in various congenital conditions such as Rothmund-Thomson syndrome, Bloom syndrome, and dyskeratosis congenita. Long-term topical corticosteroid injection produces cutaneous atrophy.

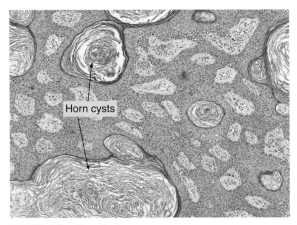

FIGURE 8.9   Horn Cysts

Horn Cysts

Horn cysts are seen commonly in seborrheic keratosis. These are well-formed cystic spaces containing keratinous material. They are seen interspersed within islands of proliferated keratinocytes in seborrheic keratoses.

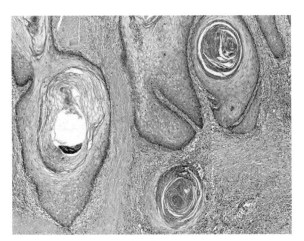

FIGURE 8.10   Squamous Pearls

Squamous Pearls

This is a term used to define the excess keratin formed in malignant squamoproliferative diseases such as squamous cell carcinoma. In a well-differentiated squamous cell carcinoma, squamous pearls are seen as a prominent feature. In H&E sections, it is usually seen as whorled keratin within a cystic space.

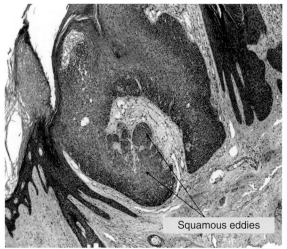

FIGURE 8.11   Squamous Eddies in Inverted Follicular Keratosis

Squamous Eddies in Inverted Follicular Keratosis

Squamous eddies are a feature identifiable in inverted follicular keratosis, also termed as irritated follicular keratosis. The eddies are seen as concentric whorls of keratinocytes around a central area of keratinization. Squamous eddies should not be mistaken for squamous pearls in malignant proliferation.

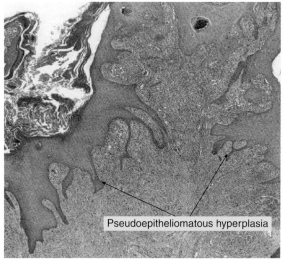

FIGURE 8.12   Pseudoepitheliomatous Hyperplasia

Pseudoepitheliomatous Hyperplasia

This is the term used to describe the marked acanthosis of the epidermis with downgrowths into the underlying dermis. The epidermal downgrowths are seen in a disorderly pattern with pointed spikes. The keratinocytes involved in the proliferation shows no evidence of atypia. Pseudoepitheliomatous hyperplasia is seen overlying neoplastic conditions such as granular cell tumor, at the edge of chronic ulcerating squamous cell carcinoma and granulomas associated with fungal infections.

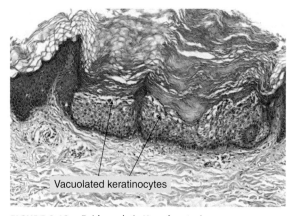

FIGURE 8.13   Epidermolytic Hyperkeratosis

Epidermolytic Hyperkeratosis

Epidermolytic hyperkeratosis is an abnormality of epidermal keratinization. It is characterized by compact hyperkeratosis and vacuolation of granular and spinous cell layer. This is a pattern seen in a number of congenital (e.g., bullous ichthyosiform erythroderma, palmoplantar keratoderma, systematized or linear epidermal nevi) and acquired conditions (epidermolytic acanthoma, associated with actinic keratoses, epidermolytic leukoplakia).

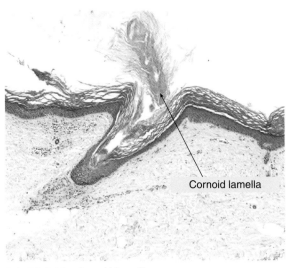

FIGURE 8.14   Cornoid Lamella

Cornoid Lamella

This is a tissue reaction pattern seen in a variety of inflammatory and neoplastic conditions. Histologically, this is seen as a thin column of parakeratotic cells with an underlying absent or decreased granular layer. Cornoid lamella is considered as the diagnostic feature in porokeratosis and its variants. It is thought to be caused by localized faulty keratinization.

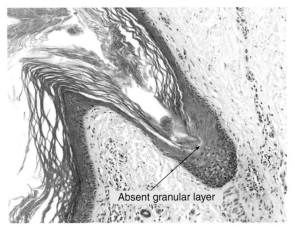

FIGURE 8.15   Cornoid Lamella—Note the Absent Granular Layer

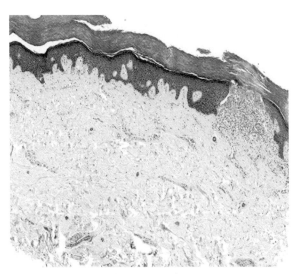

FIGURE 8.16   Palmoplantar Keratoderma

Palmoplantar Keratoderma

This is a heterogeneous group of congenital and acquired disorders of keratinization. As the name implies, it is a disorder confined to the palms and soles manifested as localized hyperkeratosis. Keratodermas are categorized based on their mode of inheritance and clinical presentation (occurring in isolation or part of a syndrome).

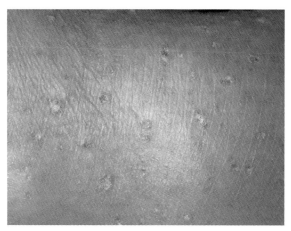

FIGURE 8.17   Flegel's Disease

Flegel's Disease

This disease, which is a rare abnormality of keratinization, is also known as hyperkeratosis lenticularis perstans. Clinically manifests as multiple discrete 1-5-mm–sized keratosis most commonly on the dosra of the feet and lower limbs (Fig. 8.17).

Under the microscope, the lesions of Flegel's disease show discrete areas of compact hyperkeratosis with focal areas of parakeratosis. The epidermis may be thinned out, and the granular layer becomes less prominent. There is vacuolation of the basal layer. The dermis may show a band-like infiltrate of lymphocytes.

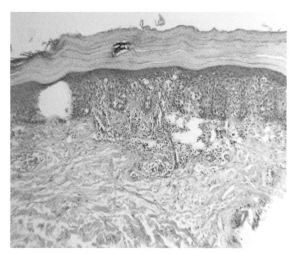

FIGURE 8.18   Flegel's Disease

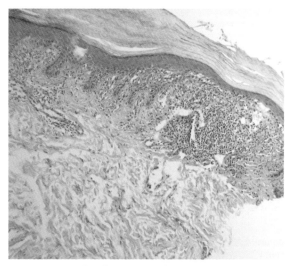

FIGURE 8.19   Flegel's Disease-High Power View

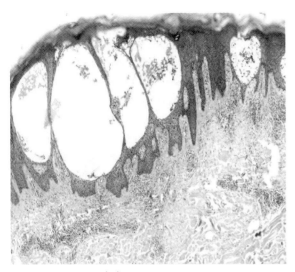

FIGURE 8.20   Pompholyx

Pompholyx

Pompholyx (acral vesicular dermatitis or dyshidrotic eczema) is an acute eczematous condition commonly seen on palms and soles. The stratum corneum is thickened and vesicles form in a sub-corneal location initially, which later displaces the spinous layer. Some of the vesicles develop into pustules with neutrophils within them. In such conditions, the possibility of a dermatophyte infection should be ruled out using a periodic acid schiff (PAS) stain. Allergic contact dermatitis of palms and soles should also be excluded. Spongiosis of the epidermis adjacent to the vesicle is a clue to diagnosis of this condition.

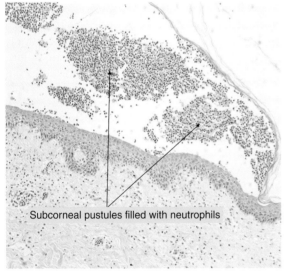

Subcorneal pustules filled with neutrophils

FIGURE 8.21   Subcorneal Pustular Dermatosis

Subcorneal Pustular Dermatosis

Clinically there are many conditions that present with pustules. On microscopy, the neutrophil-filled vesicles (or pustules) are characteristically subcorneal in location and appear to sit on the epidermis. The adjacent epidermis may or may not show any diagnostic features. A mixed inflammatory infiltrate may be seen in the dermis. Subcorneal pustules may be seen in impetigo, dermatophytosis, IgA pemphigus, early pustular psoriasis, and in drug reactions such as acute exanthematous generalized pustulosis (AGEP).

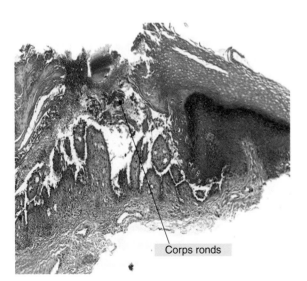

Corps ronds

FIGURE 8.22   Darier's Disease

Darier's Disease

Darier's disease is a rare autosomal dominant genodermatosis, which appears in adolescence. Individual lesions histologically show suprabasal clefting with acantholysis of cells. Projections of papillary dermis into the cleft lined by a single layer of basal cells (described as "tomb stone appearance") can sometimes be seen. The characteristic dyskeratotic cells seen in Darier's disease are described as "corps ronds and grains." Corps ronds are single cells or small groups of cells seen in the upper spinous layer or stratum corneum. These cells have intensely eosinophilic cytoplasm and pyknotic nuclei with a perinuclear halo. Grains resemble parakeratotic cells and are seen in the superficial part of the epidermis.

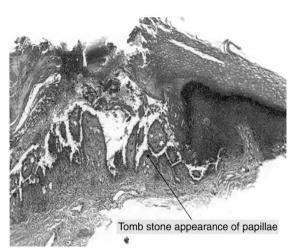

FIGURE 8.23   Darier's Disease—Tomb Stone Appearance

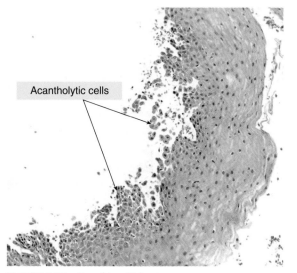

FIGURE 8.24   Pemphigus Vulgaris

Pemphigus Vulgaris

Pemphigus vulgaris usually manifests as oral blisters, which later extends to involve the trunk with characteristic widespread flaccid blisters and crusted erosions. Pemphigus characteristically demonstrates a positive Nikolsky's sign where extension of blistering can be elicited by applying pressure to the immediate clinically normal appearing adjacent perilesional skin.

On microscopy, the characteristic feature is the extensive intraepidermal split above the basal layer of the epidermis with "tomb stoning" appearance and acantholysis. The blister cavity usually contains the acantholytic cells (rounded cells, which are drifting free in the fluid of the blister). The dermis may show very nonspecific changes such as mild perivascular infiltrate of lymphocytes and may be some eosinophils.

Direct immunofluorescence shows IgG and less frequently C3c in the intercellular regions of the epidermis in a sieve-like pattern. About 80–90% of patients have circulating intercellular antibodies.

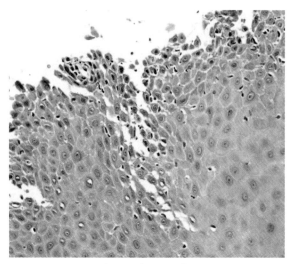

FIGURE 8.25   Pemphigus Vulgaris-High Power

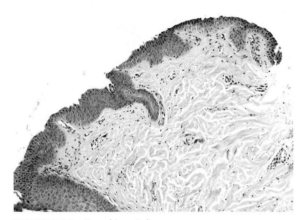

FIGURE 8.26   Pemphigus Foliaceus

Pemphigus Foliaceus

This is very uncommon and less severe form of pemphigus. Clinically, it presents with flaccid blisters and crusted erosions however, mucosal involvement is uncommon. Pemphigus foliaceus can occur in conjunction with other inflammatory/ autoimmune conditions and may be induced by various drugs such as penicillamine and ACE inhibitors (captopril, enalapril).

On microscopy, the lesions demonstrate an intraepidermal split usually high up in the granular layer. The bulla may contain acantholytic cells and some neutrophils. Neutrophilic spongiosis may rarely occur. The underlying dermis shows nonspecific changes.

Direct immunofluorescence shows intercellular staining of IgG and C3c in a sieve-like pattern.

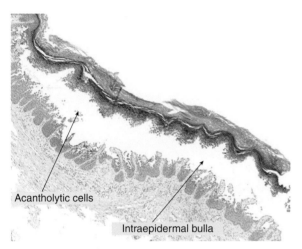

FIGURE 8.27   Hailey-Hailey Disease-Low Power

Hailey-Hailey Disease

Hailey-Hailey disease (familial benign chronic pemphigus) is an autosomal dominant condition with incomplete penetrance. Clinically, it presents as recurrent erythematous plaques that progress to flaccid bullae, which in turn rupture and form crusting plaques. Typically, Hailey-Hailey disease affects the body folds (groins, axilla, between buttock and other flexural areas of the body) starting in the third to fourth decades of life. Nikolsky's sign may be positive. The acantholysis in Hailey-Hailey disease results from the deficiency of the intercellular adhesion proteins desmoplakin 1 and 11 and plakoglobin.

On microscopy, there is intraepidermal clefting with acantholytic cells lying free within the clefts. The adjacent epidermis may show intercellular edema with partial acantholysis within the epidermis described as "dilapidated brick wall" appearance.

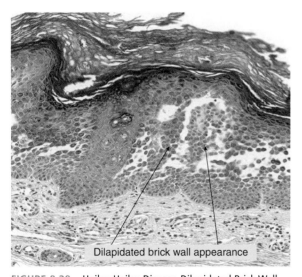

FIGURE 8.28   Hailey-Hailey Disease-Dilapidated Brick Wall Appearance

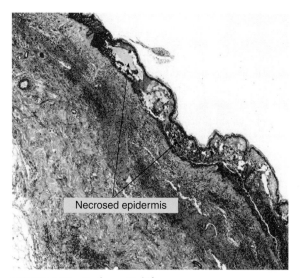

FIGURE 8.29   Erythema Multiforme

Erythema Multiforme

Erythema multiforme is a self-limiting disease involving the mucous membrane as well. The disease results from a cell-mediated immune response to a variety of agents. Several causative factors have been implicated including bacterial and viral agents (herpes simplex infection), drugs, and neoplastic conditions.

On microscopy, erythema multiforme has been divided into epidermal, dermal, and mixed varieties based on the predominant pattern of involvement. In the epidermal type, there is prominent epidermal damage with necrosis of the keratinocytes. In the dermal type there is lichenoid infiltrate of lymphocytes, which also show exocytosis. Dermal edema is also a feature.

Direct immunofluorescence show positive staining for IgM and C3c within the epidermis demonstrating the necrotic keratinocytes.

Similar histological and immunofluorescence features are also seen in paraneoplastic pemphigus, which has to be distinguished clinically.

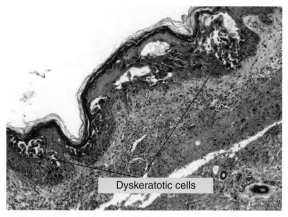

FIGURE 8.30   Dyskeratotic Cells in Erythema Multiforme

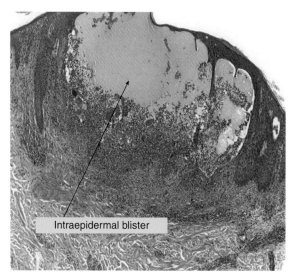

FIGURE 8.31   Intraepidermal Blister in Herpes

Herpes Simplex

There are two different types of herpes simplex viruses (HSV-1 and HSV-2). HSV-1 causes herpes labialis (cold sore), and HSV-2 causes genital herpes. The commonest presentation is groups of clear vesicles that heal without scarring.

On microscopy, well-established lesions show an intraepidermal vesicle containing swollen or ballooned keratinocytes containing intranuclear inclusions. Acantholytic keratinocytes are also seen. This is accompanied by accumulations of neutrophils and lymphocytes. The inflammatory cells are also seen in the underlying dermis.

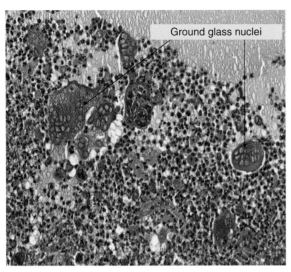

FIGURE 8.32   Ground Glass Nuclei in Herpes Simplex Infection

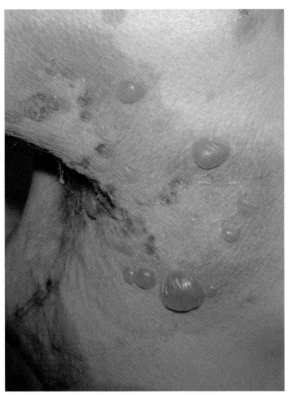

FIGURE 8.33   Bullous Pemphigoid Axilla

Bullous Pemphigoid

Bullous pemphigoid is a typically blistering disease of the elderly (although it can occur in children very rarely). Clinically, it presents as multiple tense bullae on normal skin or more commonly on the background of erythematous (red) urticated (i.e., skin lesions resembling urticaria) plaques. The pathogenesis of bullous pemphigoid involves the binding of IgG antibodies to the hemidesmosome proteins bullous pemphigoid antigen (BPAg1 and BPAg2) with resultant disruption of adherence of the basal keratinocytes to the basement membrane.

On microscopy, a unilocular subepidermal blister is the commonest presentation. The bulla contains eosinophils as the predominant cell type in the blister fluid. The epidermis often exhibits eosinophilic spongiosis. The underlying dermis shows interstitial infiltration of eosinophils.

Direct immunofluorescence show linear deposition of IgG and or C3c at the basement membrane zone. Using the salt-split skin, immune deposits are seen in the epidermal side (or "roof") of the bulla. Fluorescence overlay antigen mapping is another method that can be used to increase the sensitivity of conventional immunofluorescence microscopy. The level of split can also be confirmed by staining for type IV collagen, which is seen in the base of the blister. About 60–80% of patients have circulating IgG antibodies.

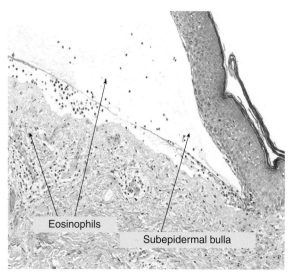

FIGURE 8.34   Bullous Pemphigoid

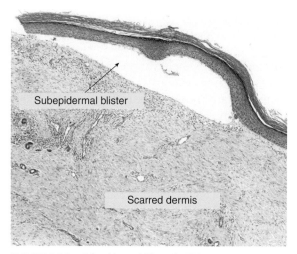

FIGURE 8.35   Subepidermal Blister in EBA

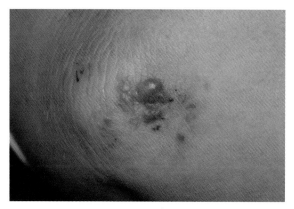

FIGURE 8.36   Dermatitis Herpetiformis-Elbow

Dermatitis Herpetiformis

Dermatitis herpetiformis is an intensely pruritic autoimmune blistering disease. The lesions occur on extensor surfaces of arms and legs, very commonly as symmetric excoriated papules and vesicles. Intact blisters are sometimes not seen clinically. Intense pruritus or burning sensation usually precede or may be the only manifestation of the disease. Almost all the patients who develop dermatitis herpetiformis are known to have clinical or subclinical small bowel villous atrophy. Dermatitis herpetiformis is considered as a cutaneous manifestation of gluten sensitivity (coeliac disease). Ingestion of gluten results in chemotaxis and activation of complement. The sole criterion for diagnosis is the demonstration of granular IgA in the dermal papillae. A quarter of patients on gluten-free diet may loose the IgA deposit after clearance of the rash.

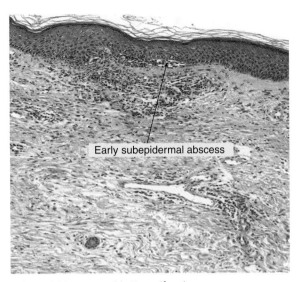

FIGURE 8.37   Dermatitis Herpetiformis

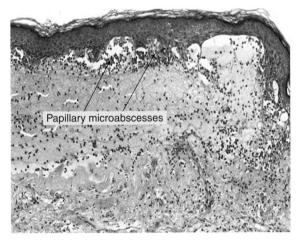

FIGURE 8.38   Dermatitis Herpetiformis-Papillary
Microabscesses

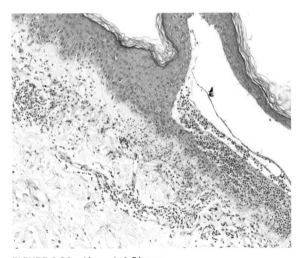

FIGURE 8.39   Linear IgA Disease

Dermatitis herpetiformis is considered an immunologic reaction to gluten found in wheat, barley, and rye. Patients with dermatitis herpetiformis have circulating antibodies against endomysium and tissue glutaminase (tTG) and epidermal glutaminase (eTG).

On microscopy, the skin biopsy shows papillary dermal microabscesses. The biopsy may also show unrelated features such as changes secondary to excoriation or nonspecific inflammation. This should prompt examination of a skin specimen under the immunofluorescence microscope.

Linear IgA Disease

Linear IgA bullous dermatoses is a rare disease that occurs in young children (chronic bullous disease of childhood) or in adults (linear IgA disease). It classically presents in children as a tense blisters in a polycyclic pattern ("cluster of jewels" sign) with predominance for the perioral and groin regions. In adults, it resembles dermatitis herpetiformis or bullous pemphigoid. It differs from dermatitis herpetiformis in the absence of gluten sensitivity and IgA antiendomysial antibodies. The condition is associated with many inflammatory and neoplastic diseases and has variety of clinical appearances and associations.

On microscopy, a subepidermal blister is the commonest feature. Neutrophils are the main component of the content of the blister and inflammatory infiltrate associated with a subepidermal split in the epidermis. In comparison, dermatitis herpetiformis shows deposition of fibrin and papillary microabscesses in the dermal papillae, with leukocytoclasia of the overlying epidermis. These features help to distinguish the two conditions.

The consistent finding seen on direct immunofluorescence is the linear homogenous deposition of IgA along the basement zone of nonlesional skin, which is seen in 80–90% of cases.

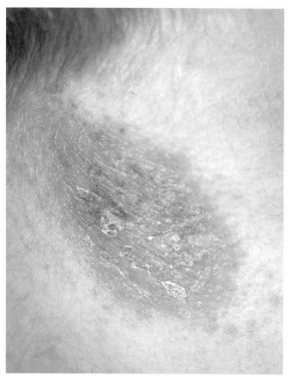

FIGURE 8.40   Lichen Simplex Chronicus

Lichen Simplex Chronicus

Lichen simplex chronicus is an idiopathic disorder characterized clinically by thickened scaly lichenified (i.e., the epidermis is thickened with prominent skin crease) plaques that develop at the site of constant rubbing or sites of pruritus.

On microscopy, there is a thick layer of compact hyperkeratosis overlying a markedly acanthotic and irregular epidermis. There is marked thickening of the papillary dermis with thickening of the dermal collagen seen as vertical streaks. The papillary and reticular dermis also shows mild perivascular infiltrate of lymphocytes.

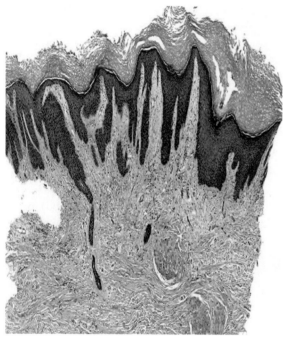

FIGURE 8.41   Lichen Simplex Chronicus

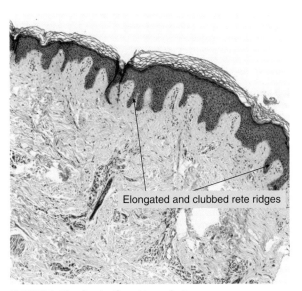

FIGURE 8.42   Psoriasiform Hyperplasia

Psoriasiform Hyperplasia

Psoriasiform hyperplasia is a reaction pattern seen in a number of cutaneous diseases but classically seen in psoriasis. This is described as regular elongation and clubbing of rete ridges. The dilated vessels in the papillary dermis releases the serum and leucocytes intermittently, which results in parakeratosis and formation of suprapapillary exudates. The vessels also release various mediators, which results in increased mitotic activity of the keratinocytes within the hyperplastic epidermis.

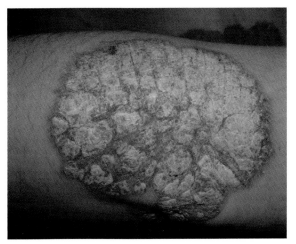

FIGURE 8.43   Plaque of Psoriasis

Psoriasis

Psoriasis is a chronic relapsing inflammatory condition of the skin, typically occurring on the extensor surfaces of the elbows and knees but may also involve the scalp, umbilicus, nails, and flexural areas (axilla, inframammary areas, groin, and between the buttocks). Lesions on the scalp and extensor surfaces present as well-demarcated plaques with silvery scale on an erythematous background, which is sharply demarcated from the surrounding skin (Fig. 8.43). In the flexures, the skin lesions lack scale.

The microscopic appearances of psoriasis vary depending on the stage of biopsy of the lesion (as the psoriatic plaques evolve with time) and vary with where the biopsy was taken. Early lesions of chronic plaque psoriasis show dilatation of papillary dermis vessels, mild perivascular lymphocytic infiltrate, and sometimes mild overlying epidermal spongiosis. Early classical psoriatic lesions show mild neutrophil migration (exocytosis) to the epidermis with formation of parakeratosis, and in some cases formation of small collections of neutrophils in the epidermis in the corneal region (Munro microabscesses) or spinous layer (pustules of Kogoj). Typical developed lesions of chronic plaques psoriasis show marked regular psoriasiform hyperplasia with a thickened epidermal layer with confluent parakeratosis, thin suprapapillary plates, and dilated papillary vessels.

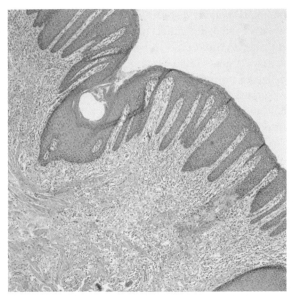

FIGURE 8.44   Psoriasis-Low Power

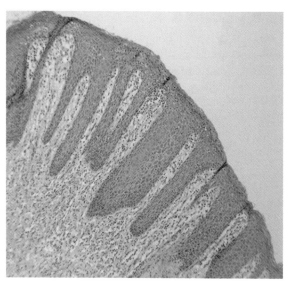

FIGURE 8.45 Psoriasis-High Power

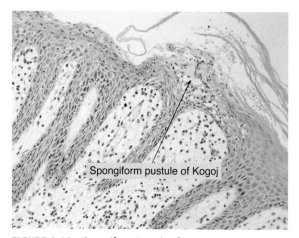

FIGURE 8.46 Spongiform Pustule of Kogoj

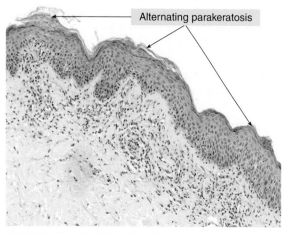

FIGURE 8.47 Pityriasis Rubra Pilaris Low Power

Pityriasis Rubra Pilaris

Pityriasis rubra pilaris is a rare disorder clinically characterized by the development of small folliculocentric papules with central area of keratin plugging that tend to become confluent to form widespread red scaly areas often resembling psoriasis but with islands of unaffected normal skin. Periumbilical sparing is often seen, unlike psoriasis. The eruption often becomes generalized with a cephalocaudal (head to toe) progression and spread to become erythrodermic (or near erythrodermic). Patients often develop marked palmoplantar keratoderma. There are a number of distinct clinical variants.

On microscopy, there is marked hyperkeratosis with parakeratosis. The parakeratotic areas show typical alternation with hyperkeratosis in the vertical and horizontal pattern. Irregular acanthosis is also seen. The dermis shows mild perivascular and perifollicular lymphocytic infiltrate.

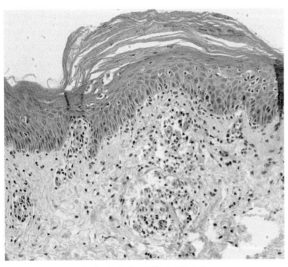

FIGURE 8.48   Pityriasis Rubra Pilaris-High Power

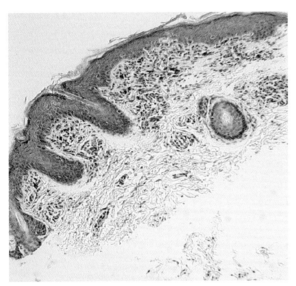

FIGURE 8.49   Nekam's Disease

Nekam's Disease

This condition also known as keratosis lichenoides chronica is a very rare inflammatory disease that affects patients with seborrheic dermatitis such as rash over the scalp and face, with numerous violaceous-purpuric (sometimes scaly) papules arranged in symmetrical, bilateral, parallel, linear patterns over the dorsa of the hands, feet, extremities, and buttock. This disorder is associated with many systemic diseases, and they heal without leaving a scar. It is thought to be a variant of hypertrophic lichen planus.

On microscopy, there is variable acanthosis and epidermal atrophy. The basal cells show vacuolar degeneration, and civatte bodies may be seen. There is usually a band-like infiltrate of lymphocytes and melanophages in the underlying dermis. In addition, perivascular and perifollicular infiltrate of lymphocytes may be seen.

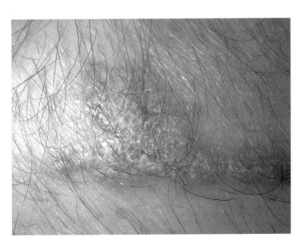

FIGURE 8.50   Lichen Planus

Lichen Planus

Lichen planus is an inflammatory disease of unknown etiology. Clinically, lichen planus presents as groups of small itchy violaceous, flat-topped papules often affecting the wrists, back, and lower legs (but can affect any area). Skin lesions often demonstrate a fine lace-like pattern on the surface (Wickham striae) and can be developed as a delayed response to scratching/trauma (Köebner phenomenon). Flexures are sometimes involved. Nails may be variably affected ranging from single digit involvement to multiple digit involvement to pan-nail involvement (20-nail dystrophy) either in conjunction with skin involvement or as isolated nail involvement. Scalp involvement (lichen planopilaris—see Chapter 13) and mucosal involvement (oral or genital) may occur as part of skin involvement or in isolation without classical skin lesions.

On microscopy of classical skin lesions, there is mild acanthosis of the epidermis with wedge-shaped hypergranulosis. There is basal cell vacuolation and typically very dense "band-like" infiltrate of lymphocytes and histiocytes in the papillary dermis. The epidermis characteristically may demonstrate a "sawtooth" appearance. Plasma cells may be present in the infiltrate in oral lesions. The basal cell vacuolation may produce cleft-like spaces called Caspary-Joseph space. Civatte bodies are prominently seen.

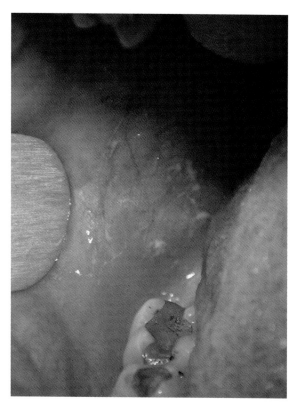

FIGURE 8.51   Oral Lichen Planus

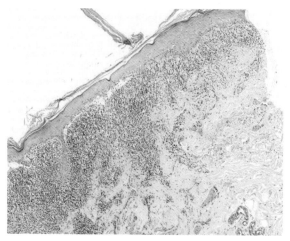

FIGURE 8.52   Lichen Planus

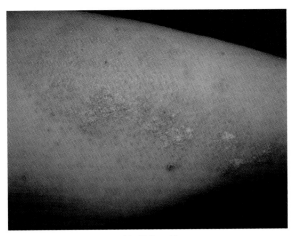

FIGURE 8.53   Hypertrophic Lichen Planus

Hypertrophic Lichen Planus

Hypertrophic lichen planus is a variant of lichen planus classically seen on the shin. It presents markedly hyperkeratotic/scaly plaques. Very rarely squamous cell carcinoma may develop in these lesions.

On microscopy, there is marked hyperkeratosis and acanthosis of the epidermis. Psoriasiform hyperplasia may be seen in occasional cases. The band-like infiltrate may not be as prominent as classical lichen planus.

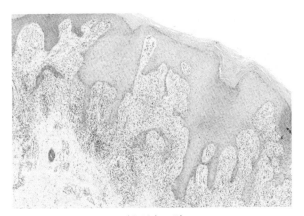

FIGURE 8.54   Hypertrophic Lichen Planus

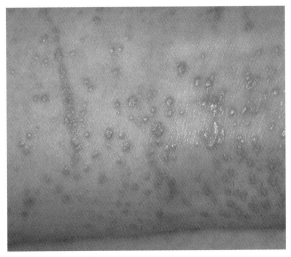

FIGURE 8.55   Lichen Nitidus

Lichen Nitidus

Lichen nitidus is a chronic eruption of multiple monomorphic 1–2-mm diameter flesh colored papules affecting the upper extremities and the trunk.

On microscopy, it shows a dense subepidermal infiltrate with a characteristic claw-like epidermal collarette on either side of the infiltrate. The infiltrate is composed of lymphocytes, histiocytes, epithelioid histiocytes, and multinucleated giant cells reminiscent of a granuloma.

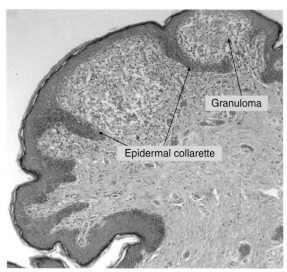

FIGURE 8.56   Lichen Nitidus

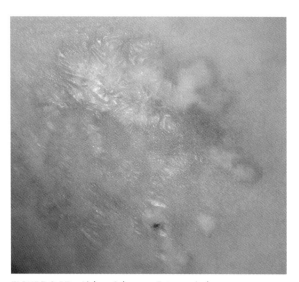

FIGURE 8.57   Lichen Sclerosus-Extragenital

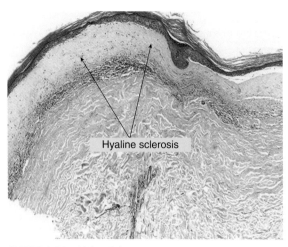

FIGURE 8.58   Lichen Sclerosus

Lichen Sclerosus Et Atrophicus

Lichen sclerosus is a chronic disorder with a predilection for anogenital region, which occurs more commonly in women. In women, it exhibits a bimodal age distribution—prepubertal girls and women in the fifth decade and older. Extragenital lesions can occur alone or concomitantly with anogenital lesions. The extragenital lesions occur more commonly on the trunk. Clinically, extragenital lesions are characterized by patches of atrophic skin with characteristic "cigarette paper" wrinkled atrophic, pale appearance. Genital lesions in women present with itch, irritation, pain, or discomfort with sexual intercourse. Clinical findings may include erosions, leukoplakia or atrophy of the epidermis, disappearance of the clitoris, labia, or vaginal narrowing. Penile lesions have similar appearances but may be associated with urethral meatal stenosis or phimosis (marked narrowing of foreskin). Squamous cell carcinoma may develop in chronically inflamed untreated genital lesions.

On microscopy, well-established lesions show hyperkeratosis and follicular plugging with thinning of the epidermis. Vacuolar degeneration of the basal cells will be seen. The dermis shows a broad zone of homogenized collagen. A variable infiltrate consisting of lymphocytes and eosinophils in a band-like pattern ("interface dermatitis") may be seen in early lesions.

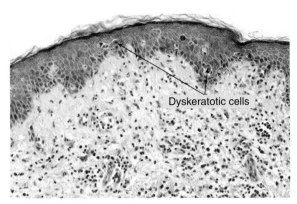

FIGURE 8.59   Drug Reaction

Drug Reaction

Cutaneous drug reactions are difficult to diagnose clinically since many patients will be on several drugs at the same time and attribution to a particular drug may not be possible. The clinical and histological appearances are not specific for a drug. The commonly encountered patterns are granulomatous drug reaction, exanthematous (spongiotic) drug reaction, urticarial reaction, fixed drug eruption, erythema multiforme, and toxic epidermal necrolysis. The mechanisms involved could be allergic, toxic, and immunologic. On microscopy, the appearances are variable depending on the mechanism involved and the pattern of drug reaction. The epidermis is mildly acanthotic with focal spongiosis and many dyskeratotic keratinocytes. The dermis shows an interstitial infiltrate of mixed inflammatory cells with a predominance of eosinophils.

Graft versus Host Disease

Graft versus host disease (GVHD) is seen in patients who have received allogenic immunocompetent lymphocytes in the course of bone marrow transplants. Acute graft versus host disease presents with a flat erythematous rash affecting the hands and feet that may spread and coalesce to involve the whole body. It typically occurs in the first 100 days after allogenic bone marrow transplantation and is associated with diarrhea, jaundice, and deranged liver function tests. Rarely it resembles a severe rash called toxic epidermal necrolysis. Chronic graft versus host disease may develop following acute graft versus host disease or de novo. It may present as dryness of the skin, lichen planus–like lesions, or with thickening and scarring of the skin (scleroderma). Graft versus host disease may be associated with internal organ involvement (e.g., liver, lung, gastrointestinal tract).

The pathogenesis of graft versus host disease is complex. The key factor is the interaction of donor cytotoxic T lymphocytes with the recipient minor histocompatibility antigens. The keratinocytes appear to be the preferred targets.

On microscopy, GVHD is graded using the Horn grading system.

Grade 0: Normal skin

Grade 1: Basal vacuolar change

Grade 2: Dyskeratotic cells in the epidermis and/or follicle
    Dermal lymphocytic infiltrate

Grade 3: Fusion of basal vacuolated cells to form clefts and microvesicles

Grade 4: Dermoepidermal separation

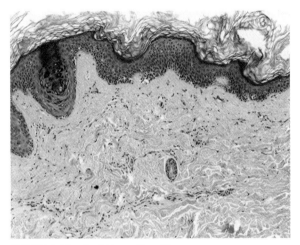

FIGURE 8.60   Graft Versus Host Disease

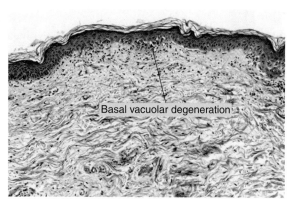

FIGURE 8.61   Dermatomyositis

Dermatomyositis

Dermatomyositis is the coexistence of inflammatory changes in the skin and nonsuppurative changes in the skeletal muscle. Cutaneous lesions without involvement of muscle are also known to occur ("amyopathic dermatomyositis"). Characteristic clinical findings include the heliotrope rash (purplish discoloration and edema of the periorbital tissue) and Gottron's papules (violaceous erythematous papules or plaques over knuckles) which are diagnostic. Proximal muscle weakness of the upper and lower limbs is typically seen. Approximately 10% of patients have an underlying systemic malignancy.

On microscopy, the histological changes are variable. The changes could be subtle and there might be changes in the basal layer such as vacuolar degeneration, which is indistinguishable from lupus erythematosus.

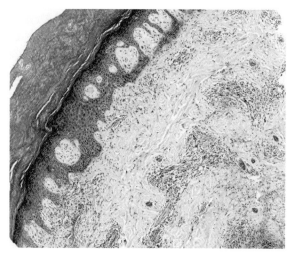

FIGURE 8.62   Chill Blain Lupus

Chill Blain Lupus

Chill blain (or perniotic) lupus results from microvascular injury and is one of the many manifestations of lupus erythematosus. Lesions usually develop in the digits as tender erythematous inflamed plaques, sometimes with a slightly bluish/purpuric central area with or without ulceration. Patients may have associated nailfold capillary abnormalities and Raynaud's phenomenon.

On microscopy, the changes are those of lupus erythematosus with basal cell changes and periadnexal, perifollicular, and perivascular lymphocytic infiltrate and subepidermal edema. Red cell extravasation can be seen.

Direct immunofluorescence shows deposition of IgG and C3c at the basement membrane zone.

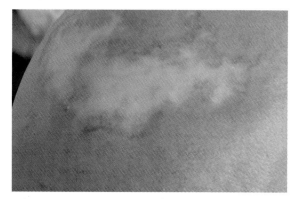

FIGURE 8.63   Scarring in Discoid Lupus Erythematosus. Courtesy of Mark Goodfield, The General Infirmary at Leeds, UK

Discoid Lupus Erythematosus

Discoid lupus typically presents as well-demarcated erythematous scaly plaques with follicular plugging, often affecting face (often in a malar or "butterfly" distribution overt both cheeks), scalp, and rarely the mucosa. Lesions may undergo atrophy and scarring with associated postinflammatory hypo or hyperpigmentation. In the scalp, these lesions may be associated with scarring alopecia. Sometimes the lesions are very hyperkeratotic (hypertrophic variant).

On microscopy, lesions of discoid lupus erythematosus show follicular plugging and dermal infiltrate of lymphocytes in a typical perifollicular and periadnexal distribution. A lichenoid infiltrate of lymphocytes is a prominent feature that results in liquefaction degeneration of the basal cells in a large majority of cases. Follicular plugging is seen in many cases.

Direct immunofluorescence shows deposition of IgG and IgM at the basement membrane zone. C3c is found less frequently.

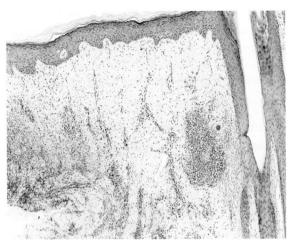

FIGURE 8.64   Discoid Lupus Erythematosus

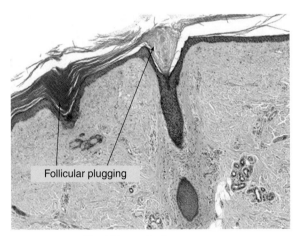

Follicular plugging

FIGURE 8.65   Discoid Lupus Erythematosus

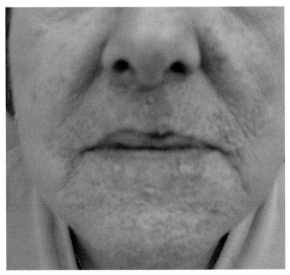

FIGURE 8.66   Subacute Lupus Erythematosus. Courtesy of Mark Goodfield, The General Infirmary at Leeds, UK

Lupus Erythematosus

Subcutaneous lupus erythematosus is a variant of lupus erythematosus and is characterized by annular polycyclic lesions or papulosquamous lesions on the upper trunk, upper arms, face, and neck. Patients may exhibit photosensitivity, mild systemic illness, and musculoskeletal symptoms. The histopathological features show less follicular plugging and hyperkeratosis and more basal vacuolar changes, epidermal atrophy, mucin deposition in the superficial dermis, and dermal edema compared with discoid lupus erythematosus.

Systemic lupus erythematosus shows much more extensive systemic involvement and cutaneous manifestations compared to with subacute lupus erythematosus. It typically includes variable renal and joint involvement and serositis. Cutaneous manifestations classically present as erythematous malar "butterfly" rash (photosensitivity). Other cutaneous lesions may be urticarial, purpuric, or bullous or vasculitic in nature. Discoid lupus-like lesions and chilblain lupus lesions can occur in systemic lupus erythematosus. Lupus profundus is a variant of lupus erythematosus and presents as subcutaneous nodules in the head and neck area and the trunk. On microscopy, the predominant feature is a lobular panniculitis composed of lymphocytes.

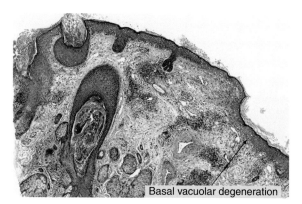

FIGURE 8.67   Lupus Erythematosus

On microscopy, acute cutaneous lesions of systemic lupus erythematosus show conspicuous vacuolar degeneration of the basal layer as a prominent feature. There could be basement membrane thickening and basal cell vacuolation with infiltration of lymphocytes in a perifollicular distribution.

The lupus band test is considered an ancillary diagnostic tool. Involved skin is positive in 100% of cases; 90% of biopsies from uninvolved sun-exposed skin is positive. One third of cases from uninvolved sun-protected sites are positive. The lupus band test may be negative in remissions.

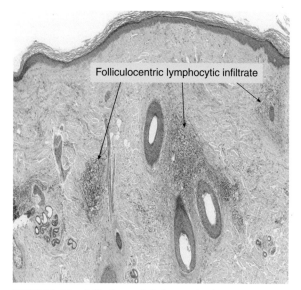

FIGURE 8.68   Folliculocentric Inflammation in Lupus

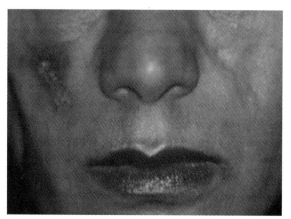

FIGURE 8.69   Lupus Profundus. Courtesy of Mark Goodfield, The General Infirmary at Leeds, UK

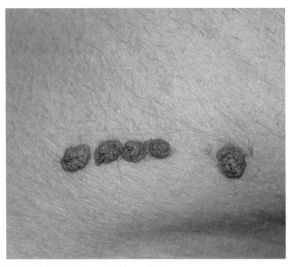

FIGURE 8.70   Linear Epidermal Nevus

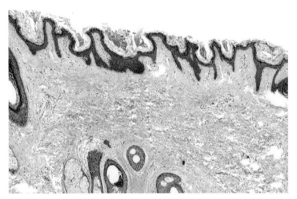

FIGURE 8.71   Epidermal Nevus

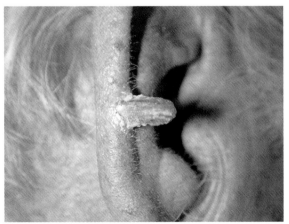

FIGURE 8.72   Keratin Horn

Linear Epidermal Nevus

Epidermal nevus has a predilection for the head and neck and extremities and is a developmental abnormality in which there is excess production of keratinocytes. Most often, the nevus takes a zosteriform or linear arrangement of brown warty lesions.

On microscopy, a variety of histological appearances are identified. Most cases are a combination of features. Hyperkeratosis, acanthosis, and papillomatosis are consistent histological findings.

Keratin Horn (Cutaneous Horn)

Cutaneous or keratin horns usually present as hard yellow-brown keratotic projection arising from a normal epidermis or overlying a small pinkish papule, typically associated with surrounding sun-damaged skin.

On microscopy, horns are composed of tiers of keratinous material, which may be amorphous or lamellated. The underlying epidermis usually lacks atypia, but occasionally on a sun-exposed site the keratinocytes can exhibit dysplasia of the keratinocytes in varying degrees of severity ranging from mild to severe. Up to 10–15% may have squamous cell carcinoma in situ or a small focus of well-differentiated squamous cell carcinoma at the base of the lesions arising in sun-damaged skin. Very rarely, horns may develop on nail groove, and they show trichilemmal type of keratinization. These lesions have been called onycholemmal horns.

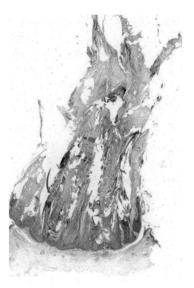

FIGURE 8.73   Cutaneous Horn-Low Power

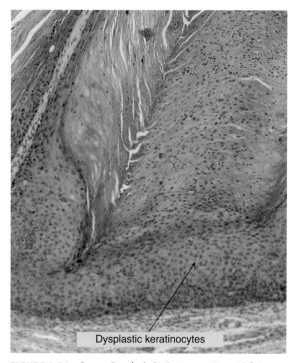

Dysplastic keratinocytes

FIGURE 8.74   Severe Dysplasia in Cutaneous Horn-High Power

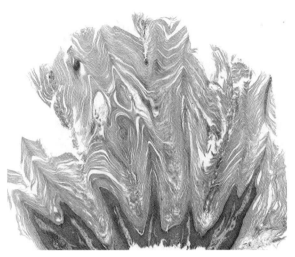

FIGURE 8.75   Squamous Papilloma

Squamous Papilloma

This is a reaction pattern seen in a number of inflammatory and neoplastic conditions. There is undulation of the epidermis with marked hyperkeratosis. The papillomatous architecture may be seen as spikes or in a broad pattern covered by parakeratotic epidermis.

Seborrheic Keratoses

Seborrheic keratosis (senile wart) is a benign tumor that may appear after middle age. Typically it presents with flat tan-colored macules (solar lentigo) and becomes progressively raised flat plaques; eventually they become brown-black markedly verrucous and warty, often with keratin horn cysts and a "stuck on" appearance (Figs. 8.76 and 8.77).

On microscopy, they exhibit a variety of features. Classically, there is proliferation of basaloid cells accompanied by horn cysts, which are keratin-filled invaginations. A small proportion of these tumors may be pigmented. Fig. 8.81 demonstrates the clonal variant of seborrheic keratosis, which shows nested proliferation of basaloid cells exhibiting the Borst-Jadassohn phenomenon. Very rarely, malignant change occurs in seborrheic keratosis manifested as in situ or invasive changes.

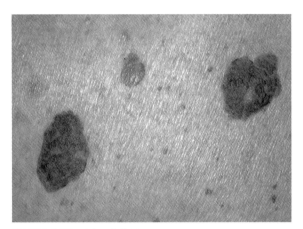

FIGURE 8.76   Seborrheic Keratoses

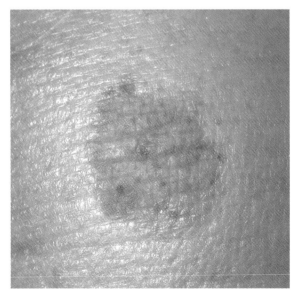

FIGURE 8.77   Seborrheic Keratoses

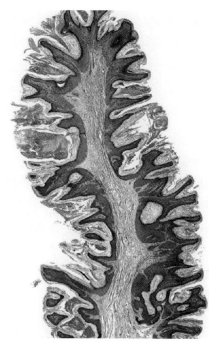

FIGURE 8.78   Seborrheic Keratoses as Fibroepithelial Polyp

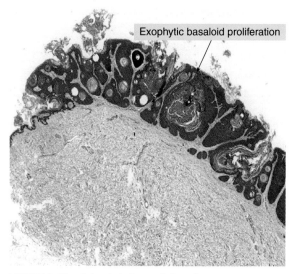

Exophytic basaloid proliferation

FIGURE 8.79   Seborrheic Keratosis-Low Power

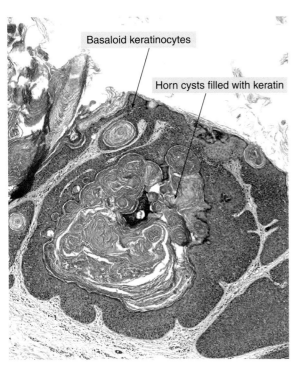

FIGURE 8.80   Seborrheic Keratoses-High Power

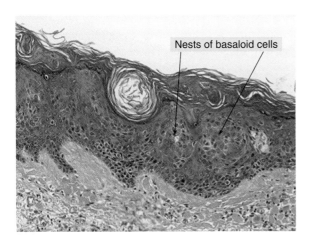

FIGURE 8.81   Clonal Seborrheic Keratoses

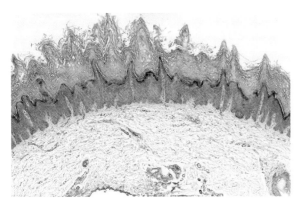

FIGURE 8.82   Stucco keratosis

Stucco Keratosis

Stucco keratosis is variant of seborrheic keratoses presenting as multiple often numerous small white (hence "stucco") verrucous plaques on the lower legs.

On microscopy, they demonstrate hyperkeratosis, parakeratosis, and mild papillomatosis.

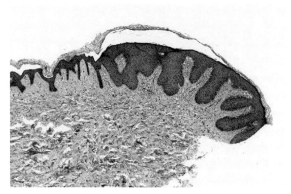

FIGURE 8.83   Dermatosis Papulosis Nigra

Dermatoses Papulosis Nigra

This lesion is found exclusively in dark-skinned races with a female preponderance. It presents with multiple small, pigmented papules and plaques on the face. This is considered a variant of seborrheic keratosis.

On microscopy, the appearances are reminiscent of reticulate variant of seborrheic keratosis, except that the cell proliferation is not of basaloid type.

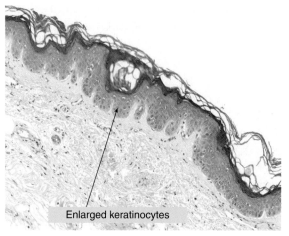

Enlarged keratinocytes

FIGURE 8.84   Large Cell Acanthoma

Large Cell Acanthoma

Large cell acanthoma occurs on sun-exposed sites of middle-aged and elderly individuals.

On microscopy, there is acanthosis of the epidermis, and it is composed of enlarged keratinocytes. The changes are confined to the epidermis with sparing of the adnexal epithelium. Malignant transformation is not known to occur in large cell acanthoma.

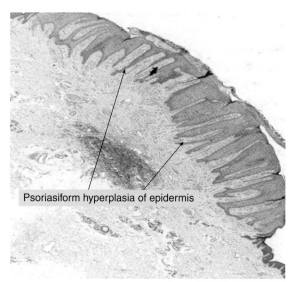

Psoriasiform hyperplasia of epidermis

FIGURE 8.85   Clear Cell Acanthoma-Low Power

Clear Cell Acanthoma

Clear cell acanthoma also known as pale cell acanthoma is a benign epidermal neoplasm. Clinically it presents as solitary and very rarely multiple papules on the lower limbs of elderly female individuals.

On microscopy, the epidermis shows well-demarcated acanthosis and psoriasiform hyperplasia. The keratinocytes appear to have pale staining cytoplasm, hence, the term clear cell acanthoma. The adnexal epithelium is spared. The underlying dermis shows a mixed inflammatory infiltrate with variable numbers of neutrophils.

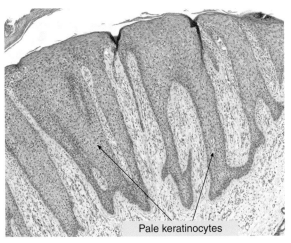

FIGURE 8.86   Clear Cell Acanthoma-High Power

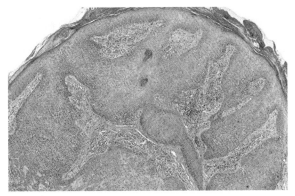

FIGURE 8.87   Inverted Follicular Keratosis

Inverted Follicular Keratosis

Inverted follicular keratosis occurs as flesh colored nodules on the head and neck skin.

On microscopy, this is a predominantly endophytic tumor with proliferation of basaloid and squamous keratinocytes. Squamous eddies composed of whorls of central squamous cells and peripheral basaloid cells are characteristically seen in inverted follicular keratosis.

PREMALIGNANT AND MALIGNANT EPITHELIAL TUMORS

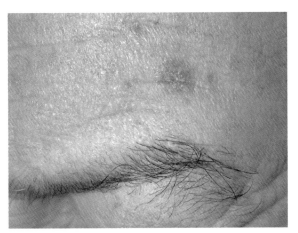

FIGURE 8.88   Actinic Keratosis

Actinic Keratosis

Actinic keratosis is a very common scaly erythematous lesion found on sun-exposed sites of individuals who have had chronic sun exposure. It typically occurs on the head and neck but occurs anywhere there has been chronic sun exposure. Occasionally, actinic keratoses may progress to squamous cell carcinoma in situ and squamous cell carcinoma.

On microscopy, there is focal parakeratosis and mild acanthosis of the epidermis. Actinic keratosis is characterized by disordered arrangement of keratinocytes with atypia ranging from mild to severe. When the atypia is of full thickness, the term bowenoid actinic keratosis is used. The underlying dermis show solar elastosis and lymphocytic infiltration to a variable degree.

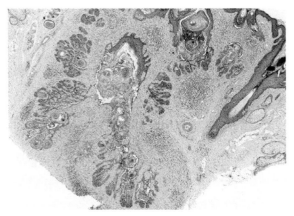

FIGURE 8.89   Proliferative Actinic Keratosis-Low Power

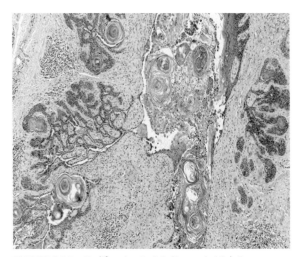

FIGURE 8.90   Proliferative Actinic Keratosis-High Power

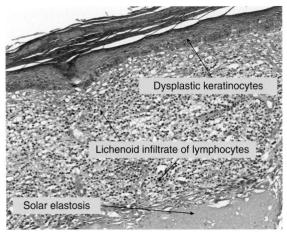

FIGURE 8.91   Actinic Keratosis with Mild Dysplasia-High
Power

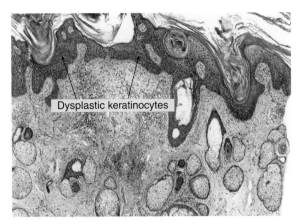

FIGURE 8.92   Moderately Dysplastic Actinic Keratosis

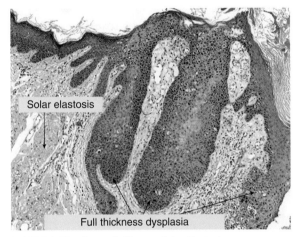

FIGURE 8.93   Bowen's Disease, Solar Elastosis

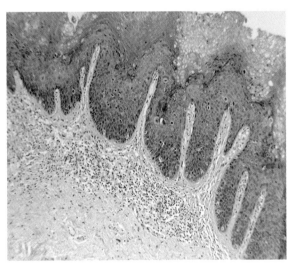

FIGURE 8.94   Bowenoid Papulosis

Bowenoid Papulosis

Bowenoid papulosis clinically presents as solitary or multiple plaque–like areas on genital skin. Majority of cases are due to human papilloma virus 16 (HPV 16) and a small number develop due to HPV 18 and 35. A very small number of cases may develop malignant transformation to squamous cell carcinoma.

On microscopy, the features are essentially that of Bowen's disease, characterized by full-thickness dysplasia of the keratinocytes. Koilocytes are not a conspicuous feature. In the female genital skin, the lesions are classified as vulvar intraepithelial neoplasia 1–111.

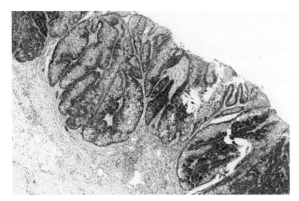

FIGURE 8.95   Clear Cell Bowen's Disease

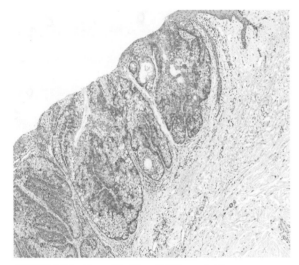

FIGURE 8.96   Berep4 in Clear Cell Bowen's Disease

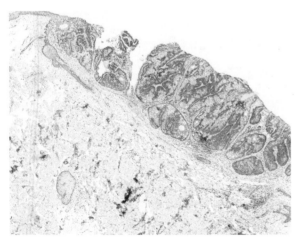

FIGURE 8.97   CK7 in Clear Cell Bowen's Disease

Clear Cell Bowen's Disease

Bowen's disease denotes full-thickness intraepithelial neoplasia of the epidermis, a premalignant condition. Clinically, it manifests as well-defined erythematous scaly plaques, somewhat larger than actinic keratoses on chronically sun-exposed sites, often the lower legs.

On microscopy, there is full-thickness dysplasia of the keratinocytes without invasion below through the basement membrane.

Several histological variants of Bowen's disease have been described, of which clear cell type is demonstrated in the images. Immunohistochemical stains become necessary in clear cell Bowen's disease as it includes differential diagnosis of melanoma in situ and Paget's disease. Specific antibodies targeted against high–molecular-weight cytokeratins such as Cytokeratin 14 (CK14) and epithelial membrane antigen (EMA) are positive in Bowen's disease. Melanocytic tumors are positive for S100 and Melan A. For differentiation of clear cell Bowen's from Paget's disease, see section on Paget's disease (Figs. 8.147–8.149).

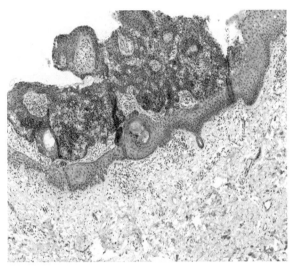

FIGURE 8.98   Clear Cell Bowen's Disease—CK14

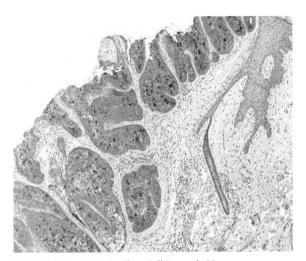

FIGURE 8.99   EMA in Clear Cell Bowen's Disease

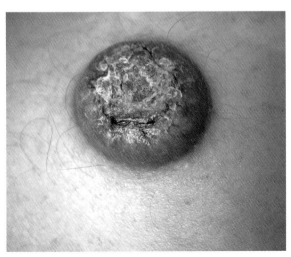

FIGURE 8.100   Keratoacanthoma

Keratoacanthoma

Keratoacanthomas clinically presents as rapidly growing solitary dome-shaped nodules with a central keratotic plug. Keratoacanthomas are thought to be of follicular infundibular origin. Invasive tumors arising from this area include squamous cell carcinomas of varying degrees of differentiation. Keratoacanthomas are predominantly seen on sun-exposed sites although less frequently other sites of the body may be involved. Clinically and histologically, it may be difficult or even impossible to clearly differentiate a keratoacanthoma from a squamous cell carcinoma in some cases as a result, they are best considered a variant of a squamous cell carcinoma.

Subungual keratoacanthoma, a rare variant, behaves in a very destructive fashion, and they are known to be associated with incontinentia pigmenti.

Very rare syndromes have been documented where patients present with multiple keratoacanthomas-like lesions including self-healing epitheliomas (Ferguson-Smith syndrome), Muir-Torre syndrome, and Grzybowski's syndrome. Clinical features and clinicopathological correlation are needed to differentiate these conditions. Multiple eruptive keratoacanthomas may also occur with immunosuppression, in association with underlying malignancy and with sorafenib (tyrosine kinase inhibitor) treatment.

On microscopy, keratoacanthomas have characteristic crateriform architecture with a central keratin plug. The epidermis is markedly hyperkeratotic and acanthotic. The keratinocytes are enlarged with ample amount of pink cytoplasm characteristically described as glassy due to excessive amounts of glycogen. Not uncommonly, there is dysplasia of these cells with increased mitotic activity. Detached islands of these dysplastic cells invade into the underlying dermis, qualifying for the designation of a squamous cell carcinoma. Perineural invasion and lymphovascular space permeation are seen. Lesions that demonstrate perineural invasion and lymphovascular permeation are probably best treated/regarded as a squamous cell carcinoma.

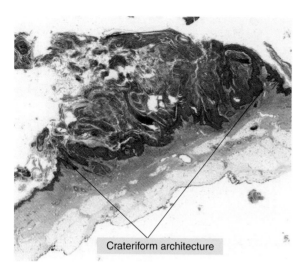

Crateriform architecture

FIGURE 8.101   Keratoacanthoma-Low Power

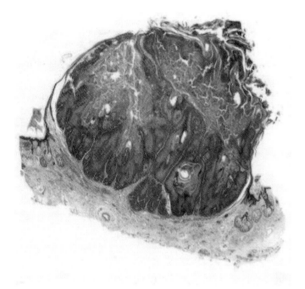

FIGURE 8.102   Keratoacanthoma—Crateriform Architecture

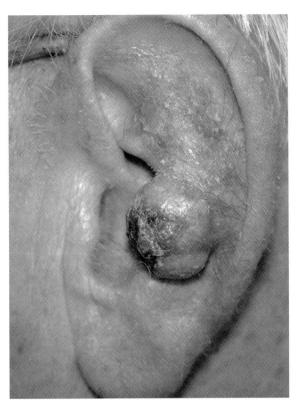

FIGURE 8.103   Squamous Cell Carcinoma

Squamous Cell Carcinoma

Squamous cell carcinoma is the second most common epithelial malignancy of the skin. A large majority of the tumors arise on sun-exposed sites. Other sites include nail bed and anogenital region (associated with HPV 16 infection).

On microscopy, squamous cell carcinoma is a tumor of the keratinocytes. The dysplastic keratinocytes invade the underlying dermis and differentiates toward abnormal keratinization. The tumor is classified into well, moderate, and poorly differentiated, based on the extent of keratinization. The site of the tumor, macroscopic size, microscopic tumor thickness, lymphovascular space permeation, and subcutaneous fat involvement are the key factors predicting the prognosis. Immunohistochemical markers aid the diagnosis only in poorly differentiated tumors. Broad spectrum cytokeratins such as MNF116 (Fig. 8.111) or high–molecular-weight cytokeratins such as CK14 and CK5/6 stain the neoplastic keratinocytes.

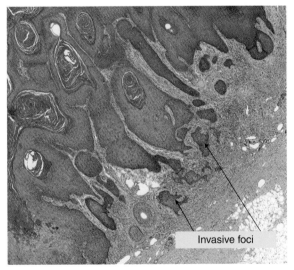

Invasive foci

FIGURE 8.104   Squamous Cell Carcinoma Arising in a Keratoacanthoma-Low Power

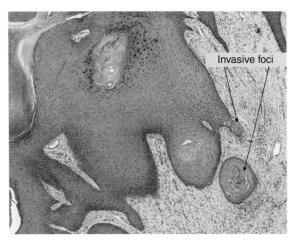

FIGURE 8.105   Well Differentiated Squamous Cell Carcinoma-High Power

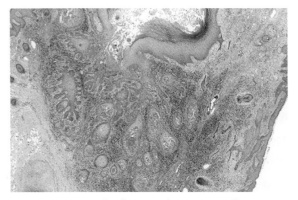

FIGURE 8.106   Well Differentiated Squamous Cell Carcinoma

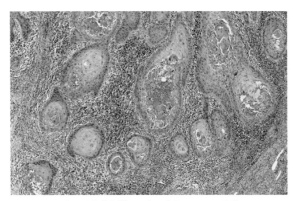

FIGURE 8.107   Well Differentiated Squamous Cell Carcinoma-High Power

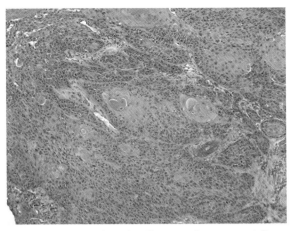

FIGURE 8.108   Moderately Differentiated Squamous Cell Carcinoma

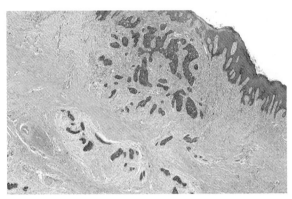

FIGURE 8.109   Poorly Differentiated Squamous Cell Carcinoma

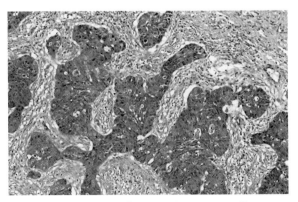

FIGURE 8.110   Poorly Differentiated Squamous Cell Carcinoma-High Power

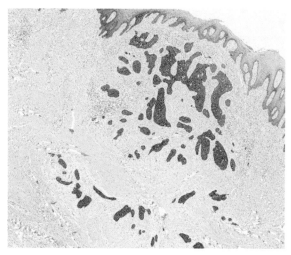

FIGURE 8.111   Poorly Differentiated Squamous Cell Carcinoma—MNF116

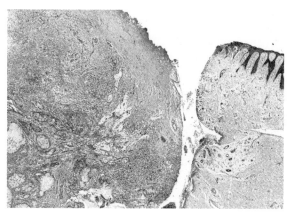

FIGURE 8.112   Mucoepidermoid Carcinoma

Mucoepidermoid Carcinoma

This is a very rare variant of squamous cell carcinoma. The tumor shows glandular differentiation admixed with neoplastic areas. The glandular component is positive for carcino embryonic antigen (CEA). Mucoepidermoid carcinoma of the skin is an aggressive tumor with high chance of nodal and distant metastasis.

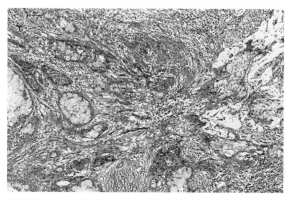

FIGURE 8.113   Mucoepidermoid Carcinoma-High Power

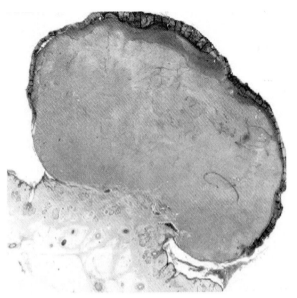

FIGURE 8.114   Carcinosarcoma-Scanning View

Carcinosarcoma

Carcinosarcoma or metaplastic carcinoma of the skin is a very rare tumor that presents as a nodule on the scalp or face of elderly individuals. Carcinosarcoma are biphasic tumors showing malignant epithelial and mesenchymal components. The epithelial components range from squamous cell carcinoma, basal cell carcinoma, or malignant adnexal tumors. Mesenchymal component may include tumors of osteoblastic, chondroblastic, smooth muscle, and skeletal muscle differentiation. The epithelial components stain with cytokeratins (Fig. 8.116), and the mesenchymal spindle cells stain variably with markers for smooth muscle or skeletal muscle differentiation. Considering the biphasic nature of the tumor, extensive sampling is required to identify the individual components.

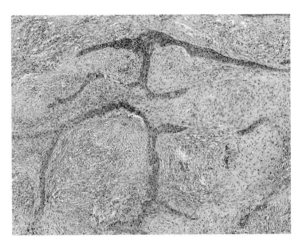

FIGURE 8.115   Carcinosarcoma-High Power

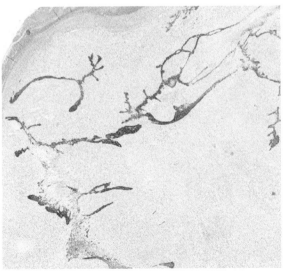

FIGURE 8.116   Carcinosarcoma—CK14

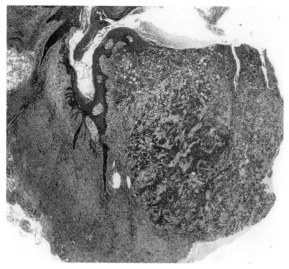

FIGURE 8.117   Squamous Cell Carcinoma with Vacuolated Cytoplasm-Low Power

Squamous Cell Carcinoma with Vacuolated Cytoplasm

This is not an uncommon variant of squamous cell carcinoma. The vacuolated cells raises the differential diagnosis of other primary clear cell tumors such as sebaceous carcinoma, malignant clear cell hidradenoma, clear cell change in a basal cell carcinoma, or metastatic tumors such as renal cell carcinoma. In situ changes in the adjacent epidermis and relevant clinical history should help in arriving at the right diagnosis.

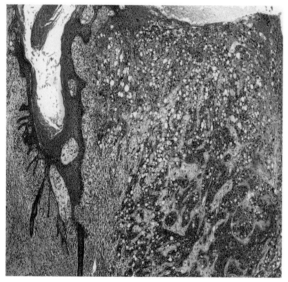

FIGURE 8.118   Squamous Cell Carcinoma with Vacuolated Cytoplasm-High Power

Verrucous Carcinoma

This is a variant of squamous cell carcinoma, most commonly arising on the sole of foot and also at other sites such as anogenital region (Buschke-Lowenstein tumor). The usual clinical presentation is that of hyperkeratotic warty growths associated with cleft formation. Longstanding tumors lead to erosion of the underlying bone. Anogenital tumors grow in a predominantly exophytic pattern, and they arise from pre-existing condyloma acuminatum. Viral etiology particularly associated with HPV 1, 2, 11, 16, and 18 have been implicated in plantar and anogenital verrucous carcinoma. They are also known to arise from sites of chronic inflammation such as osteomyelitis and tuberculosis.

On microscopy, the tumors are exophytic and endophytic. The exophytic areas show marked hyperkeratosis and acanthosis of the epidermis. Parakeratosis and koilocytosis may also be seen. The endophytic areas show bulbous downgrowths of acanthotic epidermis composed of enlarged keratinocytes with mild nuclear pleomorphism. The enlarged keratinocytes exhibit marked intracellular edema resulting in glassy appearance of the keratinocytes. Intercellular bridges are also a prominent feature of the tumor. Mitotic figures and nuclear pleomorphism are confined to the base of the tumor. The massive hyperkeratosis accompanied by necrosis is a characteristic feature resulting in the histological appearance of sinus formation. The bland nature of the keratinocytes and the growth pattern raises the differential diagnosis of an exuberant viral wart that can be difficult to distinguish. Rarely pleomorphic keratinocytes can infiltrate into the underlying dermis, when the tumor should be designated as conventional squamous cell carcinoma and treated as such. Extensive sampling of the tumor is of paramount importance in assessing such invasive foci.

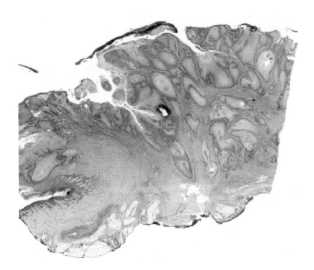

FIGURE 8.119   Verrucous Carcinoma-Low Power

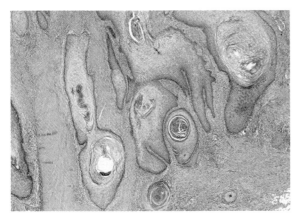

FIGURE 8.120   Verrucous Carcinoma-High Power

Spindle Cell Squamous Carcinoma

Spindle cell squamous carcinoma is a histological variant of squamous carcinoma. The microscopic appearance is predominated by pleomorphic spindle cells, and this raises a myriad of differential diagnoses. This includes spindle cell melanoma, desmoplastic melanoma, and spindle cell sarcoma, which includes leiomyosarcoma, angiosarcoma, spindle cell rhabdomyosarcoma, pleomorphic sarcoma not otherwise specified, and atypical fibroxanthoma. The diagnosis of atypical fibroxanthoma should be considered only when the tumor is strictly dermal in location. Extensive sampling and careful examination of the sections for in situ keratinocytic and melanocytic atypia aid the diagnosis. It is also prudent to consider the above-mentioned entities in a metastatic setting. Please refer to Table 8.1 for the immunohistochemical stains used in the diagnostic armamentarium.

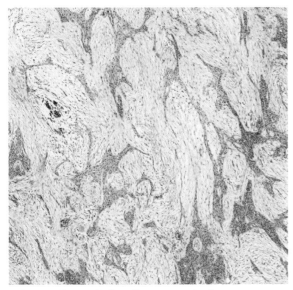

FIGURE 8.121   Spindle Cell Squamous Carcinoma

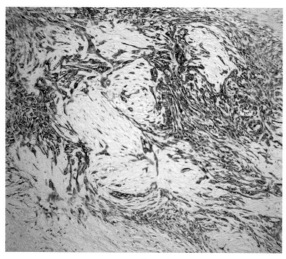

FIGURE 8.122   CK14 in Spindle Cell Squamous Carcinoma

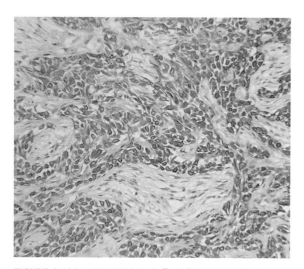

FIGURE 8.123   AE1/AE3 in Spindle Cell Squamous Carcinoma

Table 8.1								

Differential diagnosis of cutaneous spindle cell tumors

Diagnosis	Broad Spectrum Cytokeratins MNF116, AE1/AE3	High mol. wt Cytokeratins CK14, CK5/6	Melano-cytic Marker S100	Melanocytic Markers HMB-45, Mart 1 (Melan A)	Smooth Muscle Markers SMA, Desmin, h-caldesmon	Skeletal Muscle Marker Desmin, Myogenin	Vascular Markers CD-34, CD-31	Other Markers CD-10, CD-117, CD-68, CD-163
Spindle cell carcinoma	+	+	−	−	−	−	−	−
Spindle cell melanoma	±	−	+	+	−	−	−	+ CD-117
Desmoplastic melanoma	−	−	+	−	−	−	−	−
Leiomyosarcoma	+	−	−	−	+	−	−	−
Spindle cell rhabdomyo-sarcoma	−	−	−	−	−	+	−	−
Pleomorphic sarcoma NOS	−	−	−	−	SMA+	−	−	−
Spindle cell angiosarcoma	−	−	−	−	−	−	+	−
Atypical fibroxanthoma	−	−	−	−	SMA+	−	−	CD-10+, CD-68+, CD-163+

NOS, not otherwise specified; SMA, smooth muscle actin.

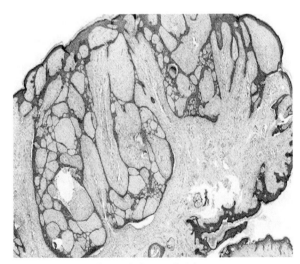

FIGURE 8.124   Fibroepithelioma of Pinkus-Low Power

Fibroepithelioma of Pinkus

Fibroepithelioma of Pinkus is an uncommon tumor and is considered a variant of basal cell carcinoma. They present as single or multiple pink-, yellow-, brown-, or skin-colored dome-shaped papules with a broad base or as pedunculated tumors, most commonly occurring on the lower back.

On microscopy, strands of interconnected basaloid cells are seen growing down into the dermal stroma, which is rather fibrotic in appearance. Very rarely, additional features such as amyloid may be seen within the tumor as an incidental finding (Fig. 8.126).

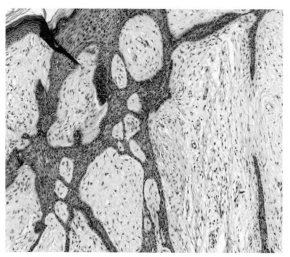

FIGURE 8.125   Fibroepithelioma of Pinkus-High Power

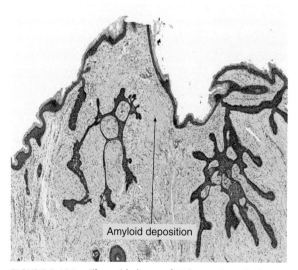

Amyloid deposition

FIGURE 8.126   Fibroepithelioma of Pinkus and Amyloid

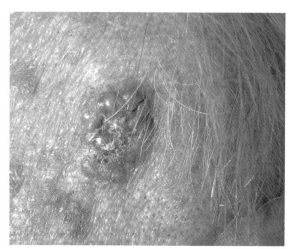

FIGURE 8.127   Basal Cell Carcinoma

Basal Cell Carcinoma

Basal cell carcinoma is the most common cutaneous malignant tumor seen on sun-exposed site. Although metastasis is exceptionally rare, the tumor is notorious for destructive local recurrence, hence the name rodent ulcer. Basal cell carcinoma can occur as single or multiple lesions and may be sporadic or familial. Multiple basal cell carcinomas at an early age are seen in patients with Gorlin-Goltz syndrome. Germline mutations in the human homologue of the Drosophila gene patched (*PTCH1*) located on chromosome 9q22,23 are the underlying defect in Gorlin-Goltz syndrome. This mutation is also identified in 30% of sporadic basal cell carcinoma. Overexposure to ultraviolet rays is considered as the single most important causative factor. *PTCH1* is a member of the sonic hedgehog signaling pathway that controls cell proliferation. Mutations in p53 have also been identified as one of the factors involved in the tumorigenesis of basal cell carcinoma.

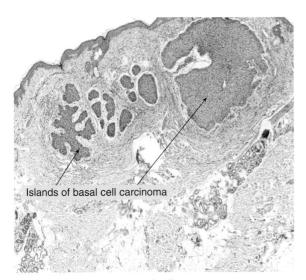

FIGURE 8.128   Nodular Basal Cell Carcinoma

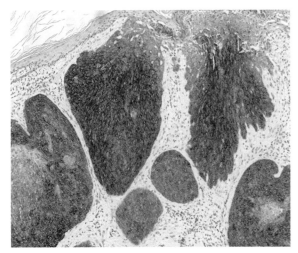

FIGURE 8.129   BerEP4 in Basal Cell Carcinoma

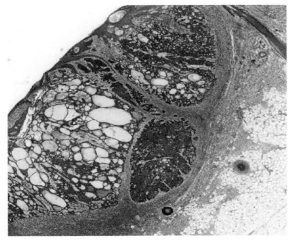

FIGURE 8.130   Nodulocystic Basal Cell Carcinoma

Clinically, the tumor presents with a small pinkish, semi-translucent papule or plaque with a pearly rolled edge exhibiting characteristic arborizing telangiectasia. Central ulceration may or may not be present. There are several clinical variants of basal cell carcinoma described. The tumor has a tendency to be locally destructive. High-risk areas of tumor recurrence include central face, postauricular region, and forehead. Morphoeic or infiltrative basal cell carcinoma presents with a scar- or plaque-like appearance.

On microscopy, a variety of histological patterns have been described. The most common pattern is nodular basal cell carcinoma. Nodules of basaloid cells of varying sizes are seen growing down into the dermis. The nodules or islands exhibit peripheral palisading and many apoptotic bodies or mitotic figures. Clefting at the periphery of the islands and mucinous degeneration of the stroma are the classical features. Basal cell carcinomas at risk of recurrence include high-risk site (periocular, ears, lips, nasolabial folds); morphoeic, infiltrative, and micronodular subtypes; recurrent tumors following prior treatment; size >2 cm in high-risk sites; perineural spread; and immunocompromised patients.

Morphoeic and infiltrative basal cell carcinoma are challenging diagnostically. These subtypes show thin strands, or small groups of basaloid cells infiltrating into the dermis. Morphoeic basal carcinomas are associated with sclerosed or fibrosed dermal stroma in a diffuse pattern. Morphoeic and infiltrative basal cell carcinoma may coexist with other subtypes. The distinct histological appearances of morphoeic basal cell carcinoma raise the differential diagnosis of desmoplastic trichoepithelioma and microcystic adnexal carcinoma. Desmoplastic trichoepithelioma can be impossible to differentiate particularly on a punch biopsy. Papillary mesenchymal bodies, keratocysts, and foci of calcification favor a desmoplastic trichoepithelioma over morphemic basal cell carcinoma. Infiltration into deep dermis and/or subcutaneous fat with identification of duct formation differentiates a microcystic adnexal carcinoma from a morphemic basal cell carcinoma. Perineural infiltration is a characteristic feature seen in morphoeic basal cell carcinoma and is considered one of the adverse prognostic features.

Another variant with high rates of recurrence is the micronodular variant of basal cell carcinoma. In this variant, basaloid cells are seen in small aggregates of 15–20 cells with an infiltrative pattern.

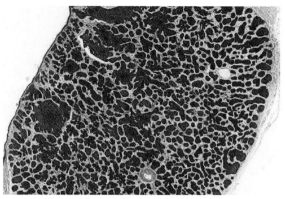

FIGURE 8.131   Nodular Basal Cell Carcinoma

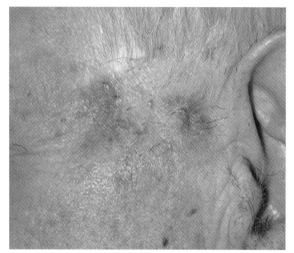

FIGURE 8.132   Morpheic Basal Cell Carcinoma

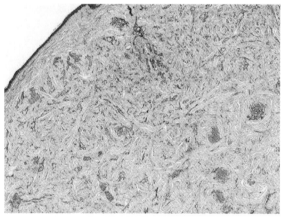

FIGURE 8.133   Morpheic Basal Cell Carcinoma-Low Power

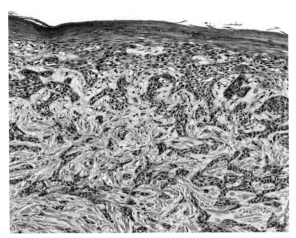

FIGURE 8.134   Morpheic Basal Cell Carcinoma-High Power

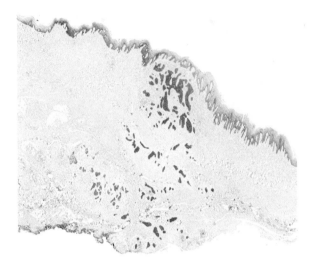

FIGURE 8.135   BerEp4 in Morpheic Basal Cell Carcinoma

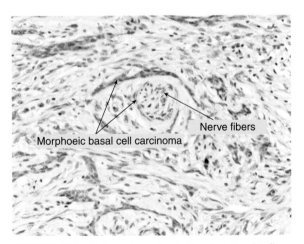

FIGURE 8.136   Perineural invasion in Morpheic Basal Cell Carcinoma S100 Stain

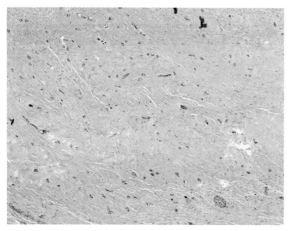

FIGURE 8.137   Micronodular Basal Cell Carcinoma-Low Power

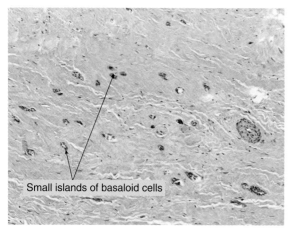

Small islands of basaloid cells

FIGURE 8.138   Micronodular Basal Cell Carcinoma

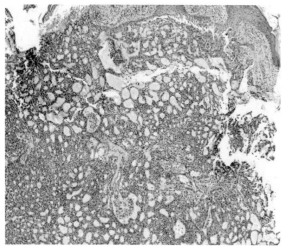

FIGURE 8.139   Adenoid Basal Cell Carcinoma

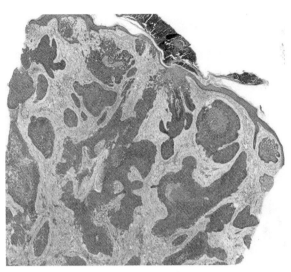

FIGURE 8.140   Metatypical Basal Cell Carcinoma

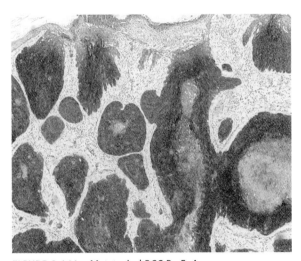

FIGURE 8.141   Metatypical BCC BerEp4

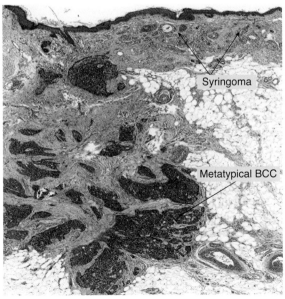

FIGURE 8.142   Metatypical Basal Cell Carcinoma and Syringoma-Low Power

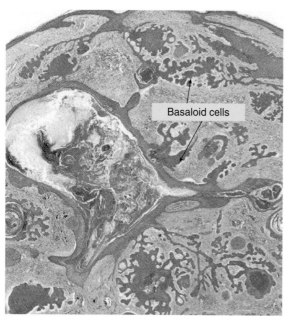

FIGURE 8.143 Keratotic Basal Cell Carcinoma

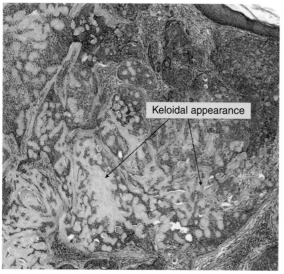

FIGURE 8.144 Keloidal Basal Cell Carcinoma

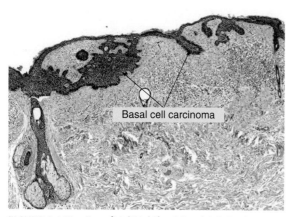

FIGURE 8.145 Superficial Multifocal Basal Cell Carcinoma

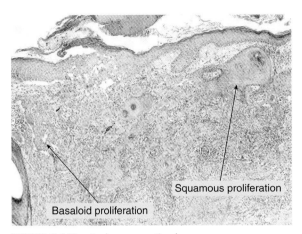

FIGURE 8.146   Basisquamous Carcinoma

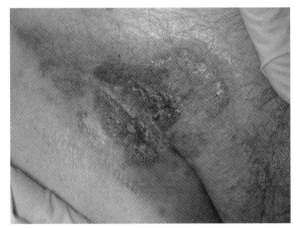

FIGURE 8.147   Extramammary Paget's Disease

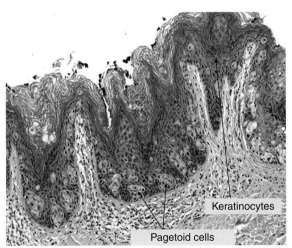

FIGURE 8.148   Extramammary Paget's Disease HE

Extramammary Paget's Disease

Mammary and extramammary Paget's disease shows infiltration of pale staining cells in the epidermis. Mammary Paget's disease results from an underlying carcinoma. In exceptional cases, the tumor may not be found. Extramammary Paget's disease as the name implies can present in other locations, but most commonly in the genital and perianal areas. They are seen as erythematous and moist lesions (Fig. 8.147). Once the diagnosis of extramammary Paget's disease is established, the challenge is to identify whether it is primary or secondary extramammary Paget's disease. Primary extramammary Paget's disease is the result of invasion into the epidermis of an adnexal adenocarcinoma. Secondary extramammary paget's disease results from a primary elsewhere such as gastrointestinal tract, gynaecological tract, breast or prostate. Immunohistochemical studies (Tables 8.2–8.3) and clinicopathological correlation will help to confirm the diagnosis.

Table 8.2

Extramammary Paget's disease–differential diagnosis

Diagnosis	CK7	Cam 5.2	S100	Melan A	CK14
EMPD	+	+	−	−	−
Bowen's disease	−	−	−	−	+
Melanoma in situ	−	−	+	+	−

EMPD, extramammary Paget's disease.

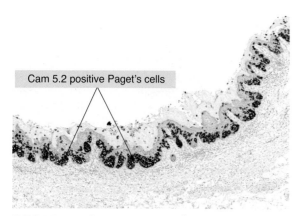

FIGURE 8.149   Extramammary Paget's Disease Cam 5.2

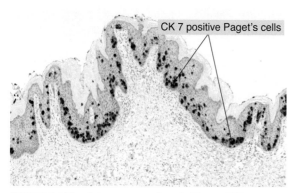

FIGURE 8.150   Extramammary Paget's Disease CK7

Table 8.3

Extramammary Paget's disease–panel of immunohistochemical antibodies

Diagnosis	CK7	CK20	CdX2	Urothelin	Villin	PSA/PSAP	GCDPF
Breast	+	−	−	−	−	−	+
Gynecological tract	+	−	−	−	−	−	−
GIT	+	+	+	−	+	−	−
Urological tract	+	+	−	+	−	−	−
Prostate	+	−	+	+	+	−	+
Prostate	+	−	−	−	−	+	−

EMPD, extramammary Paget's disease; GCDPF, gross cystic disease protein fluid; GIT; PSA, prostate specific antigen; PSAP, prostate specific acid phosphatase.

CUTANEOUS PIGMENTED LESIONS

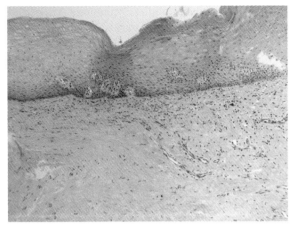

FIGURE 8.151   Mucosal Melanotic Macule

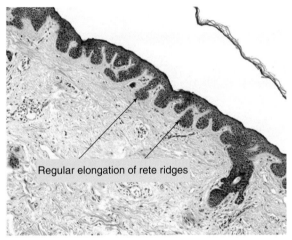

FIGURE 8.152   Solar Lentigo-Low Power

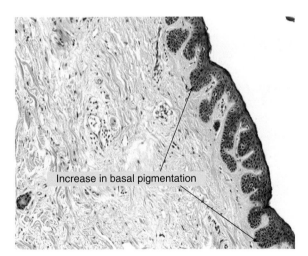

FIGURE 8.153   Solar Lentigo-High Power

Mucosal Melanotic Macule

These are commonly solitary or multiple macules seen at mucosal sites. Mucosal melanotic macules are a manifestation of functionally hyperactive melanocytes. These are known to be associated with melanonychia striata (longitudinal pigmented bands on nails) and pigmentation of genitalia.

On microscopy, there is pigmentation of the basal layer with no or minimal melanocytic hyperplasia. Pigment incontinence of the papillary dermis is a constant feature. Differential diagnosis includes postinflammatory hyperpigmentation and syndromes associated with increased pigmentation such as Peutz-Jeghers syndrome and Albright's syndrome. These are distinguished by their clinical features since the histological appearances are similar.

Solar Lentigo (Senile Lentigo, Senile Freckle)

Solar lentigo clinically presents as tan-, brown-, or black-colored macular lesions on sun-damaged skin of middle-aged and elderly individuals. Some variants such as "ink spot" lentigo have an irregular, reticulate outline that resembles the pattern an ink spot makes on the skin.

On microscopy, the epidermis may be mildly acanthotic. There is regular elongation of rete ridges with increased pigmentation at the base of the rete ridges. These are classically described as "hanging dirty feet." There is mild keratinocyte and melanocytic hyperplasia as a reflection of photoactivation. The dermis shows solar elastosis of the collagen and mild lymphocytic infiltration. Pigment incontinence is also seen.

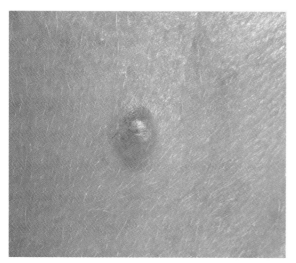

FIGURE 8.154 Mature Dome Shaped Normal Mole. Courtesy of Julia Newton-Bishop, St. James's University Hospital, Leeds, UK

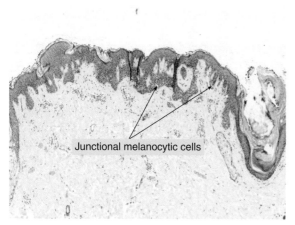

Junctional melanocytic cells

FIGURE 8.155 Junctional Melanocytic Nevus

Benign Melanocytic Nevi

Melanocytic nevi are hamartomatous proliferation of nevus cells. They are common in Caucasians and less common in Asians and Afro-Caribbean races. The nevi usually start to develop in childhood and increase in numbers by the mid 30s. Intense intermittent sun exposure is an important etiological factor in the development of nevi. Malignant transformation of nevi can occur.

Clinically, they appear as regular round-oval, dome-shaped lesions that are light or dark brown in color. Some lesions have a warty appearance. Intradermal nevi are devoid of pigment and occur more commonly on the face.

On microscopy, the earliest feature is the proliferation of melanocytes at the dermoepidermal junction in a lentiginous pattern or as nests. This appearance is seen in a junctional melanocytic nevus. The nests are usually regular. The melanocytes or nevus cells that form these nests are bland cells with scanty cytoplasm. They have fine melanin pigment in their cytoplasm, and the nuclei appear rounded or oval. These cells are designated as type A nevus cells. Nuclear pleomorphism is not a feature, but mitotic activity may be seen. Macrophages containing melanin pigment, which are termed melanophages may be seen in the dermis.

Compound melanocytic nevi exhibit proliferation of bland melanocytes into the papillary and reticular dermis in conjunction with a junctional component. The nevus cells are seen to be arranged as nests, cords, and sheets. As the cells mature, they get smaller and have very densely stained nuclei similar to lymphocytes and are designated "type B nevus cells." These cells lack melanin in their cytoplasm and are typically seen toward the deeper part of the lesion.

Intradermal melanocytic nevi lack any junctional component. The dermal nevus cells are seen as nests, cords, and sheets, and they get smaller or spindle shaped and are termed "type C nevus cells." Mitotic activity and melanin pigment are not seen in the deep aspect of the nevi. Intradermal nevi could show true evidence of neurotization (i.e., resembling nerve fibers) with spindle-shaped cells distributed in a neurofibrillary background. Not uncommonly intradermal or compound melanocytic nevi exhibit papillomatous architecture with proliferation of nevus cells within exuberant dermal papillae. Seborrheic keratosis may coexist with melanocytic nevi. Clinically, the term ancient nevus refers to the presence of multinucleation and smudged appearance of the nucleus in longstanding intradermal nevi, pseudovascular spaces are sometimes seen in the intradermal component, and these nevi are designated as angiomatous nevi. This is considered an artifactual change.

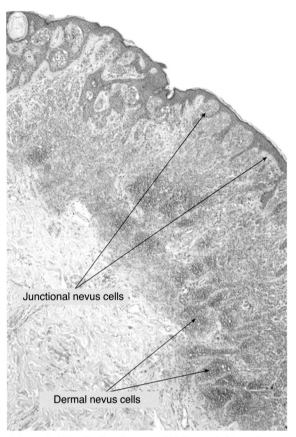

FIGURE 8.156   Benign Compound Melanocytic Nevus-Low Power

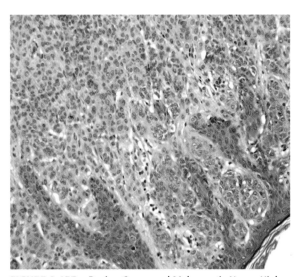

FIGURE 8.157   Benign Compound Melanocytic Nevus-High Power

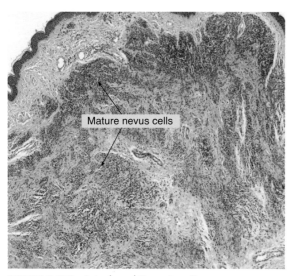

FIGURE 8.158   Intradermal Nevus-Low Power

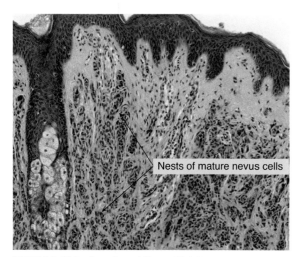

FIGURE 8.159   Intradermal Nevus-High Power

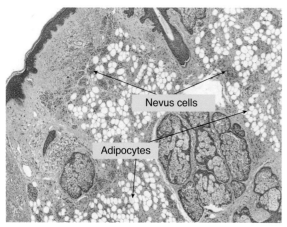

FIGURE 8.160   Intradermal Melanocytic Nevus with
Adipocytic Differentiation-Low Power

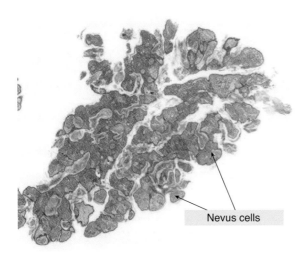

FIGURE 8.161 Keratotic Nevus-Low Power

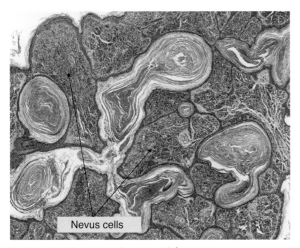

FIGURE 8.162 Keratotic Nevus-High Power

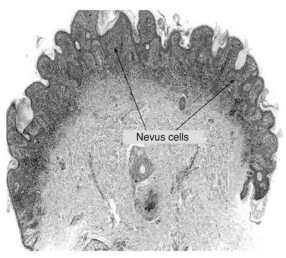

FIGURE 8.163 Nevus with Seborrheic Keratosis Like Architecture-Low Power

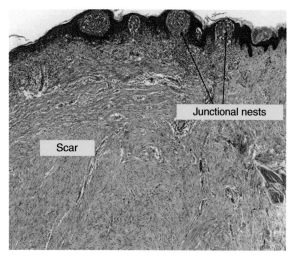

FIGURE 8.164   Recurrent Nevus Overlying Scar

Recurrent Nevus Overlying Scar

Recurrence of a nevus may occur in nevi that have been incompletely excised or removed by shave excision. The recurrence of the melanocytic proliferation is seen just above the scar, and they are junctional in majority of cases. The nevus cells appear enlarged and may exhibit mild nuclear pleomorphism. The presence of a dermal scar and the clinical history should be the clue to the diagnosis of a recurrent nevus.

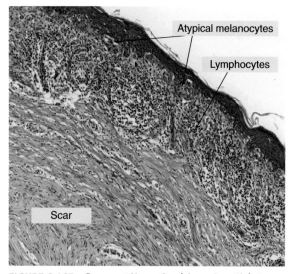

FIGURE 8.165   Recurrent Nevus Overlying a Scar High Power

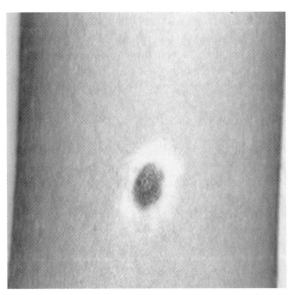

FIGURE 8.166   Halo Nevus, Courtesy of Julia Newton-Bishop, St. James's University Hospital, Leeds, UK

Halo Nevus

A depigmented halo around a pigmented lesion characterizes halo nevus. This is considered a manifestation of the lymphocytes destroying the nevus cells around the periphery.

On microscopy, the nevus cells are almost entirely masked by the dense infiltrate of lymphocytes. The surviving nevus cells appear swollen. Some histiocytes may be seen in the infiltrate. It is very unusual to have such dense infiltrate in a melanoma.

The positive staining with S100 protein helps to identify the nevus cells. The lymphocytes are known to be CD-8 positive T-cells.

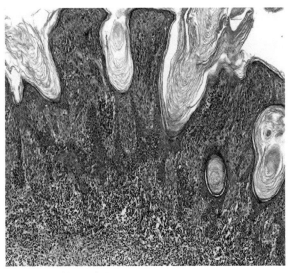

FIGURE 8.167   Halo Nevus

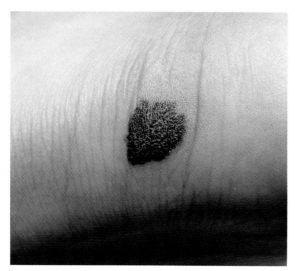

FIGURE 8.168   Acral Nevus

Acral Nevus

Acral nevi are well-circumscribed, regularly shaped, densely pigmented lesions occurring on the extremities of limbs (often on the palms and soles). These often have pigment distributed in a linear pattern in the furrows of the skin markings (parallel furrow pattern), sometimes with pigmented lines that cross the skin creases perpendicularly (lattice-like pattern) or at an angle (fibrillar pattern).

On microscopy, acral nevi are circumscribed and symmetrical. They show dense proliferation of bland melanocytes in a lentiginous pattern and as nests of varying sizes. A retraction artifact may be seen as a characteristic feature. Prominent transelimination of nevus cells is noted. This feature has earned acral nevi the acronym MANIAC (melanocytic acral nevi with intraepidermal ascent of cells). Melanin pigmentation is also seen in a large majority of cells. The nevus cells tend to be bland with no nuclear pleomorphism. Mitotic activity is not a feature.

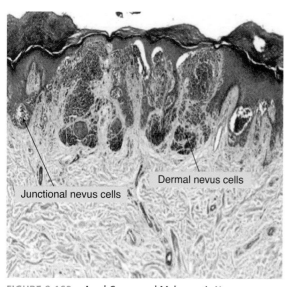

FIGURE 8.169   Acral Compound Melanocytic Nevus

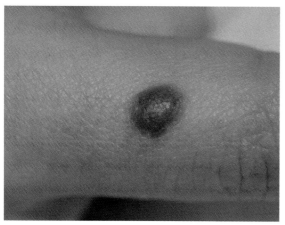

FIGURE 8.170   Spitz Nevus

Spitz Nevi

Spitz nevi are most commonly seen in children and young adults and present as solitary pink-, reddish-, or flesh-colored papules on the trunk, face, or extremities (especially the lower limbs). Ulceration is rarely seen. Older lesions may be pigmented. Multiple grouped (or "agminated") lesions have been reported.

On microscopy, Spitz nevi show epidermal hyperplasia with hyperkeratosis and acanthosis in addition to junctional and compound melanocytic proliferation. The nevus is generally symmetrical and circumscribed. The junctional component is seen as well-formed regular nests. Upward migration of the melanocytes into the epidermis as single cells and small nests is a prominent feature. Spitz nevi classically show proliferation of spindle and epithelioid cell types or a mixture of both. Nuclear pleomorphism is uniformly seen in all the cells. The epithelioid cell type also may show many multinucleated giant cells. A common feature seen in majority of Spitz nevi are Kamino bodies. These are eosinophilic globules seen in the superficial epidermis. Kamino bodies are formed of basement membrane substance and hence they stain with PAS and collagen 1V. The presence of Kamino bodies is considered a sign of benignity. The dermal component in Spitz nevi mature toward the base. The nevus cells are seen as single cells infiltrating the dermal collagen. Sparse lymphocytic infiltrate may be seen. Uniform nuclear atypia is noted in the dermal nevus cells. Occasional mitoses (<2) in the entire lesion may be seen within 0.25 mm of the lesional edge.

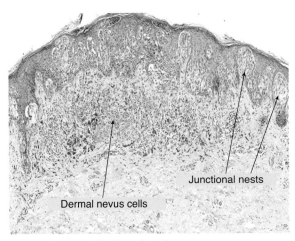

FIGURE 8.171   Spitz Nevus-Low Power

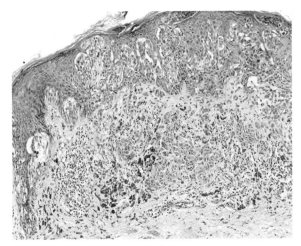

FIGURE 8.172   Spitz Nevus-High Power

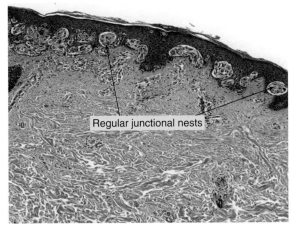

FIGURE 8.173   Regular Junctional Nests of Melanocytes in Spitz Nevus

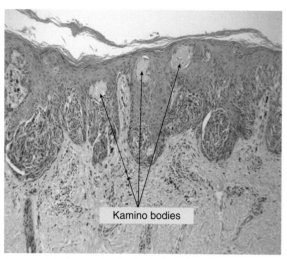

FIGURE 8.174   Kamino Bodies in Spitz Nevus

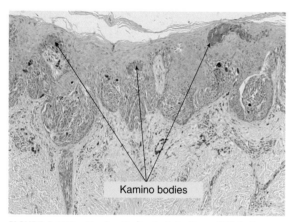

FIGURE 8.175   Kamino Bodies in Spitz Nevus PAS Stain

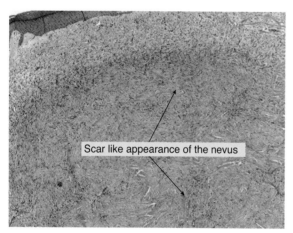

FIGURE 8.176   Desmoplastic Spitz-Low Power

Desmoplastic Spitz Nevus

Desmoplastic Spitz nevus is a variant of Spitz nevus.

On microscopy, the junctional component is inconspicuous, or the epidermis may be thinned out. The dermal melanocytes are small and spindle shaped and are seen to infiltrate the dermal collagen diffusely. Nuclear pleomorphism is seen in a uniform pattern. Ganglion-like cells with ample eosinophilic cytoplasm and prominent nucleoli may be seen. Dermal mitoses are absent or very infrequent. S100 protein and Melan A or Mart1 are positive in the melanocytes.

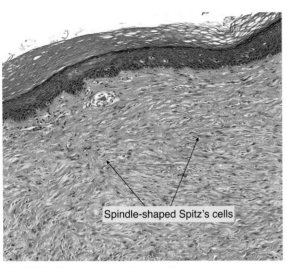

FIGURE 8.177   Desmoplastic Spitz-High Power

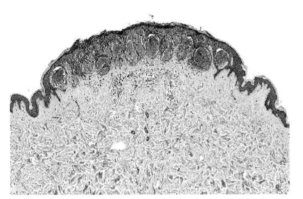

FIGURE 8.178   Spindle Cell Nevus of Reed

Spindle Cell Nevus of Reed

This is a variant of Spitz nevus. Clinically, the nevus presents as an acquired intensely darkly pigmented papule on the thigh of young to middle-aged women.

On microscopy, the spindle cell nevus of Reed may be junctional or compound in pattern, usually well circumscribed and symmetrical. The infiltration into the dermis is in a regular and orderly pattern. The nevus cells are heavily pigmented and are arranged in a raining down pattern. The cell type is predominantly spindle type. Kamino bodies are infrequently seen.

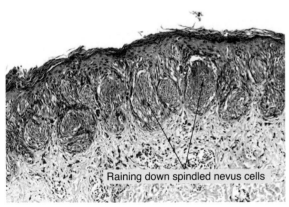

FIGURE 8.179   Spindle Cell Nevus of Reed.-High Power

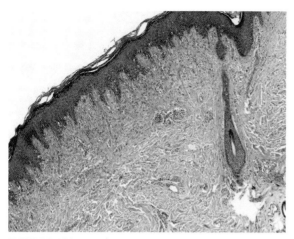

FIGURE 8.180 Sparks Nevus

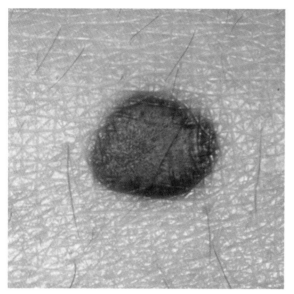

FIGURE 8.181 Blue Nevus. Courtesy of Julia Newton-Bishop, St. James's University Hospital, Leeds, UK

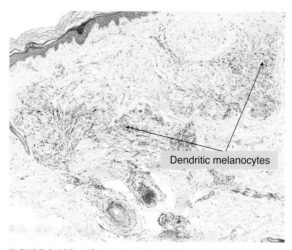

Dendritic melanocytes

FIGURE 8.182 Blue Nevus-Low Power

Spark's Nevus

Spark's nevus is a recently described variant of Spitz nevus showing features of Spitz nevus and dysplastic nevus (Clark's nevus). The clinical appearance is usually that of Spitz nevus.

On microscopy, Spark's nevus shows a combination of features of shouldering, and elongation of rete ridges with dermal fibroplasia as seen in dysplastic nevus. The cell type is either spindle or epithelioid type. Nuclear atypia is not seen.

Blue Nevus and its Variants

The blue nevus is a common lesion occurring on the hands, feet, and buttocks. The nevus is also known to occur in other extracutaneous sites such as oral mucosa, conjunctiva, lymph nodes, and breast. The nevus appears blue-black in color, particularly on dermoscopy because of the light scattering due to Tyndall effect. Malignant transformation to malignant blue nevus is a rare occurrence.

On microscopy, a large majority of common blue nevi are dermal lesions, which may extend to the subcutaneous fat. A small minority may show a junctional component. The dermal component is the result of proliferation of cells originating from premelanosomes. The premelanosomes originate in the neural crest and travel to the epidermis during embryological development. These cells get arrested in the dermis during their travel and develop into blue nevi. The nevus cells are spindle shaped and dendritic in appearance and intersect collagen bundles in a pattern parallel to the overlying epidermis. Majority of the cells contain melanin within their cytoplasm. Nuclear pleomorphism and mitotic activity are not features of this tumor.

Several histological variants have been described. These include epithelioid blue nevus where the cells appear larger with eosinophilic cytoplasm and vesicular nuclei. The cells show the same pattern of infiltration as ordinary blue nevi. Epithelioid blue nevus is known to be associated with Carney complex. Amelanotic blue nevus, as the name implies, does not exhibit the excessive pigmentation and clinically they present as scar. On microscopy, they exhibit the same histological features as an ordinary blue nevus.

Cellular blue nevus is not an uncommon variant of blue nevus. It is usually bigger than an ordinary blue nevus. Scalp and sacrococcygeal area tend to be the commonest sites. On microscopy, there is a central dense and compact cellular area. The peripheral aspects toward the superficial and the deep aspects exhibit thickened collagen and desmoplasia. The cells in the center exhibit scanty cytoplasm and spindle-shaped nuclei. Epithelioid cell forms are also seen. These cells are admixed with many dendritic cells in the periphery of the lesion.

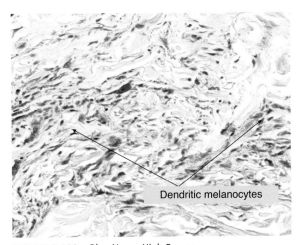

FIGURE 8.183   Blue Nevus-High Power

Pigment-laden cells are seen in abundance at the center and periphery of the lesion. Nuclear pleomorphism is not a feature of this nevus. Up to two mitoses per 10 HPFs may be seen. Necrosis is not seen.

Blue nevi are positive for S100 and HMB-45. In heavily pigmented lesions, a different colored chromogen used along with the immunohistochemical antibody helps to highlight the positive staining (Fig. 8.184). Increased numbers of mitoses or areas of necrosis are features suggestive of atypical cellular blue nevus or even malignant blue nevus.

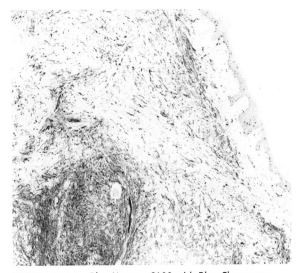

FIGURE 8.184   Blue Nevus—S100 with Blue Chromogen

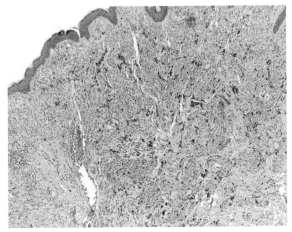

FIGURE 8.185   Epithelioid Blue Nevus

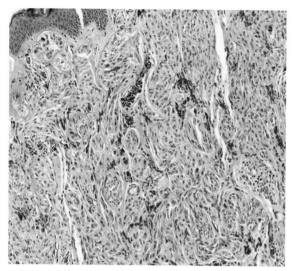

FIGURE 8.186   Epithelioid Blue Nevus-High Power

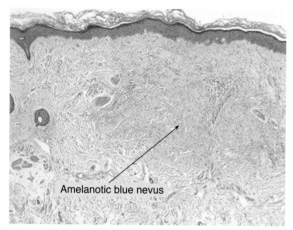

Amelanotic blue nevus

FIGURE 8.187   Amelanotic Blue Nevus

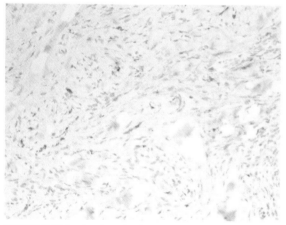

FIGURE 8.188   Amelanotic Blue Nevus—S100

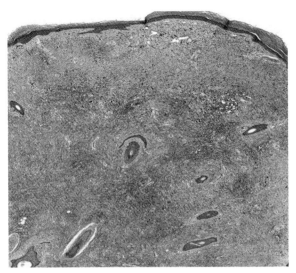

FIGURE 8.189   Cellular Blue Nevus-Low Power

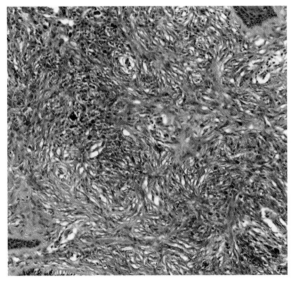

FIGURE 8.190   Cellular Blue Nevus-High Power

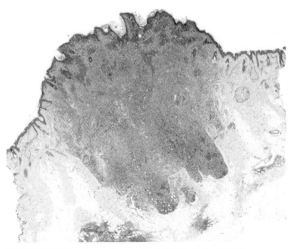

FIGURE 8.191   Deep Penetrating Nevus-Low Power

Deep Penetrating Nevus

Deep penetrating nevus has been considered as a variant of blue nevus. Clinically, the nevus has the appearance of ordinary blue nevus. Face and trunk are the common areas involved.

On microscopy, the nevus occupies the dermis and the subcutaneous fat, with a dumbbell-shaped architecture seen in the subcutaneous fat. The cells are a combination of dendritic cells as in ordinary blue nevus and epithelioid and pale staining cells. Multinucleated giant cells may be seen. Large numbers of melanophages and melanocytes containing pigment are seen. An ordinary nevus may be seen in combination with deep penetrating nevus.

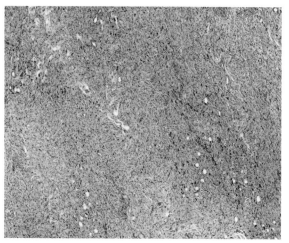

FIGURE 8.192   Deep Penetrating Nevus-High Power

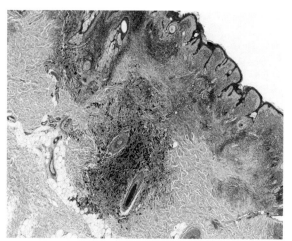

FIGURE 8.193   Combined Nevus

Combined Nevus

Combined nevus is the term used when two or more cytologically different combination of cells are seen in a nevus. Clinically, combined nevus appears in early childhood or in young adults. A large majority of these nevi are acquired ones, but combinations of congenital nevi with cell types of other nevi can also be seen.

On microscopy, the cell types seen could be a combination of congenital nevus with blue nevus and Spitz nevus or Spitz nevus with blue nevus, deep penetrating nevus with blue nevus, and ordinary nevus with blue nevus or Spitz nevus.

Combined nevus could be mistaken for a melanoma histologically and clinically and hence it is important to identify the features correctly.

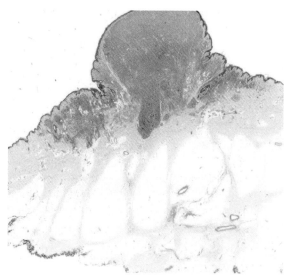

FIGURE 8.194   Atypical Proliferative Nodule in a Congenital Nevus-Scanning View

Atypical Proliferative Nodule in a Congenital Nevus

Proliferative nodules appear as nodules and plaques in a congenital nevus. They stand out in the background of a congenital nevus as deeply pigmented lesions. Lightly colored ones may also occur. They are generally longstanding lesions, and once they attain their growth potential they are stable.

On microscopy, the proliferative nodules show distinct features. They are dermal nodules and well circumscribed. They can show blue nevus–like, Spitz nevus–like, or deep penetrating nevus–like appearances. The cells forming the nodule may be large oval cells with pale staining cytoplasm and vesicular nuclei or small cells with hyperchromatic nuclei. Mitotic figures are variable and could be numerous. Atypical mitoses are not a feature and when they are seen, the possibility of melanoma should be considered. Necrosis is conspicuously absent. The peripheral border of the proliferative nodule merges with the congenital nevus with intermediate cell forms in between. This is a feature that can be used to differentiate from a melanoma arising in a congenital nevus where the border is much more sharply defined.

The prognostic features are difficult to predict due to the lack of long-term studies. Genetically, proliferative nodules are known to show loss or gain of whole chromosomes rather than focused losses and gains of chromosomes as seen in melanomas.

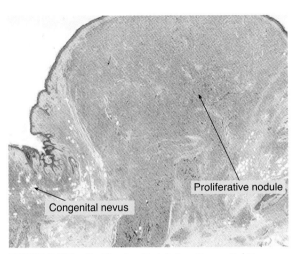

FIGURE 8.195   Proliferative Nodule in a Congenital Nevus-Low Power

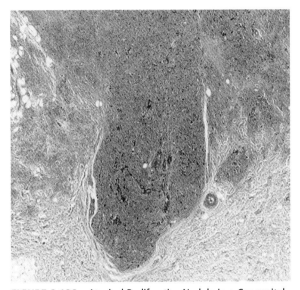

FIGURE 8.196   Atypical Proliferative Nodule in a Congenital Nevus-Deep Penetrating Naevus Like Pattern

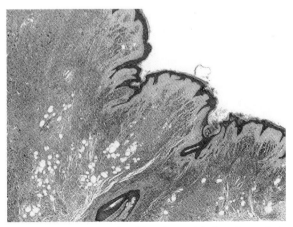

FIGURE 8.197   Atypical Proliferative Nodule in a Congenital Nevus-Low Power

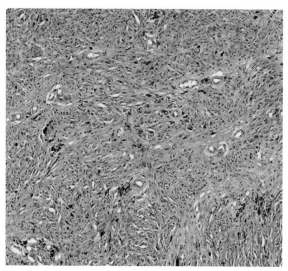

FIGURE 8.198   Atypical Proliferative Nodule in a Congenital Nevus-High Power of the Nodule

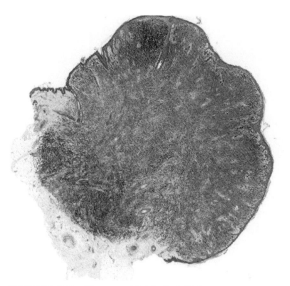

FIGURE 8.199   Pigmented Epithelioid Melanocytoma-Low Power

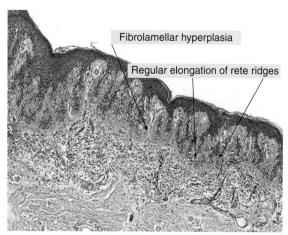

FIGURE 8.200   Mildly Dysplastic Nevus Compound Melanocytic Nevus

Pigmented Epithelioid Melanocytoma

Pigmented epithelioid melanocytoma is a recently described low-grade variant of melanoma that metastasizes to lymph nodes with an indolent clinical course. They are seen as deeply pigmented lesion most commonly in the extremities, although other sites are well known to be involved.

On microscopy, the lesions extend to the deep dermis and subcutaneous fat. The cells are either spindle shaped or epithelioid and are closely packed admixed with cells with heavy melanin pigmentation. Combined nevus may be seen in a small number of cases and so is ulceration of the overlying epidermis. Pigmented epithelioid melanocytoma has lot of similarities to epithelioid blue nevus and animal type melanoma, and this is considered as a lesion encompassing the two entities. In a recent series (Martin Mihm et al), 46% of cases metastasized to regional lymph nodes.

Dysplastic Nevus

Dysplastic nevi occur as solitary, sporadic, or familial cases. The importance of identifying a dysplastic nevus is that it recognizes a group of individuals with a potential for developing subsequent melanoma. The association is well established in familial and sporadic multiple dysplastic nevi. The relationship between single dysplastic nevi and melanoma is not yet established. Evidence suggesting the development of melanoma in the background of dysplastic nevus establishes the importance of dysplastic nevus as a premalignant condition. Familial dysplastic nevus syndrome is an autosomal dominant condition and is associated with *CDKN2A* gene in 50% of cases.

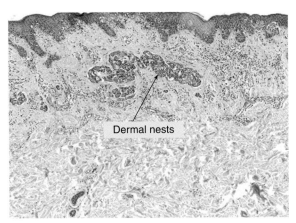

FIGURE 8.201   Mildly Dysplastic Compound Melanocytic Nevus with Dermal Nests-Low Power

On microscopy, dysplastic nevi show similar features regardless of whether they are familial or sporadic. Dysplastic nevi are classically known to show lentiginous proliferation of melanocytes at the dermoepidermal junction and form junctional nests of varying sizes. The melanocytes are known to proliferate along elongated rete ridges in a lentiginous pattern. The tips of the rete shows nested melanocytes. The rete ridges may also exhibit fusion or bridging. The papillary dermis shows concentric lamellar hyperplasia or dermal fibroplasias. The nevus cells in the dermis are typically seen in a nested pattern. Dermal mitoses are not seen. There is scattered perivascular and interstitial distribution of lymphocytes.

Dysplastic nevi are graded as mild, moderate, or severe based on architectural or cytological atypia.

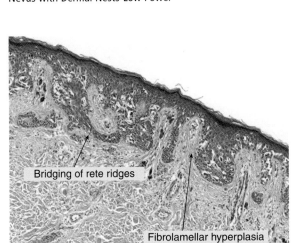

FIGURE 8.202   Moderately Dysplastic Nevus

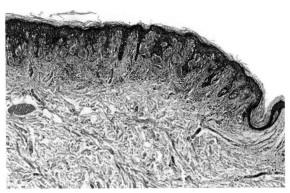

FIGURE 8.203   Severely Dysplastic Nevus

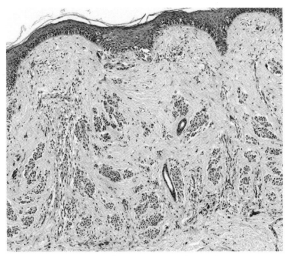

FIGURE 8.204   Dermal Nests in Severely Dysplastic Nevus

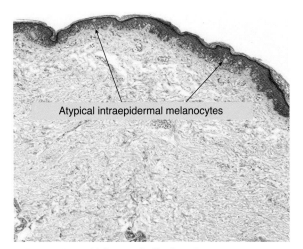

FIGURE 8.205   Melanoma in Situ-Low Power

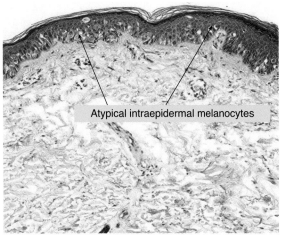

FIGURE 8.206   Melanoma in Situ-High Power

Melanoma-in-situ

Melanoma in situ is the term used when the proliferation of atypical melanocytes is confined to the epidermis. Various patterns of proliferation may be seen such as nested or lentiginous patterns. The cells exhibit moderate to severe atypia. The underlying dermis may show varying degrees of lymphocytic infiltration ranging from mild perivascular to lichenoid pattern. Serial sectioning of the specimen should be carried out to exclude the possibility of invasion into the underlying dermis. In cases of doubtful invasion and when the papillary dermis is heavily infiltrated by melanophages, Melan A (Mart1) should be useful in identifying the atypical melanocytes in the dermis.

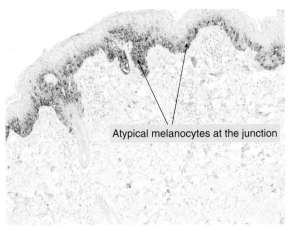

FIGURE 8.207   Melan A with Blue Chromagen in Melanoma in Situ-High Power

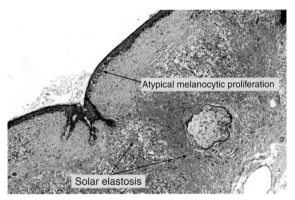

FIGURE 8.208   Lentigo Maligna

Lentigo Maligna

Lentigo maligna is essentially in situ melanoma in sun-damaged skin. The clinical appearances are also characteristic in that they are seen in chronically sun-damaged skin as variably pigmented macule with ill-defined and often irregular margins. Longstanding lesions may develop areas of hyperpigmentation or pigmented nodules indicating the development of lentigo maligna melanoma.

On microscopy, the earliest change is the proliferation of melanocytes along the dermoepidermal junction in a lentiginous pattern. The melanocytes are seen to be arranged one next to each other as in a "picket fence." The cells exhibit only very minimal nuclear pleomorphism in the early stages. At this stage, it is usually difficult to differentiate lentigo maligna from increased proliferation of photoactivated melanocytes in a chronically sun-damaged skin. Moderate to marked cytological atypia, upward migration of atypical melanocytes in the epidermis, hyperchromasia of the nuclei and nesting of the melanocytes, and proliferation of atypical melanocytes along the follicular epithelium are features that favor the diagnosis of lentigo maligna over changes of photoactivation. The underlying dermis shows extensive solar elastosis and lymphocytic infiltration of variable degree. The junctional melanocytes show variable degree of pigmentation. Melanophages may be seen in the papillary dermis.

Dermal invasion of atypical melanocytes warrants a diagnosis of lentigo maligna melanoma in severely sun-damaged skin. The proliferation of atypical melanocytes can be very florid in occasional cases, and the invasive focus may be seen adjacent to the follicle involved. In such instances, it is important to note that the Breslow thickness should be measured from the follicular epithelium to the deepest point of invasion in a horizontal direction rather than in the conventional vertical method.

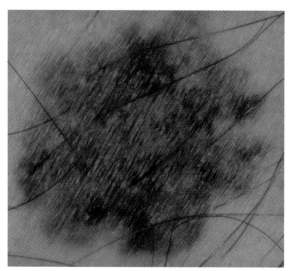

FIGURE 8.209   Early Melanoma. Courtesy of Julia Newton-Bishop, St. James's University Hospital, Leeds, UK

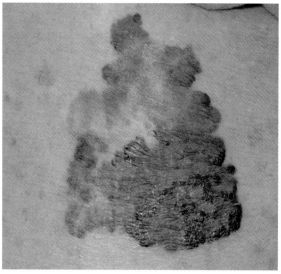

FIGURE 8.210   Melanoma in Type 1V Skin. Courtesy of Howard Peach, St. James's University Hospital, Leeds, UK

Superficial Spreading Malignant Melanoma

Invasive melanoma has two broad patterns of growth, the commonest being the superficial spreading type. Here the predominant pattern of growth is seen in a horizontal pattern along the epidermis and the dermoepidermal junction. The invasive component in the dermis could be in the radial or vertical growth phase. Radial growth phase melanoma shows a dermal component where there might be single cells invading the dermis or nests smaller than the junctional nests. Dermal mitoses are not seen in a radial growth phase melanoma. Vertical growth phase melanoma shows dermal nests larger than junctional nests in addition to dermal mitoses. The junctional activity in a superficial spreading melanoma should extend to three rete ridges or more on one or either side of the dermal component. As is obvious from the growth pattern, superficial spreading melanoma offers a better prognosis than does nodular melanoma.

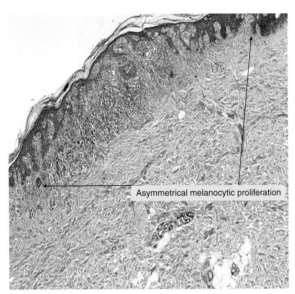

FIGURE 8.211   Superficial Spreading Malignant Melanoma
Showing Asymmetry of the Lesion

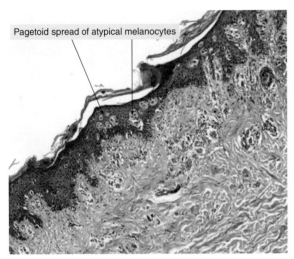

FIGURE 8.212   Superficial Spreading Malignant Melanoma-
Pagetoid Spread

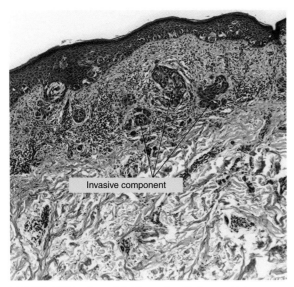

FIGURE 8.213   Superficial Spreading Malignant Melanoma in Vertical Growth Phase

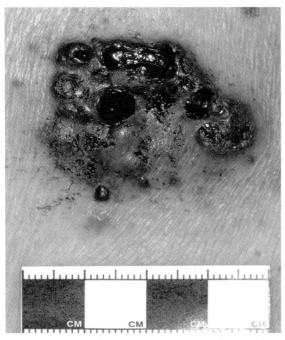

FIGURE 8.214   Nodular Melanoma. Courtesy of Howard Peach, St. James's University Hospital, Leeds, UK

Nodular Malignant Melanoma

Nodular melanoma is the second most common growth pattern seen in melanoma. It characteristically presents as rapidly growing dark brown, black, or occasionally reddish amelanotic nodule. The lesions may have ulceration present. It may present in unusual locations as Sister Mary Joseph's nodule (Fig. 8.216).

On microscopy, the invasive dermal component is predominant and the junctional activity is not seen beyond the dermal component. Majority of the nodular melanomas are ulcerated.

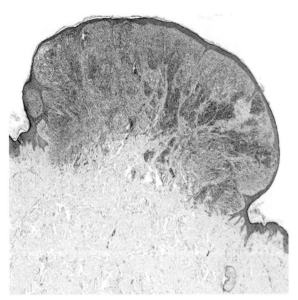

FIGURE 8.215   Nodular Melanoma

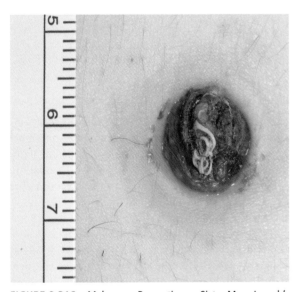

FIGURE 8.216   Melanoma Presenting as Sister Mary Joseph's Nodule. Courtesy of Howard Peach, St. James's University Hospital, Leeds, UK

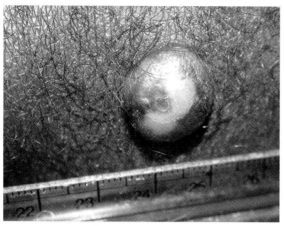

FIGURE 8.217 Melanoma in Type 1V Skin. Courtesy of Howard Peach, St. James's University Hospital, Leeds

Melanoma in Type V Skin

Melanoma in Afro-Caribbean skin is very rare with an incidence of 1 in 100,000 population. Subungual and mucosal melanomas are the types identified than cutaneous melanoma.

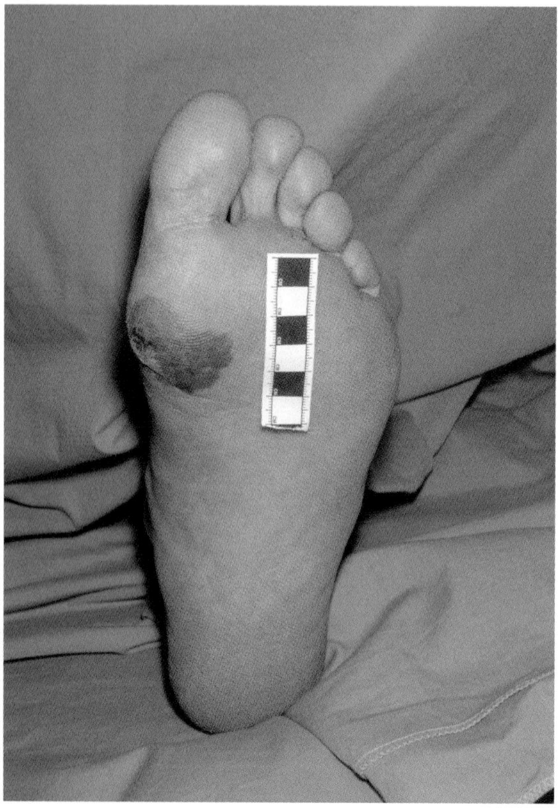

Acral Melanoma

Acral lentiginous melanomas arise most commonly on sun-exposed sites of the dorsum of hands and feet or in the subungual location and non–hair-bearing parts of hands and feet. The latter type is more common in Asian and Afro-Caribbean population. Lesions present as a slowly growing patches or plaques that develop into darkly pigmented nodules.

On microscopy, the epidermis is hyperplastic and hyperkeratotic, and the proliferation of atypical melanocytes is seen in a florid pattern. In the earliest phase, the melanocytes are arranged in a lentiginous pattern with single cells arranged in the dermoepidermal junction. In the later stages, the cells are seen invading the entire epidermis and then invading into the dermis as nests of variable sizes and single cells. The cells usually have perinuclear halo, and the nuclei are either elongated or cuboidal. Nuclear pleomorphism and mitotic activity can be prominent. The melanocytes are variably pigmented.

FIGURE 8.218 Acral Melanoma. Courtesy of Howard Peach, St. James's University Hospital, Leeds, UK

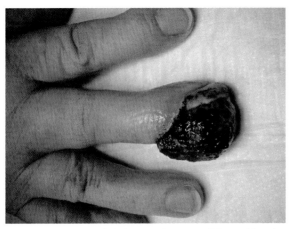

FIGURE 8.219 Acral Melanoma. Courtesy of Howard Peach, St. James's University Hospital, Leeds, UK

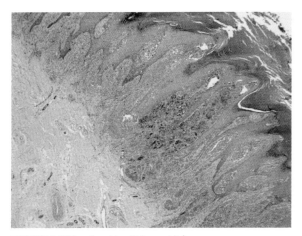

FIGURE 8.220 Acral Lentiginous Melanoma

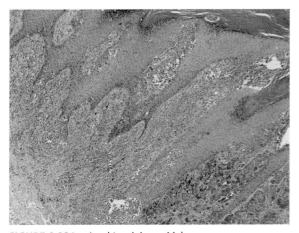

FIGURE 8.221 Acral Lentiginous Melanoma

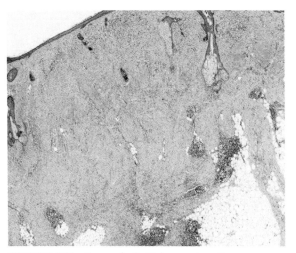

FIGURE 8.222   Desmoplastic Melanoma-Low Power

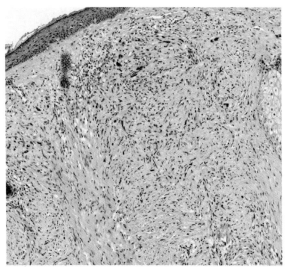

FIGURE 8.223   Desmoplastic Melanoma-High Power

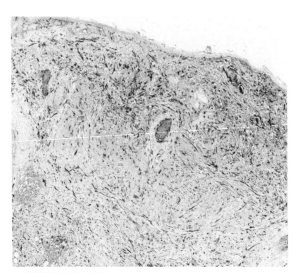

FIGURE 8.224   S100 in Desmoplastic Melanoma

Desmoplastic Melanoma

Desmoplastic melanoma is an unusual variant of melanoma that poses diagnostic challenge clinically and histologically. The majority of lesions present in elderly individuals on sun-exposed sites such as head and neck, as infiltrated plaques or tumors. Some lesions are associated with a lentigo maligna overlying or adjacent to the desmoplastic melanoma. Desmoplastic melanomas are deeply infiltrative tumors, and they have a special predilection for neurotropism (predilection for spreading to the nerves). The tumors in the scalp may spread to involve the cranial nerves. Because of the lack of pigmentation and epidermal involvement, the clinical presentation can be varied, which often leads to a delay in diagnosis. Superficial shave biopsies of lentigo maligna should be interpreted with caution as a deeper desmoplastic melanoma can be easily missed completely. Recurrences are common due to the ill-defined margins in many of the cases.

On microscopy, junctional activity is not a conspicuous feature. The dermis shows diffusely infiltrative tumor composed of spindle-shaped cells that exhibit mild nuclear pleomorphism. The cells resemble fibroblasts, smooth muscle cells, or occasionally Schwann cells. Interstitial fibrosis, collagenization, and lymphoid aggregates are commonly seen. Lymphovascular permeation may be seen. Perineural and endoneural involvement is commonly seen.

The tumor is positive for S100 protein in a diffuse and strong pattern. The dermal component of the tumor is negative for HMB-45 and Melan A or Mart1. Epithelial membrane antigen (EMA) may be present in small numbers of cases. Smooth muscle actin (SMA) positivity reflects the myofibroblastic differentiation. The positivity for S100 raises the possibility of a low-grade malignant peripheral nerve sheath tumor. However, careful examination of the junctional component should reveal the atypical melanocytes at the junction. Perineural invasion is an additional clue.

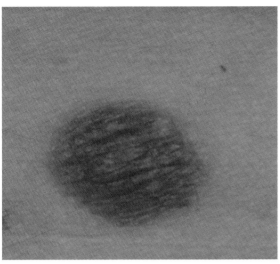

FIGURE 8.225   Spitzoid Melanoma. Courtesy of Julia Newton-Bishop, St. James's University Hospital, Leeds, UK

Spitzoid Melanoma

Spitzoid melanoma is rather unusual and arises in the setting of a Spitz nevus in majority of the cases. Clinically, it presents as nodules with minimal pigmentation.

Nevoid Melanoma

Nevoid melanoma is a rare variant of melanoma mistaken for benign nevus. As the name implies, the tumor has clinical and histological similarities to nevus.

On microscopy, the junctional and dermal proliferations of cells are in a regular pattern. Keratotic pattern of growth is commonly encountered. The cells are small resembling type A nevus cells with scanty cytoplasm, rounded nuclei, and speckled chromatin. Epithelioid cells may also be seen. Dermal mitoses may be inconspicuous but may be seen in the deep part of the nevus. Tumor infiltrating lymphocytes are usually absent or nonbrisk and focal.

The diagnosis is challenging and immunohistochemical stains may be helpful in the diagnosis. Cyclin D1 and MIB-1 (proliferation marker) show diffuse positivity of the melanocytes in nevoid melanoma as opposed to superficial scattered cells in benign nevi. HMB-45 stains the atypical nevus cells in the superficial aspect of the benign nevi, but they stain the deeper cells in nevoid melanoma.

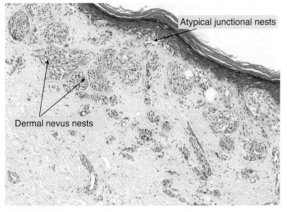

FIGURE 8.226   Nevoid Melanoma-Low Power

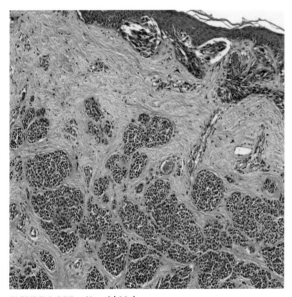

FIGURE 8.227   Nevoid Melanoma

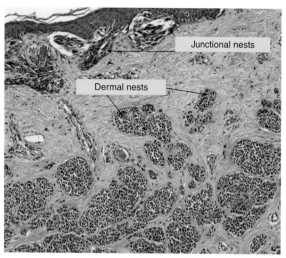

FIGURE 8.228   Nevoid Melanoma

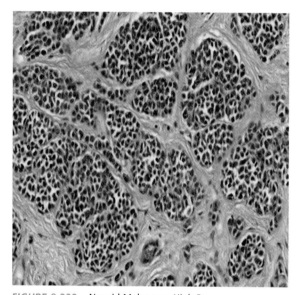

FIGURE 8.229   Nevoid Melanoma-High Power

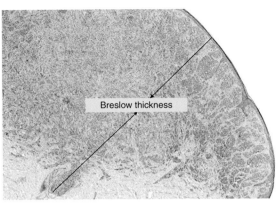

FIGURE 8.230   Breslow Thickness

Breslow Thickness

First described by Alexander Breslow, pathologist at George Washington University in 1970. Breslow's depth is determined using an ocular micrometer in millimeters and is measured vertically from the granular layer to the deepest point of invasion of the melanoma cells in the dermis. The proliferation of cells along adnexal structures is not taken into account. In lentigo maligna melanoma, the Breslow thickness may be measured in a horizontal pattern from the adnexal epithelium to the horizontal point of invasion. Breslow thickness is considered as the single most important prognostic factor predicting lymph node metastasis in melanoma. The inclusion of microsatellites in the Breslow thickness measurement is still controversial and hence it is useful to state in the pathology report whether microsatellites have been included in the measurement or not.

The AJCC (American Joint Committee on Staging of Cancer) predicts the prognosis of melanoma based on the Breslow thickness as follows:

Breslow Thickness (mm)	Approximate 5-yr Survival (%)
<1	95–100
1–2	80–96
2.1–4	60–75
>4	50

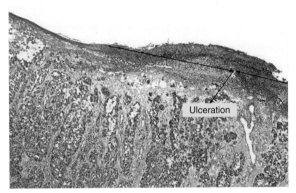

FIGURE 8.231   Ulceration in Melanoma

Ulceration in Melanoma

Ulceration overlying melanoma is defined as complete absence of epidermis and the defect covered by fibrin, neutrophils, and parakeratotic keratinocytes with associated reactive hyperplasia in the adjacent epidermis. These features help to differentiate true ulceration from trauma caused during surgical removal of the lesion. The width of the ulcer should be documented in the report since this is found to be prognostically significant.

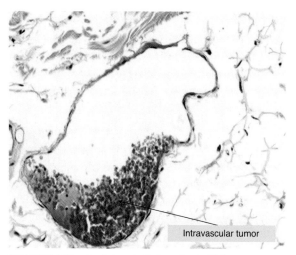

FIGURE 8.232 Angiolymphatic Invasion in Melanoma

Angiolymphatic and Perivascular Tumor Infiltration

Angiolymphatic invasion and perivascular tumor infiltration (extravascular migratory metastasis) are seen in thick melanomas and are known to be signs of lymph node involvement, although the statistical significance have not been entirely conclusive. Lyve-1 and D2-40 stain the lymphatics and CD-34 and CD-31 stains the blood vessels in doubtful cases.

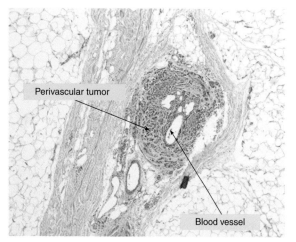

FIGURE 8.233 Perivascular Tumor Infiltration

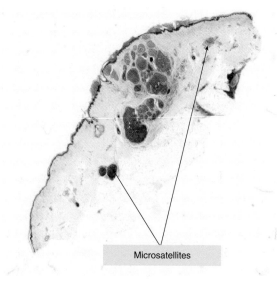

FIGURE 8.234 Microsatellites-Scanning View

Microsatellites

Microsatellites are defined as discontinuous nests of cells more than 0.05 mm in diameter that are clearly separated by normal dermis and not fibrosis or chronic inflammation from the main invasive component of melanoma cells by a distance of at least 0.3 mm. Published data have shown that the survival outcome is comparable to patients with clinically detectable metastasis (AJCC 2010).

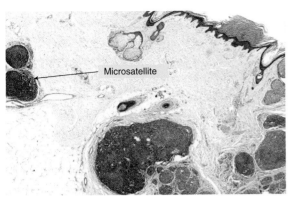

FIGURE 8.235   Microsatellites

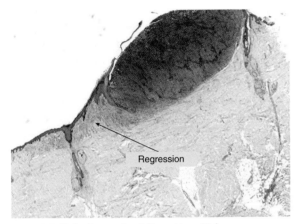

FIGURE 8.236   Regression Adjacent to a Melanoma

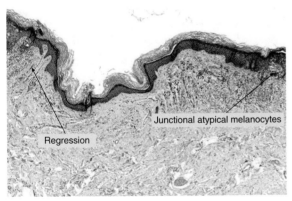

FIGURE 8.237   Stage 2 Regression in Melanoma

Regression in Melanoma

Regression is a controversial entity seen in 5% of cases of primary melanoma. Clinically, regression may present as an area of scarring or as hypopigmented areas within a melanoma.

On microscopy, regression is classified into three stages. Stage 1 regression is when the junctional and dermal components are identifiable, but the dermal nests or single cells seem to be set in a fibrotic or scarred dermis. This is accompanied by vertically orientated blood vessels and scattered lymphocytes. Many melanophages may be seen. In stage 2 regression, there is absent dermal component, but retained junctional component. The dermis beneath the junctional cells shows scarring, blood vessels, and lymphocytic infiltration with melanophages. Stage 3 regression shows complete absence of melanocytic hyperplasia with scarring of the dermis, lymphocytic infiltration, and melanophages. The overlying epidermis may appear atrophic.

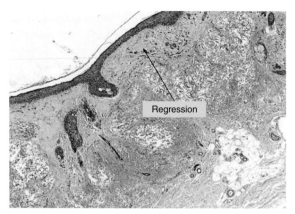

FIGURE 8.238   Regression Stage 3

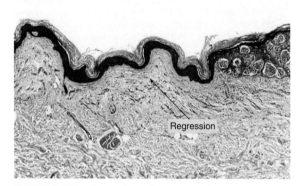

FIGURE 8.239   Regression Adjacent to Melanoma

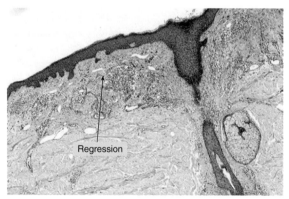

FIGURE 8.240   Stage 3 Regression

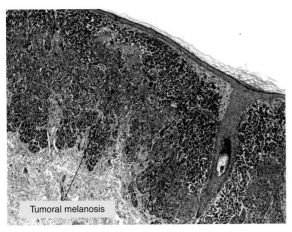

FIGURE 8.241   Tumoral Melanosis

Tumoral Melanosis

The complete replacement of viable melanocytes with melanophages is the characteristic feature seen in tumoral melanosis. This feature is considered as an evidence of stage 3 regression in melanoma.

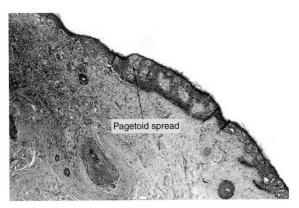

FIGURE 8.242   Pagetoid Spread

Pagetoid Spread in Melanoma

Cells within the epidermis is seen in many benign and malignant melanocytic diseases. The term Pagetoid spread of melanocytes is used when the atypical melanocytes are seen as single cells or nests within the epidermis above a line drawn at the upper level of the dermal papillae. The atypical melanocytes are also seen to destroy the keratinocytes. In all other situations, the term upward migration should be used.

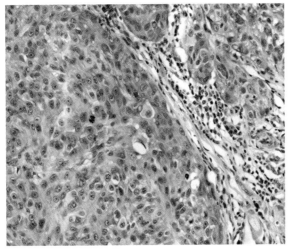

FIGURE 8.243   Epithelioid Melanoma Cells with Mitoses

Epithelioid Melanocytes with Mitoses

Melanoma is known to show several cell types histologically, of which epithelioid cells are not uncommon. These cells have ample eosinophilic cytoplasm and rounded nuclei with prominent nucleoli.

Mitotic activity in melanoma is measured per square millimeter. Mitotic activity is defined as a powerful independent predictor of survival.

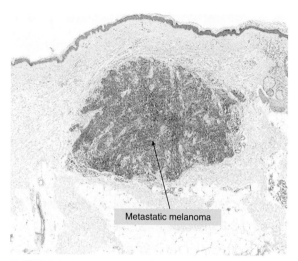

FIGURE 8.244 Metastatic Melanoma-Low Power

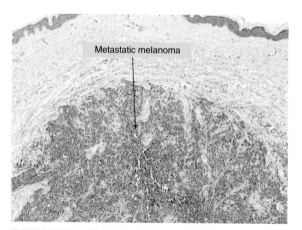

FIGURE 8.245 Metastatic Melanoma-High Power

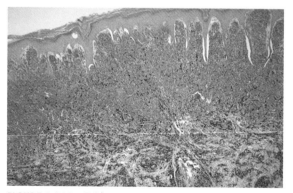

FIGURE 8.246 Epidermotropic Metastasis-Low Power

Cutaneous Metastatic Melanoma

Cutaneous metastasis in melanoma is very common. Clinically, they present as in-transit metastasis or satellite nodules.

On microscopy, the metastatic deposit is seen within the dermis and subcutaneous fat as circumscribed nodules. Uncommonly the metastasis is seen to infiltrate the overlying epidermis, and this is referred to as epidermotropic metastasis (Figs. 8.246 and 8.247). Epidermotropic metastasis can be difficult to distinguish histologically and clinically from an independent cutaneous primary melanoma.

Sentinel Lymph Node Biopsy in Melanoma

The AJCC staging committee on melanoma recommends sentinel lymph node biopsy on all patients with a Breslow thickness of more than 1 mm, with or without ulceration and clinically uninvolved regional lymph nodes. Sentinel lymph node biopsy remains a powerful prognostic tool in assessing patients for completion lymphadenectomy. Selected patients with a Breslow thickness of <1 mm, ulceration, and mitoses of more than 1 per square millimeter may also be offered sentinel lymph node biopsy. The sentinel lymph node biopsy is performed as a staging procedure where the information can be used for subsequent planning of the treatment regimes.

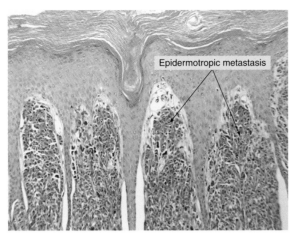

FIGURE 8.247   Epidermotropic Metastasis-High Power

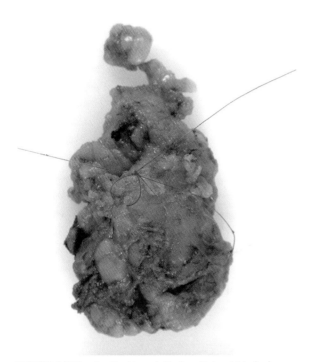

FIGURE 8.248   Sentinel Lymph Node—Hotspot Marked

Sentinel Lymph Node Biopsy for Melanoma

The sentinel lymph nodes are removed after a technetium-99m–tagged radioactive substance is injected at the site of the primary tumor. Scintigraphic imaging is started within 5 minutes of the injection, and the node appears within 5 minutes to 1 hour. This is done several hours before the actual biopsy. About 15 minutes before the biopsy, a blue dye is injected at the same site. During the biopsy, the lymph nodes are inspected using a Gamma probe to detect the radioactive substance and the "hot spots" within the lymph nodes are clearly identified. The lymph node manifesting the radioactivity is removed and the hot spots are marked with a suture. One or more sentinel lymph nodes may be removed in this procedure.

The marked sentinel lymph nodes are sent for pathological examination in 10% formalin. In the laboratory, the hot spots are marked with colored ink and bisected at the site of the hot spot. The bivalved pieces of lymph nodes are examined using the EORTC protocol, where step sections are stained with hematoxylin and eosin, and S100 and Melan A and HMB-45 are performed after every sixth level.

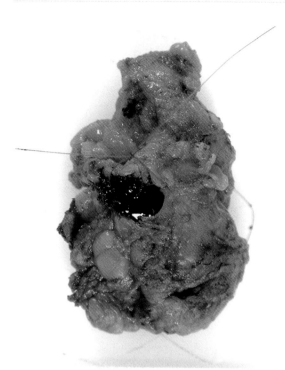

FIGURE 8.249 Sentinel Lymph Node—Hotspot Painted

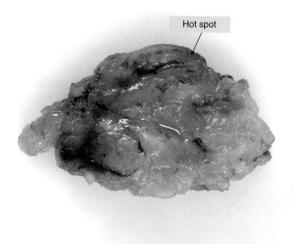

FIGURE 8.250 Bisected Sentinel Lymph Node—Paint at Hot Spot

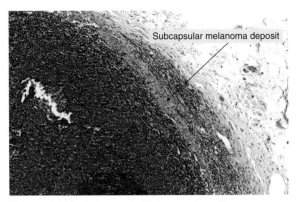

FIGURE 8.251   Subcapsular Melanoma Deposit

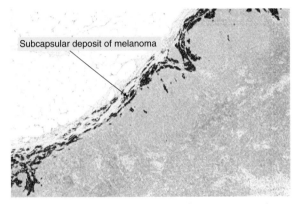

FIGURE 8.252   Subcapsular Deposit of Melanoma—Melan A

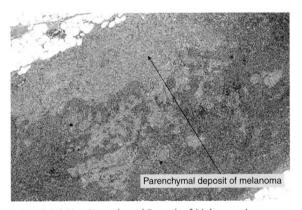

FIGURE 8.253   Parenchymal Deposit of Melanoma in a Lymph Node

Metastatic Melanoma in a Lymph Node

On microscopy, deposits of melanoma may be seen in subcapsular and parenchymal location. A single measurement of the maximum diameter of the largest lesion in any direction should be measured. Cumulative measurements of multiple foci decrease the accuracy of the measurements. A subcapsular deposit usually has a smooth curved outline at the periphery. Parenchymal deposits may be single or multiple.

The pathology report should include the sentinel lymph node burden according to the Rotterdam criteria (<0.1 mm, 0.1–1.0 mm, >1 mm) and the Dewar classification for microanatomic location of the metastasis.

Dewar Classification

Code 01—Subcapsular: (Metastasis confined to the subcapsular sinus)

Code 02—Combined: (subcapsular and parenchymal metastasis)

Code 03—Parenchymal: (Metastasis entirely in the paracortical area)

Code 04—Multifocal: (Multiple discrete deposits, must include parenchymal deposits)

Code 05—Extensive: (any metastasis >5 mm, any node with extracapsular spread)

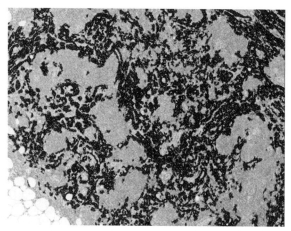

FIGURE 8.254   Parenchymal Deposit of Melanoma—Melan A

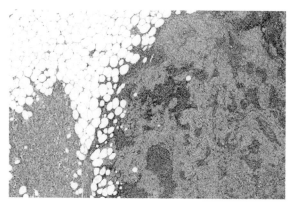

FIGURE 8.255   Metastatic Melanoma in a Lymph Node with Extracapsular Spread

BIBLIOGRAPHY

Balch CM, Gershenwald JE, Soong SJ, Thompson JF, Atkins MB, Byrd DR, Buzaid AC, Cochran AJ, Coit DG, Ding S, Eggermont AM, Flaherty KT, Gimotty PA, Kirkwood JM, McMasters KM, Mihm MC Jr, Morton DL, Ross MI, Sober AJ, Sondak VK. Final version of 2009 AJCC melanoma staging and classification. J Clin Oncol 2009;27(36):6199–6206.

Massi G, Leboit PE. Histological Diagnosis of Nevi and Melanoma, 1st Ed. Steinkopff, New York: Raven Press, 2004.

McKee PH. Pathology of the Skin, 3rd Ed. Mosby, Elsevier, 2005.

Mooi WJ, Krausz T. Pathology of Melanocytic Disorders. London: Chapman & Hall, 1992.

van Akkooi AC, Nowecki ZI, Voit C, Schäfer-Hesterberg G, Michej W, de Wilt JH, Rutkowski P, Verhoef C, Eggermont AM. Sentinel lymph node tumor burden according to Rotterdam criteria is the most important prognostic factor for survival in melanoma patients: a multicenter study in 388 patients with positive sentinel nodes. Ann Surg 2008;248(6):949–955.

van Akkooi AC, Spatz A, Eggermont AM, Mihm M, Cook MG. Expert opinion in melanoma. Eur J Cancer 2009;45(16):2736–2742.

Weedon D. Skin Pathology, 3rd Ed. Edinburgh: Elsevier, 2010.

Dermis—Inflammatory and Neoplastic Diseases

INTRODUCTION

The dermis occupies a considerable part of the structure of skin. It is composed of predominantly collagen type I and III and elastic fibers. In addition to fibroblasts, the dermis also contains dermal dendrocytes. It is composed of two zones namely papillary and reticular dermis. There is a superficial plexus of capillaries in the papillary dermis and a deep plexus in the reticular dermis. The lymphatics are mainly located in the reticular dermis. The entire dermis is supplied by a network of thin nerve fibers. Large nerve bundles are seen in the deep reticular dermis.

The pathological processes affecting the dermis involve all the structures within it. It could also be due to exogenous factors or disease processes involving other organ systems.

EPIDERMAL CYSTS

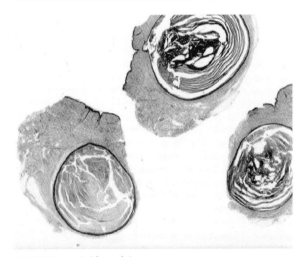

FIGURE 9.1   Epidermal Cysts

Epidermal cysts are the commonest type of cysts encountered in the dermis and are usually located in the mid and lower dermis. They are known to arise from the pilosebaceous follicle in majority of the cases and exhibit a punctum. The eccrine duct may give rise to an epidermal cyst in the palms and soles. Multiple epidermal cysts may be seen in Gardner's syndrome.

On microscopy, epidermal cysts are lined by squamous epithelium with a granular layer and contain lamellated keratin. Several histological changes have been described, which includes clear cell change, seborrheic-like change, and pigmentation. Proliferating epidermal cysts are seen as multiple cysts within the dermis with a possible connection with the overlying epidermis. In situ or invasive neoplastic changes in an epidermal cyst are rare.

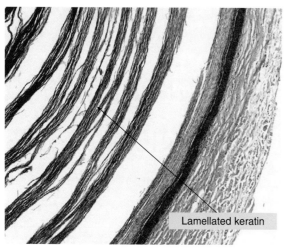

FIGURE 9.2   Lamellated Keratin in Epidermal Cysts

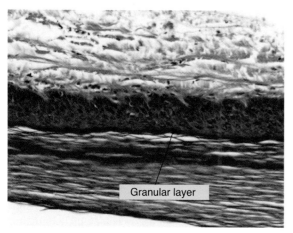

FIGURE 9.3   Granular Layer in Epidermal Cysts

SQUAMOUS CELL CARCINOMA ARISING IN AN EPIDERMAL CYST

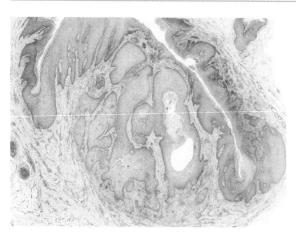

FIGURE 9.4   Squamous Cell Carcinoma Arising in an Epidermal Cyst.

Very rarely in situ changes and squamous cell carcinoma arise in an epidermal cyst. The clinical presentation is no different from an epidermal cyst. The existence of this entity has been questioned, and the alternative view is that this may represent a proliferating epidermal cyst.

On microscopy, the cyst lining is acanthotic with in situ changes that may be focal or diffuse. Buds of atypical keratinocytes are seen extending down into the surrounding tissue.

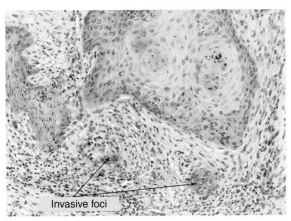

FIGURE 9.5   Squamous Cell Carcinoma Arising in an Epidermal Cyst-High Power

TRICHILEMMAL CYST

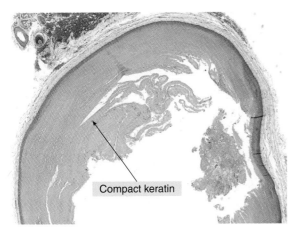

FIGURE 9.6   Trichilemmal Cyst

Trichilemmal cysts have a predilection for the scalp, although it may be seen at other locations rarely. They arise from the isthmic part of the hair follicle and show trichilemmal type of compact keratinization. A granular layer is conspicuously absent. Dystrophic calcification and cholesterol clefts are seen. Nuclear pleomorphism and mitotic activity are not seen.

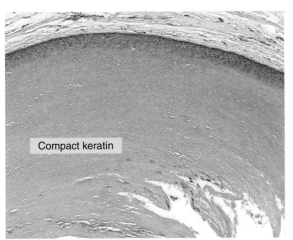

FIGURE 9.7   Compact Keratin in Trichilemmal Cyst

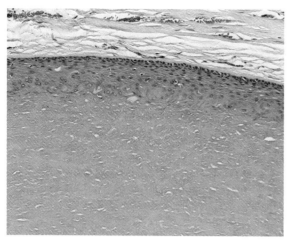

FIGURE 9.8   Absent Granular Layer in Trichilemmal Cyst

PROLIFERATING TRICHILEMMAL CYST

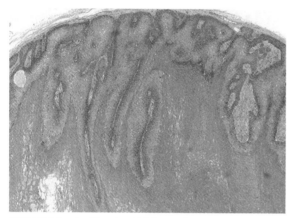

FIGURE 9.9   Proliferating Trichilemmal Cyst

Proliferating trichilemmal cysts are usually seen as solid nodules and rarely as cysts. In some instances they are ulcerated. They are commonly seen on the scalp of middle-aged or elderly individuals. Excision usually cures the lesion and recurrences and malignant transformation are rare.

On microscopy, the cyst lining is made up of squamous epithelium without a granular layer. The keratinization is compact trichilemmal type of keratinization. The lining squamous epithelium proliferates into the lumen of the cyst as broad strands. Nuclear atypia and mitotic activity are uncommon. The diagnosis of malignant trichilemmal cyst is made when there is marked nuclear atypia and invasion of the atypical epithelium into the adjacent tissue outside the cyst.

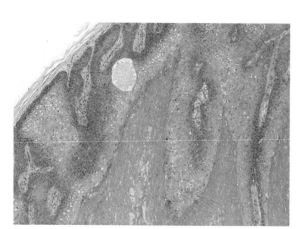

FIGURE 9.10   Trichilemmal Cyst-High Power

DERMOID CYST

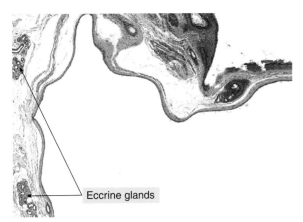
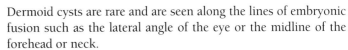

FIGURE 9.11   Dermoid Cyst-Low Power

Dermoid cysts are rare and are seen along the lines of embryonic fusion such as the lateral angle of the eye or the midline of the forehead or neck.

On microscopy, they are lined by stratified squamous epithelium. Follicular structures and sebaceous glands may be seen embedded in the wall of the cyst. Mucinous, apocrine, or conjunctival epithelium may be seen depending on the location of the cyst.

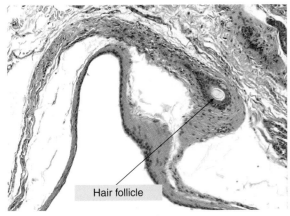

FIGURE 9.12   Dermoid Cyst-High Power

VELLUS HAIR CYST

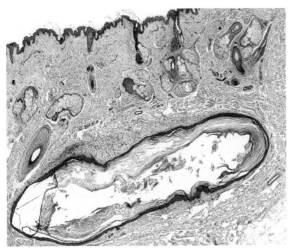

FIGURE 9.13   Vellus Hair Cyst-Low Power

Vellus hair cysts are seen as multiple small papules on the chest and axillae of young adults and children. They may occur sporadically or may have autosomal dominant inheritance.

On microscopy, these small cysts are lined by stratified squamous epithelium, which may also show trichilemmal type of keratinization. The lumen contains keratin and transversely orientated vellus hair shafts. The cysts may rupture and produce a foreign body giant cell reaction. Spontaneous regression occurs in majority of the cases.

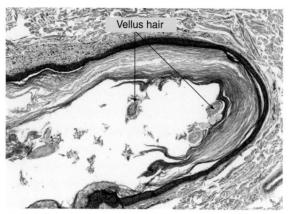

FIGURE 9.14   Vellus Hair Cyst-High Power

STEATOCYSTOMA SIMPLEX

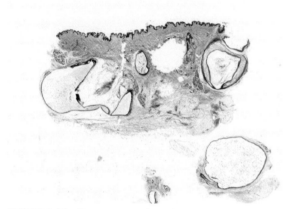

FIGURE 9.15   Steatocystoma-Scanning View

Steatocystoma simplex manifests as single or multiple skin-colored papules or nodules mainly on the chest, face, and the extremities. Majority of the cases are sporadic, but they may also be inherited as autosomal dominant. Mutation of keratin 17 has been documented in some cases of steatocystoma multiplex.

On microscopy, the cyst is lined by stratified squamous epithelium and has an undulating appearance due to the collapse of the cyst. The cyst wall shows sebaceous glands within its wall.

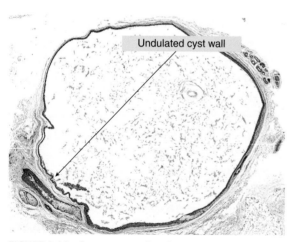

FIGURE 9.16   Steatocystoma-Low Power

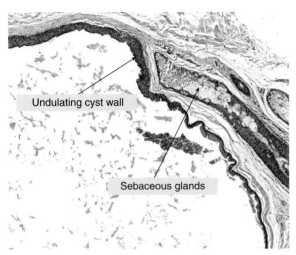

FIGURE 9.17   Steatocystoma-High Power

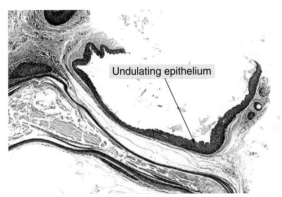

FIGURE 9.18   Steatocystoma-High Power

BRANCHIAL CLEFT CYST

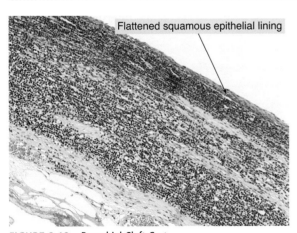

FIGURE 9.19   Branchial Cleft Cyst

Branchial cleft cyst usually arises from first or second branchial pouch. Clinically, they are seen as sinus tracts or cysts.

On microscopy, the cysts are lined by stratified squamous epithelium, and the wall contains dense lymphoid aggregates. Mucinous lining or glands could also be seen.

MORPHEA

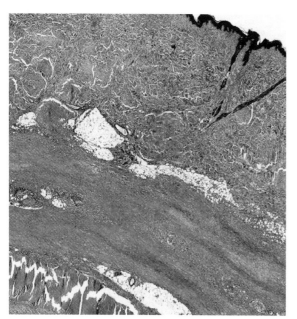

FIGURE 9.20   Morphea-Low Power

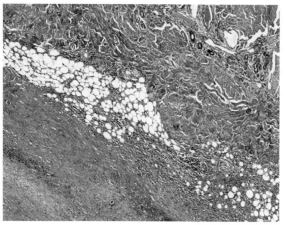

FIGURE 9.21   Morphea-Low Power

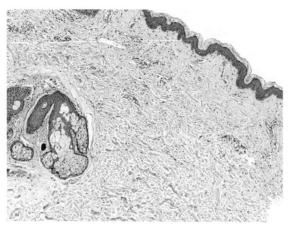

FIGURE 9.22   Inflammatory Stage of Morphea

Morphea is localized scleroderma where there is deposition of collagen in the dermis and other organs. It may occur as localized disease with involvement of the dermis or may occur in conjunction with Raynaud's phenomenon. Clinically, it presents as several plaques on trunk and extremities. The lesions are generally termed lilac rings with an ivory-colored center and violaceous border. Several clinical types of morphea have been described. Morphea is also known to coexist with lichen sclerosus et atrophicus. The etiology of morphea is still controversial. Association with *Borrelia burgdorferi* has been postulated among some patients from Germany and Austria. The increased deposition of collagen in the dermis is also postulated due to lymphokines released by the inflammatory cell infiltrate in morphea.

On microscopy, mainly three changes are identified. They are the increased deposition of collagen in the dermis and the subcutaneous fat, vascular changes, and the inflammatory cell infiltration. The epidermis may vary from being normal to atrophic. The dermis is usually markedly increased in thickness and is replaced by thick bands of collagen. This change extends to the interface between the dermis and the subcutaneous fat, replaces the fat around the sweat glands, and extends even deeper into the subcutaneous tissue. The vessels in the dermis and the subcutaneous tissue show thickening of their walls and subsequent narrowing of their lumen. The inflammatory cells are seen in the earlier stages of morphea and are mainly lymphocytes, macrophages, and some plasma cells. Few histological variants of morphea have also been described, and they show slightly different patterns in each type.

Masson's trichrome stain shows the marked increase in dermal collagen, which is stained blue in color.

Direct immunofluorescence shows negative staining pattern in majority of the cases, but occasional cases have been reported to show IgM at the basement membrane zone or around the dermal blood vessels.

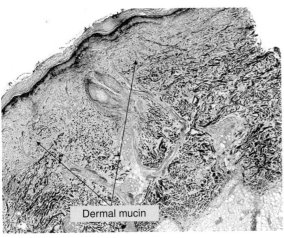

Dermal mucin

FIGURE 9.23   Masson's-Trichrome

SCLERODERMA

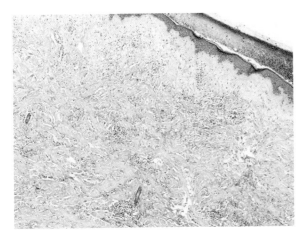

FIGURE 9.24   Scleroderma-Low Power

Systemic scleroderma is either diffuse form (progressive systemic sclerosis) or limited form. The limited variant usually affects older individuals and is preceded by Raynaud's phenomenon. The lesions are usually confined to the digits. Limited scleroderma includes CREST syndrome, which includes calcinosis, Raynaud's phenomenon, esophageal dysfunction, sclerodactyly, and telangiectasia. One or all of these features may be seen in affected patients. Pigmentary changes may also be seen. The etiology of scleroderma is still not fully understood with different theories being postulated.

On microscopy, the changes are those of thickening of the dermal collagen and extension of the collagen into the subcutaneous fat. The inflammatory changes are much less than that in morphea. The vascular changes are more prominent than that in morphea. Other changes such as calcification and increase in mast cells have been documented.

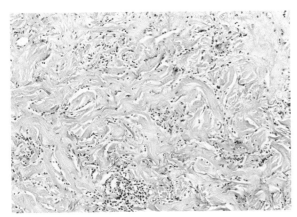

FIGURE 9.25   Scleroderma-High Power

LICHEN SCLEROSUS ET ATROPHICUS

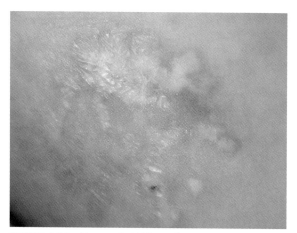

FIGURE 9.26   Extragenital Lichen Sclerosus

Extragenital lichen sclerosus et atrophicus occurs in 20% of patients with genital lichen sclerosus. The upper part of the body is more commonly affected with neck, trunk, and arms being the most common sites. The lesions are seen as flat ivory to white papules, which coalesce to form plaques. The hemorrhagic bullous form may also be seen. Lichen sclerosus is a slowly progressive disease with periods of quiescence. Spontaneous regression may occur in rare cases. A controversial relationship exists between morphea and lichen sclerosus. There are a small number of cases reported with both lesions in the same patient. Malignant transformation in an extragenital lichen sclerosus has not been reported. Around 5% of genital lichen sclerosus undergo malignant transformation to develop squamous cell carcinoma. *B. burgdorferi* has been isolated in patients with lichen sclerosus and has been reported from patients mostly from Austria.

On microscopy, the epidermis may be acanthotic or atrophic. Basal vacuolar degeneration is seen. A broad zone of homogenized collagen and edema is seen in the subepidermal zone. There might be some dilated blood vessels in this zone. The dermis beneath this shows an infiltrate of lymphocytes. A lichenoid pattern of lymphocytes may be seen in the early stages.

The elastic fibers in lichen sclerosus are pushed toward the deeper aspect by the homogenized collagen in lichen sclerosus and are subsequently destroyed. In morphea, the elastic fibers are normal or increased in number.

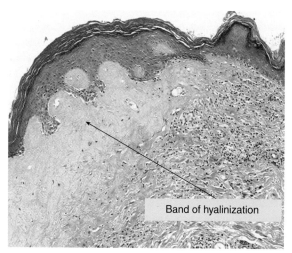

Band of hyalinization

FIGURE 9.27   Lichen Sclerosus

HYPERTROPHIC SCAR

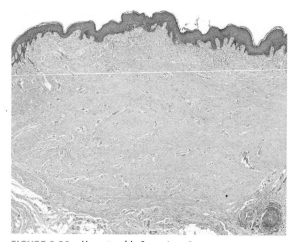

FIGURE 9.28   Hypertrophic Scare-Low Power

Hypertrophic scars usually develop over a long period of time. Clinically, they have been described as being raised beyond the original wound. This definition does not always hold true.

On microscopy, hypertrophic scar shows orientation of collagen bundles parallel to the overlying epidermis. There is increased production of fibroblasts, which may be seen in a well-defined pattern. Many thin-walled blood vessels may also be seen amongst the fibroblasts. There are scattered lymphocytes may be seen in within a scar.

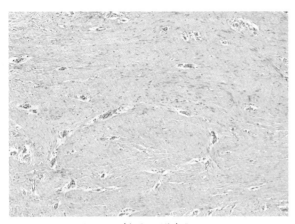

FIGURE 9.29   Hypertrophic Scar-High Power

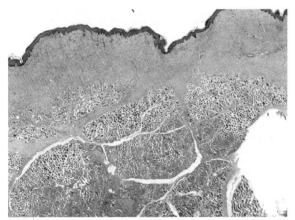

FIGURE 9.30   Scar-Scanning View

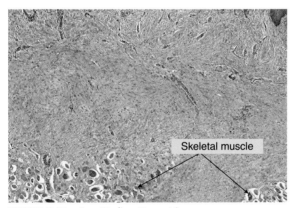

Skeletal muscle

FIGURE 9.31   Scar-Medium Power View

KELOID

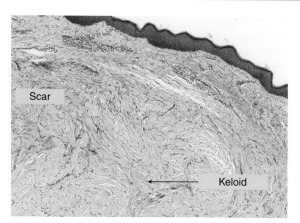

FIGURE 9.32   Scar with Keloid

Keloids develop in the background of hypertrophic scars. The tendency for keloid formation is based on the race of the patient, age, wound infection, and the site of the wound. Cytokines particularly transforming growth factor (TGF)-beta has been postulated to play an important role in the development of keloids. Excision of keloids generally produces a larger keloid.

Clinically keloids are raised above the skin surface. On microscopy, the overlying epidermis is usually stretched over the keloid. Mature keloids show broad brightly eosinophilic homogeneous bundles of collagen arranged in a haphazard pattern. There may be dilated blood vessels in the subepidermal location along with scattered lymphocytes.

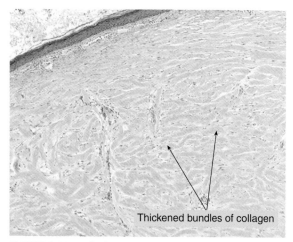

FIGURE 9.33   Keloid-Low Power

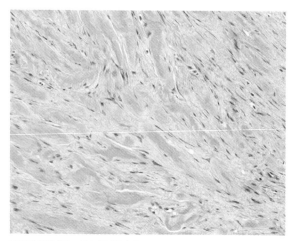

FIGURE 9.34   Keloid-High Power

PERFORATING COLLAGENOSIS

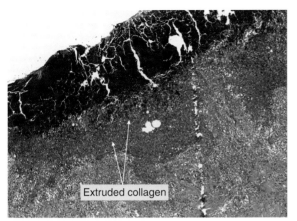

FIGURE 9.35   Perforating Collagenosis

Perforating collagenosis is rare. They are a group of diseases in which altered collagen is extruded from the dermis through damaged and ulcerated epidermis. Inherited and acquired variants have been described. Autosomal recessive and dominant modes of inheritance have been postulated, and they manifest usually in childhood. The acquired variants are seen in adult life in persons with diabetes mellitus and chronic renal failure. In this situation, there is known to be histological overlap with other perforating disorders such as reactive perforating folliculitis and Kyrle's disease.

On microscopy, there is a cup-shaped crater in the middle with ulceration of the epidermis. There is usually dense granulation tissue and inflammatory cell infiltration. Collagen and elastic fibers are seen to be extruded through the epidermis. Masson's trichrome stain demonstrates the blue-colored collagen being extruded through the epidermis.

CHONDRODERMATITIS NODULARIS HELICIS

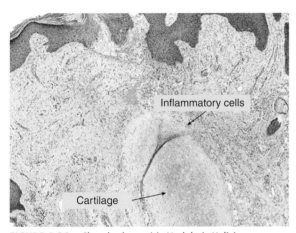

FIGURE 9.36   Chondrodermatitis Nodularis Helicis

Chondrodermatitis nodularis helicis is a chronic disorder seen in elderly males on the helix of the ear. This is a chronic crusty disorder and presents as a tender nodule. This disorder has been categorized as one of the perforating disorders. Degeneration of the collagen is the primary pathological process, and this could be triggered by inflammation, trauma, or severe solar elastosis.

On microscopy, the classical cases show a central area of epidermal ulceration with the underlying dermis showing the degenerated collagen, granulation tissue, solar elastosis, and inflammation. The inflammatory infiltrate is composed of lymphocytes, plasma cells, and some neutrophils. There may be some dilated blood vessels with some of them containing fibrin within their lumen. The inflammation and granulation tissue infiltrates the cartilage and causes degenerative changes within the cartilage. Very rarely, calcification and transepidermal elimination of degenerated collagen may be seen.

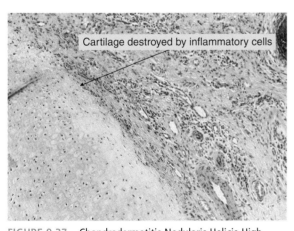

FIGURE 9.37   Chondrodermatitis Nodularis Helicis-High Power

ELASTOFIBROMA

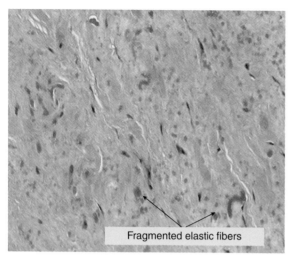

FIGURE 9.38   Elastofibroma-H&E Stain

Elastofibroma is not a true neoplasm, but a pseudotumor representing a degenerative or reactive disorder of the elastic fibers. The lesion is classically seen on the interscapular area and chest wall of middle-aged men. Rarely thigh and arm may be involved.

On microscopy, elastofibroma is an ill-defined lesion with many broken and clumped elastic fibers. Thick and globular masses of elastic fibers may also be seen.

Verhoff's elastic van-Geison stain highlights the elastic fibers, and they stain black.

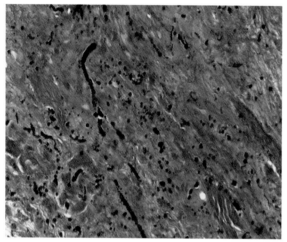

FIGURE 9.39   Elastofibroma Elastic van-Gieson Stain

SOLAR ELASTOSIS

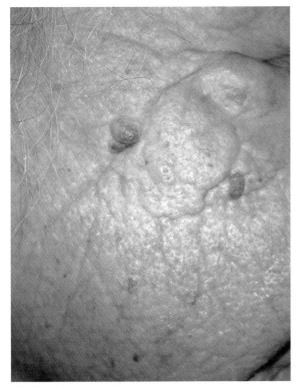

FIGURE 9.40   Solar Elastosis

Solar elastosis is the change seen in the skin due to chronic sun exposure. Ultraviolet rays are thought to cause the maximum damage. There are several clinical patterns described, some of which have distinct histological appearances. The commonest change encountered is described under the umbrella term of solar elastosis. Skin exposed to chronic sun exposure is susceptible to repeated infections and malignancy. The commonest malignant tumors encountered are basal cell carcinoma, squamous cell carcinoma, melanoma, and precursor changes such as actinic keratosis and melanoma in situ.

On microscopy, the epidermal changes are variable and ranges from atrophy to variable degrees of acanthosis. Varying degrees of keratinocyte atypia labeled as mild to severe actinic keratosis accompanied by proliferation of photoactivated melanocytes along the dermoepidermal junction is seen (see Chapter 8). The dermis shows thickened and curled masses of collagen in the early stages and in severe cases, amorphous masses of elastotic material with ill-defined margins are seen.

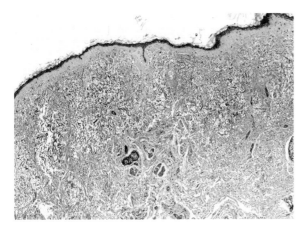

FIGURE 9.41   Solar Elastosis-Low Power

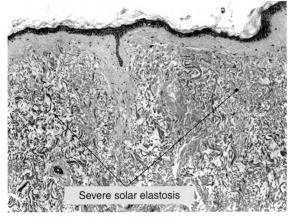

Severe solar elastosis

FIGURE 9.42   Solar Elastosis-High Power

PRETIBIAL MYXEDEMA

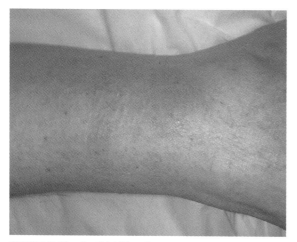

FIGURE 9.43   Pretibial Myxedema

Pretibial myxedema is seen in Grave's disease and may not manifest until after the correction of hyperthyroidism. It may occasionally be seen in patients with autoimmune thyroiditis. Clinically, the different manifestations include circumscribed nodules or diffuse nonpitting edema. The anterior aspect of the leg is the commonest site but rarely the upper trunk and face may also be involved.

On microscopy, the dermis shows excessive amounts of mucin in the mid and the lower thirds, which is highlighted by the Alcian blue stain at pH 2.5. Occasional stellate fibroblasts may be seen. The overlying epidermis may be normal to hyperkeratotic.

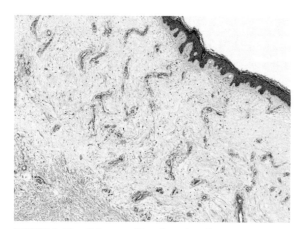

FIGURE 9.44   Cutaneous Myxedema-Low Power

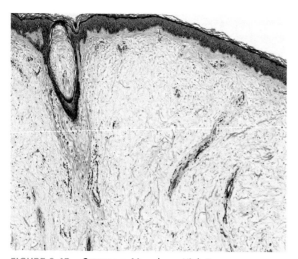

FIGURE 9.45   Cutaneous Myxedema-High Power

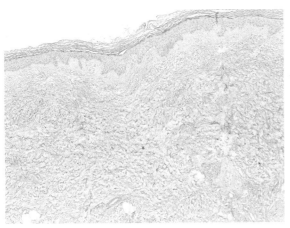

FIGURE 9.46   Cutaneous Myxedema-Mucin Stained with Alcian Blue pH 2.5

DIGITAL MUCOUS CYST

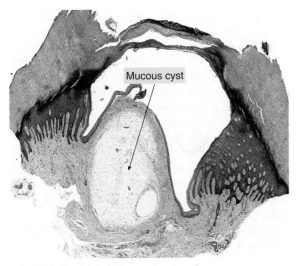

FIGURE 9.47   Digital Mucous Cyst-Low Power

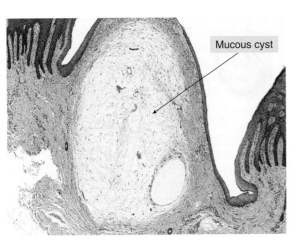

FIGURE 9.48   Digital Mucous Cyst-Medium Power

Digital mucous cysts are not uncommon lesions occurring in the middle-aged or elderly individuals with a predilection for the distal interphalangeal joints of fingers and toes.

On microscopy, a circumscribed, but unencapsulated lesion is seen in the dermis separate from the overlying epidermis. The lesion is predominantly mucinous with scattered fibroblasts within it. The mucin can be demonstrated by Alcian blue stain at pH 2.5.

CALCINOSIS CUTIS

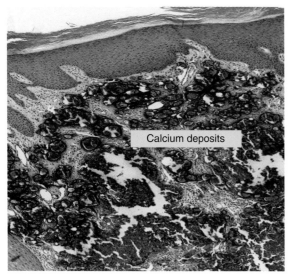

FIGURE 9.49   Calcinosis Cutis

Deposition of calcium within the skin termed calcinosis cutis is mainly due to two mechanisms. Dystrophic calcification, when the calcium deposition is in damaged or degenerated tissue or less commonly, metastatic calcification when the calcium deposition results from the derangement of calcium or phosphate metaobolism. Clinically, the deposits may manifest as subepidermal calcified nodule, idiopathic scrotal calcinosis, or tumoral calcinosis. Other rarer forms have also been described.

On microscopy, dystrophic and metastatic calcium deposition show similar appearances. The epidermis could be acanthotic or atrophic. Large areas of intense basophilic amorphous substances are deposited in the dermis and the subcutaneous fat. Foreign body giant cell reaction is seen around the deposits.

CUTANEOUS OSSIFICATION

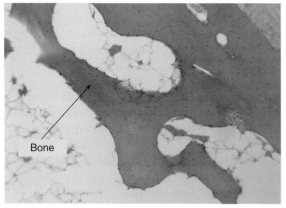

FIGURE 9.50   Cutaneous Ossification

Cutaneous ossification is broadly classified into primary and secondary types. The primary type is termed osteoma cutis, where there is an absence of a preexisting lesion, and the secondary type is termed metaplastic ossification where the ossification develops secondary to trauma, infection, or neoplasia.

On microscopy, cutaneous ossification is seen as spicules of mature bone rimmed by osteoblasts in the dermis and the subcutaneous fat. The bone develops by mesenchymal ossification without a cartilage precursor. Occasionally, hemopoietic cells and fat may be seen.

CARTILAGE

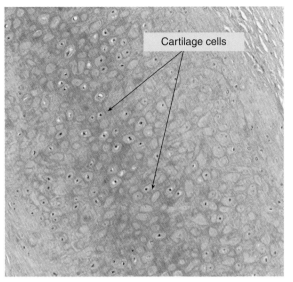

Cartilage cells

FIGURE 9.51   Cartilage

Cartilaginous deposition in the skin may be primary or secondary. Primary deposits are seen in tumors such as enchondromas, hamartomas, or mixed tumors of skin, and secondary deposits are seen as cartilaginous differentiation of a cutaneous soft tissue tumor.

GOUT

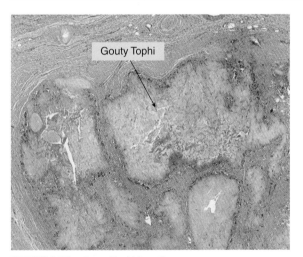

Gouty Tophi

FIGURE 9.52   Gouty Tophi-Low Power

Gout is a manifestation of altered purine metabolism resulting in elevated levels of uric acid. Clinically, gout manifests as exceedingly painful monoarticular arthritis predominantly affecting the great toe, but other joints may be involved. In the chronic state, the skin over the joint gets swollen and erythematous and in long-standing cases, the swelling discharges a chalky material. Urate nephropathy is the most common complication of gout.

On microscopy, H&E of formalin-fixed sections show gouty tophi as amorphous eosinophilic material surrounded by a granulomatous response with many foreign body giant cells. On alcohol-fixed sections, the tophi appear as needle-shaped crystals arranged as sheaves of corn. These crystals show negative birefringence.

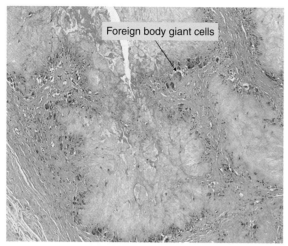

FIGURE 9.53   Gouty Tophi-Foreign Body Giant Cells

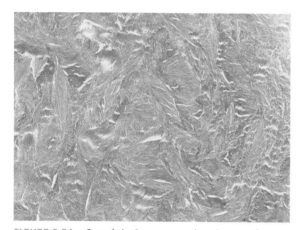

FIGURE 9.54   Crystals in Gout arranged as sheaves of corn

LICHEN AMYLOIDOSIS

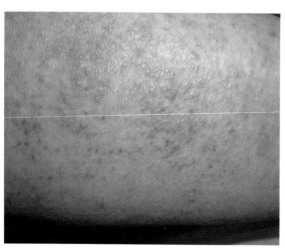

FIGURE 9.55   Lichen Amyloidosis

Clinically, lichen amyloidosis presents as multiple small discrete waxy papules on the extensor surface of the extremities.

On microscopy, there is homogenous deposition of eosinophilic material in the papillary dermis. The overlying epidermis shows acanthosis and apoptotic bodies within the epidermis. This amyloid is confirmed to be of keratinocyte origin and is designated as amyloid-K. The amyloid stains orange-red color with Congo red and Sirius red and demonstrates the apple-green birefringence on polarized light microscopy.

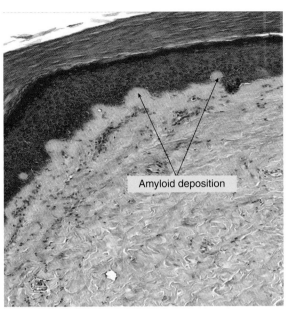

FIGURE 9.56   Lichen Amyloidosis-Low Power

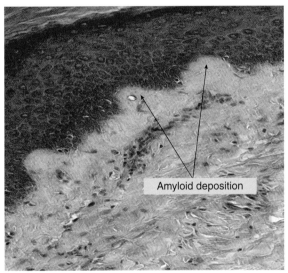

FIGURE 9.57   Lichen Amyloidosis-High Power

NODULAR AMYLOIDOSIS

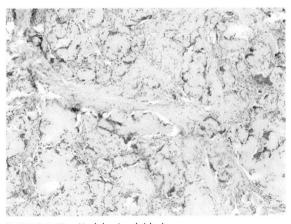

Nodular amyloidosis is uncommon and clinically presents as single or multiple nodules on scalp, lower limbs, face, or genital region. Nodular amyloidosis could be primary or secondary. Primary nodular amyloidosis is very rare. It may be seen in association with monoclonal paraproteinemia, lymphoplasmacytoid lymphoma, and incidentally in a rectal biopsy. Secondary cutaneous amyloidosis is seen in association with tumors such as basal cell carcinoma, adnexal tumors, and chronic inflammatory conditions such as tuberculosis and rheumatoid arthritis.

FIGURE 9.58   Nodular Amyloidosis

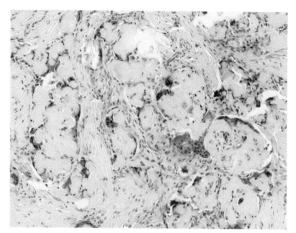

FIGURE 9.59 Nodular Amyloidosis-High Power

On microscopy, large masses of eosinophilic homogenous material are seen in the dermis and the subcutaneous fat. A granulomatous response with a foreign body giant cell reaction is seen around the deposits. The deposits may also be seen around blood vessels. Congo red and Sirius red stains show orange-red staining and apple-green birefringence on polarized light microscopy.

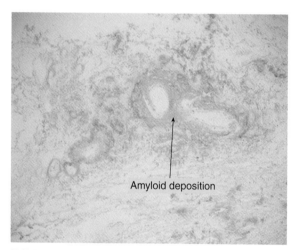

FIGURE 9.60 Amyloid in the Dermis—Congo Red Stain

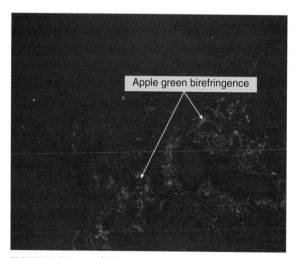

FIGURE 9.61 Amyloid on Polarized Microscopy

COLLOID MILIUM

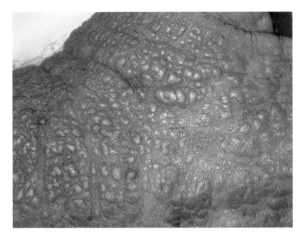

FIGURE 9.62   Adult Colloid Milium

Colloid milium is also known as papular elastosis. The adult form is much more common than the juvenile form, and the lesions are seen on sun-exposed sites. Clinically, colloid milium presents as multiple dome-shaped yellow translucent papules. Colloid milium, particularly in adults, is the result of extreme sun damage.

On microscopy, a band-like area of severely sun-damaged dermal collagen is seen. Characteristic clefting may be present within this area of collagen. Adult colloid milium shows the same staining characteristics as amyloid. It is positive for Congo red and demonstrates the apple-green birefringence. Colloid milium shows positive staining with Thioflavin T and it is PAS positive and diastase resistant.

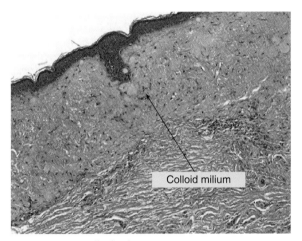

FIGURE 9.63   Colloid Milium

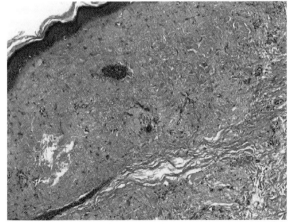

FIGURE 9.64   Colloid Milium-High Power

OCHRONOSIS

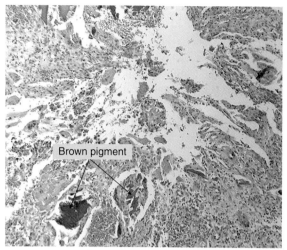

FIGURE 9.65   Ochronosis

Ochronosis refers to the deposition of ochre or yellow-brown pigment. The pigment is homogentisic acid deposited in the dermal collagen in the rare metabolic disorder called alkaptonuria. The disorder results in the deficiency of homogentisic acid oxidase. The term ochronosis is also used when there is deposition of similar colored pigment following the topical use of phenol in the treatment of leg ulcers, picric acid in the treatment of burns, intramuscular injection of antimalarial drugs, and the topical use of hydroquinone bleaching creams.

On microscopy, there is mild basophilia of the dermal collagen. Yellow-brown pigment is seen within macrophages or lying free within the collagen. Foreign body giant cell reaction may be seen. Many melanophages may be seen in hydroquinone-induced ochronosis. The pigment induced by antimalarial drugs is positive for melanin and hemosiderin.

HEMOSIDERIN

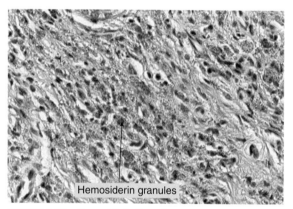

FIGURE 9.66   Hemosiderin Granules

Hemosiderin is the breakdown product of hemoglobin. Cutaneous deposition of hemosiderin occurs in a number of situations such as pigmented purpuric dermatoses, at the site of a previous injury, following application of Monsel's solution (20% aqueous ferric sulfate) for hemostasis in minor surgical procedures, and in the rare multisystem metabolic disease called hemochromatosis. The cutaneous manifestation of pigment in hemochromatosis is termed Bronze diabetes.

On microscopy, the appearances can be variable and include scattered golden yellow granules within macrophages, or lying free within the collagen. The intensity of deposition depends on the severity of the underlying diseases. The granules of hemosiderin stain blue with Perl's Prussian blue stain (see Chapter 5).

ENDOMETRIOSIS

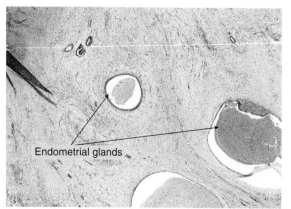

FIGURE 9.67   Endometriosis-Low Power

Endometriosis is the abnormal location of endometrial glands and stroma in a dermal or subcutaneous location. Clinically, they present at the site of previous caesarean section scars and very rarely at other sites. Different theories have been postulated regarding the cause of endometriosis. These include direct implantation, coelomic spread, and lymphatic or hematogenous spread.

On microscopy, the dermis and subcutaneous tissue are infiltrated by endometrial glands surrounded by endometrial stroma. The presence of glands alone is not sufficient for the diagnosis. The stromal cells stain strongly with CD10, which can be used to confirm the diagnosis in doubtful cases.

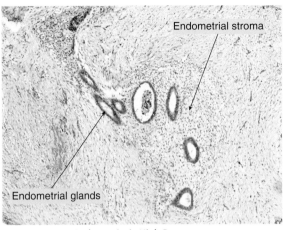

FIGURE 9.68   Endometriosis-High Power

DERMAL GRANULOMA

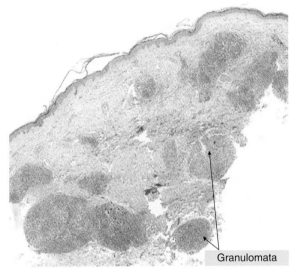

FIGURE 9.69   Dermal Granuloma

Granulomas in the dermis can be due to many causes. A granuloma is defined as a collection of histiocytes, lymphocytes, and multinucleated giant cells. The cells constituting the granuloma, the pattern of arrangement, and the presence or absence of central necrosis are features that help to arrive at a diagnosis in many of the granulomatous disorders. An infective etiology should be considered in all granulomatous disorders and necessary special stains should be carried out. A separate sample for culture should also be sent. All skin biopsies showing granulomatous reaction pattern should be examined under polarized light to detect or exclude a foreign body.

SARCOIDOSIS

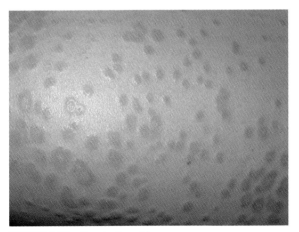

FIGURE 9.70   Papular Sarcoid

Sarcoidosis is a multisystem disease that involves skin, lymph nodes, lung, and eyes. One third of patients with systemic sarcoidosis develop cutaneous disease. Clinically, the cutaneous manifestations are very varied and include maculopapular rash with acute lymphadenopathy, nodules and papules, and plaques with marked telangiectasias.

On microscopy, the sarcoidal granulomas are distributed in the dermis or may extend to the subcutaneous fat. The granulomas are classically described as naked granulomas in that they are composed of histiocytes and multinucleated giant cells with hardly any lymphocytes around them. There is no central necrosis. The granulomas do not have any predilection for adnexal structures or nerves. Schaumann bodies that are calcium-impregnated bodies in the shape of a shell are seen but are not in any way specific for sarcoidosis.

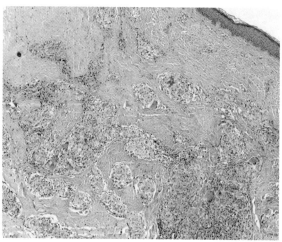

FIGURE 9.71   Sarcoidosis-Low Power

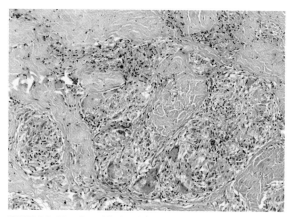

FIGURE 9.72   Sarcoidosis-High Power

GRANULOMATOUS ROSACEA

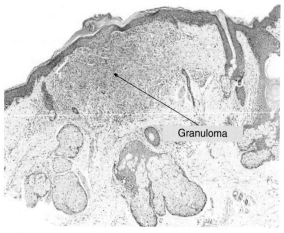

FIGURE 9.73   Granulomatous Rosacea-Low Power

Clinically, granulomatous rosacea is suspected when yellow-brown papules develop in the background of rosacea. Perioral areas and face are the commonest sites.

On microscopy, the overlying epidermis may show multiple dilated follicular ostia with *Demodex folliculorum*. The dermis shows edema, dilated dermal blood vessels, and granuloma in the interfollicular dermis, which is characteristic. The presence of *D. folliculorum* and the subsequent rupture of the follicle can give rise to granulomatous response, and care should be taken to exclude this possibility. Clinico-pathological correlation would be crucial in this setting. Special stains to exclude the possibilities of tuberculosis and fungal organisms should be done.

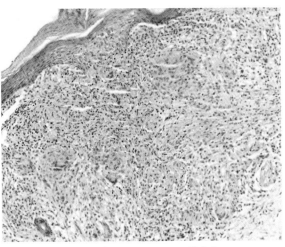

FIGURE 9.74   Granulomatous Rosacea-High Power

GRANULOMA ANNULARE

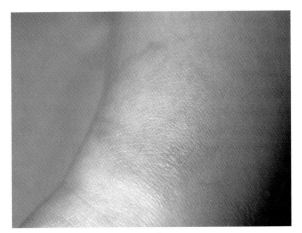

FIGURE 9.75   Granuloma Annulare

Granuloma annulare is a common disease of unknown etiology. It manifests in different clinical settings and include inflammatory conditions, drugs, autoimmune diseases, benign and malignant neoplastic diseases, and infective conditions such as HIV. Granuloma annulare associated with HIV has been termed HAGA (HIV-associated granuloma annulare).

On microscopy, the most common histological pattern seen is that of an ill-defined palisaded granuloma. There is a central area of degenerate collagen separated by mucin, surrounded by radially arranged histiocytes and fibroblasts. Very rarely lymphocytes are seen within the granuloma. Elastic fibers are absent within the granuloma. Multinucleated giant cells are seen. The central mucinous area can be demonstrated by Alcian blue at pH 2.5 (Fig. 9.78). A characteristic feature of almost all types of granuloma annulare is the presence of perivascular lymphocytic infiltration around the granuloma. Neutrophils are a feature and if present are associated with vasculitis and possible association with a systemic involvement.

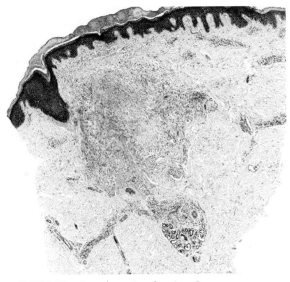

FIGURE 9.76   Granuloma Annulare-Low Power

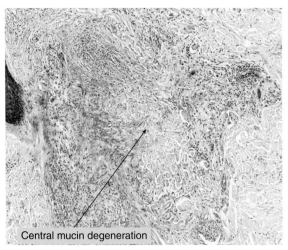

FIGURE 9.77   Granuloma Annulare-High Power

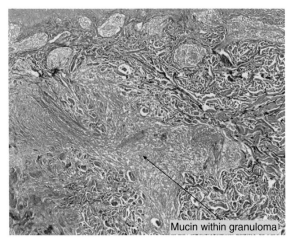

FIGURE 9.78   Alcian Blue Demonstrating Mucin in
Granuloma Annulare

DEEP GRANULOMA ANNULARE (PSEUDORHEUMATOID NODULE)

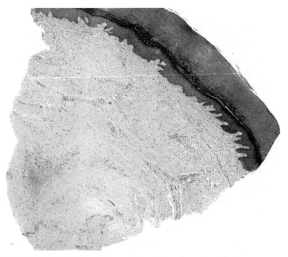

FIGURE 9.79   Deep Gyranuloma Annulare-Low Power

Deep granuloma annulare is a variant of granuloma annulare seen in younger individuals in a deeper location such as subcutaneous fat. They are commonly seen in the lower extremities.

On microscopy, granulomas with central areas of mucin degeneration and palisaded arrangement of histiocytes and fibroblasts are seen. It is also known as pseudorheumatoid nodule due to its location in the deeper tissues.

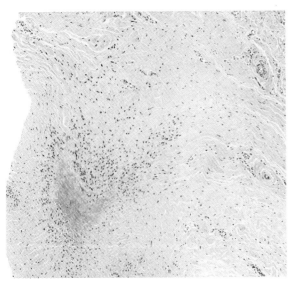

FIGURE 9.80   Deep Granuloma Annulare-High Power

RHEUMATOID NODULE

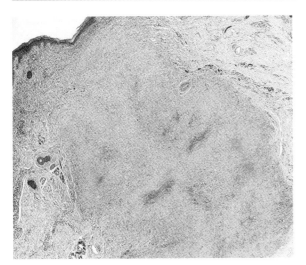

FIGURE 9.81   Rheumatoid Nodules

Rheumatoid nodules develop in patients with longstanding rheumatoid arthritis. Such patients usually have high serum rheumatoid factor. Large numbers of the nodules are located in the subcutaneous fat, but they are also seen in the dermis.

On microscopy, the classical appearance is that of multiple ill-defined palisaded granulomas with central areas of fibrin degeneration. The granulomas are composed of palisaded histiocytes, neutrophils, and some lymphocytes. Active granulation tissue is seen in the intervening dermis in occasional cases. Vasculitis has also been recorded.

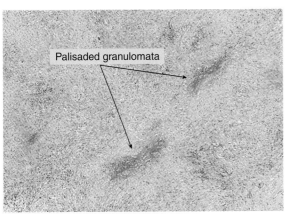

Palisaded granulomata

FIGURE 9.82   Rheumatoid Nodules-Medium Power

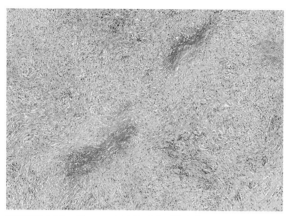

FIGURE 9.83   Rheumatoid Nodules-High Power

PALISADED NEUTROPHILIC AND GRANULOMATOUS DERMATITIS

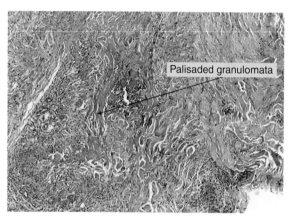

FIGURE 9.84   Palisaded Neutrophilic and Granulomatous Dermatitis

Palisaded neutrophilic and granulomatous dermatitis is a reaction pattern seen in many diseases ranging from drugs to inflammatory diseases such as vasculitis and autoimmune diseases, malignancies, HIV infection, diabetes, and viral infection. The trunk and extremities are the common sites.

On microscopy, the consistent finding is that of multiple ill-defined palisaded granulomatous foci. The granulomata usually have a central area of necrobiosis with radially arranged histiocytes and neutrophils. Karyorrhexis is a feature. Multinucleated giant cells are occasionally seen.

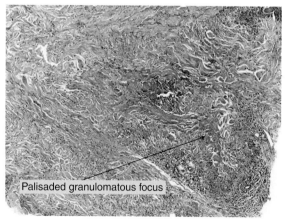

FIGURE 9.85   Palisaded Neutrophilic and Granulomatous Dermatitis

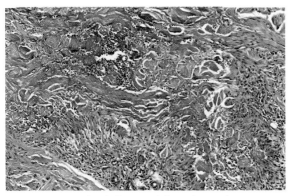

FIGURE 9.86   Palisaded Neutrophilic and Granulomatous
Dermatitis-High Power

HENOCH-SCHONLEIN PURPURA

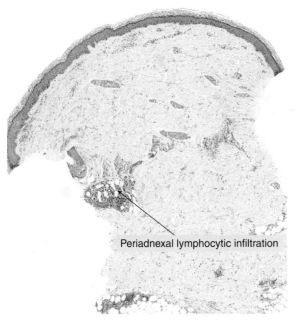

Periadnexal lymphocytic infiltration

FIGURE 9.87   Henoch–Schönlein Purpura-Low Power

Henoch-Schonlein purpura is a multisystem disorder characterized by abdominal pain, joint pains, and widespread purpura due to leucocytoclastic vasculitis. It is caused by circulating IgA immune complexes.

On microscopy, there is periadnexal and perivascular infiltration of lymphocytes and neutrophils. Leukocytoclastic vasculitis is seen.

Direct immunofluorescence shows deposition of IgA around dermal blood vessels and dermal mesangium.

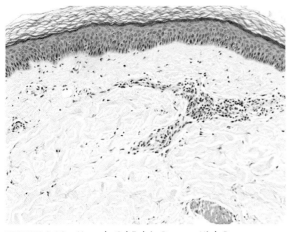

FIGURE 9.88   Henoch–Schönlein Purpura-High Power

URTICARIAL VASCULITIS

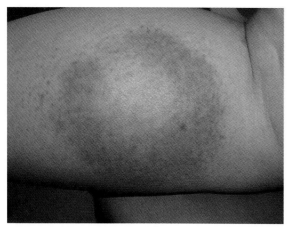

FIGURE 9.89   Urticarial Vasculitis

Urticarial vasculitis is an uncommon condition where there is clinical chronic urticaria and histological leukocytoclastic vasculitis. Patients have systemic manifestations, and they include joint pains, stiffness, angioedema, and gastrointestinal (GI) symptoms. Urticarial vasculitis could be the cutaneous manifestation of many underlying systemic diseases.

On microscopy, features of vasculitis are superimposed on a background of urticaria. The vasculitic changes are subtle and are those of leukocytoclastic vasculitis. Extravasation of red blood cells is seen. In severe cases, there might be necrotizing vasculitis, thus displaying a range of features.

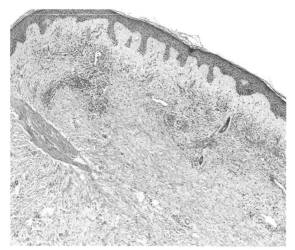

FIGURE 9.90   Urticarial Vasculitis-Low Power

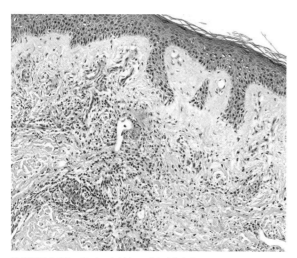

FIGURE 9.91   Urticarial Vasculitis-High Power

LEUKOCYTOCLASTIC VASCULITIS

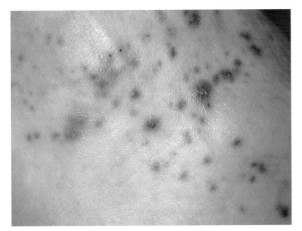

FIGURE 9.92   Vasculitis-C5a

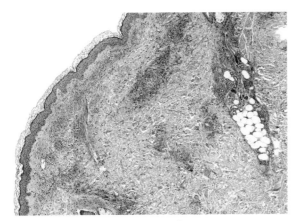

FIGURE 9.93   Leukocytoclastic Vasculitis-Low Power

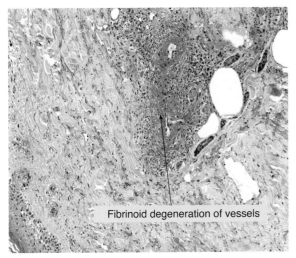

Fibrinoid degeneration of vessels

FIGURE 9.94   Leukocytoclastic Vasculitis-High Power

Leukocytoclastic vasculitis also known as hypersensitivity vasculitis is a vascular reaction pattern to circulating immune complexes. It is the commonest type of vasculitis. Systemic involvement of the GI tract and kidneys may be found. Nonblanching palpable purpura is the commonest cutaneous manifestation. Urticarial or bullous lesions may also be seen. Very rarely annular erythema or erythema gyratum repens–like lesions may occur. In extremely rare cases, the vasculitis can be asymptomatic. A number of etiological agents are involved in the development of leukocytoclastic vasculitis. These include drugs, infections, and associated diseases. Leukocytoclastic vasculitis could be a paraneoplastic manifestation of an underlying malignancy such as leukemia and lymphoma. The primary pathogenetic mechanism is the deposition of immune complexes in the walls of small blood vessels. This activates the complement cascade and the production of C5a, a neutrophil polymorph chemotactant. C5a is associated with the release of lysosomal enzymes such as elastases and collagenases. This results in blood vessel wall damage, fibrin deposition, and release of red blood cells into the adjacent connective tissue.

On microscopy, the overlying epidermis may manifest ischemic necrosis. The small dermal vessels show fibrinoid necrosis, endothelial swelling, and the infiltration of the vessel wall by neutrophils, particularly with nuclear dust. Neutrophils, eosinophils, and lymphocytes may be seen in the surrounding connective tissue. The presence of fibrin thrombi in the lumina of the blood vessels is a pointer toward an infective etiology.

CUTANEOUS POLYARTERITIS NODOSA

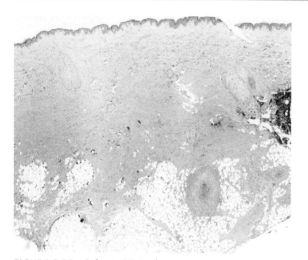

FIGURE 9.95   Polyarteritis Nodosa-Low Power

Cutaneous polyarteritis nodosa is rare, and the patients never manifest systemic symptoms. The commonest presentation is as recurrent tender painful nodules on the lower legs. Complications may include ulceration and gangrene. The etiopathogenesis of polyarteritis nodosa is poorly understood. Immune complex–mediated mechanism has been postulated triggered by viral and bacterial infections. ANCA (antineutrophilic cytoplasmic antibody) does not play any part in the pathogenesis of cutaneous polyarteritis nodosa.

On microscopy, the characteristic feature is the presence of necrotizing vasculitis in the medium-sized vessels of the deep dermis and subcutaneous fat. The fibrinoid necrosis involves the entire thickness of the vessel wall. Leukocytoclastic vasculitis is seen in almost all cases. In the later stages of the disease, scarring and fibrosis supervene.

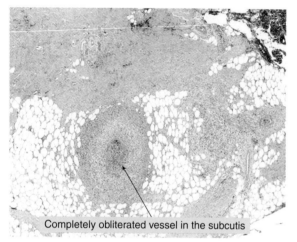

Completely obliterated vessel in the subcutis

FIGURE 9.96   Polyarteritis Nodosa-Medium Power

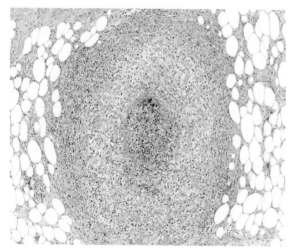

FIGURE 9.97   Polyarteritis Nodosa-High Power

ACUTE GENERALIZED EXANTHEMATOUS PUSTULOSIS

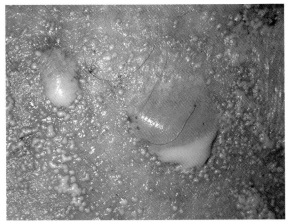

FIGURE 9.98   Acute Generalized Exanthematous Pustulosis

Acute generalized exanthematous pustulosis is also known as toxic pustuloderma. Clinically, it presents as sudden onset of numerous pustules that are nonfollicular. The lesion is pruritic and is usually seen on the face, although other areas may be involved. Systemic symptoms such as fever and facial edema are commonly seen. Very commonly, it is seen as a drug-induced lesion.

On microscopy, the pustules are seen in the intracorneal or subepidermal location. The dermal papillae are edematous and show moderate to dense infiltration of neutrophils and some histiocytes. Leukocytoclastic vasculitis may be seen in a large majority of cases.

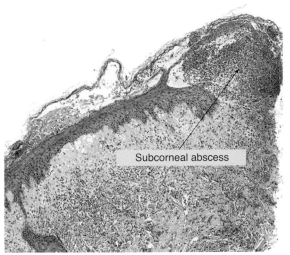

FIGURE 9.99   Acute Generalized Exanthematous Pustulosis-Low Power

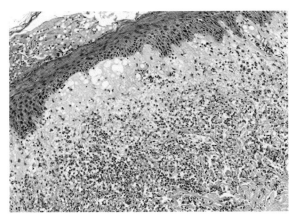

FIGURE 9.100   Acute Generalized Exanthematous Pustulosis—Edema of Papillary Dermis

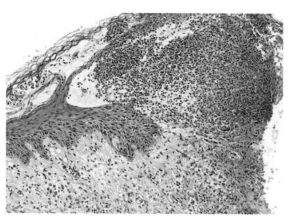

FIGURE 9.101 Acute Generalized Exanthematous Pustulosis-High Power

STASIS DERMATITIS

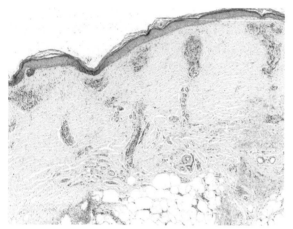

FIGURE 9.102 Stasis Dermatitis-Low Power

Stasis dermatitis results from impaired venous drainage. In the early stages, it is manifested as edema. In longstanding cases, ulceration may develop.

On microscopy, the epidermis is usually thinned out. The underlying dermis shows proliferation of dermal capillaries and edema. There is extravasation of red blood cells and hemosiderin deposition.

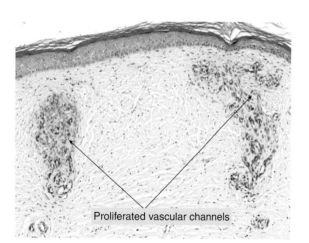

Proliferated vascular channels

FIGURE 9.103 Stasis Dermatitis-High Power

GYRATE ERYTHEMA

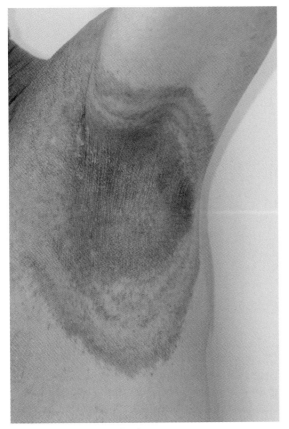

FIGURE 9.104   Gyrate Erythema

Gyrate erythemas are a heterogeneous group of disorders and manifest as arcuate and circinate lesions and include erythema annulare centrifugum, erythema gyratum repens, and erythema marginatum to include a few. Erythema gyratum repens is the most distinctive of the gyrate erythemas.

On microscopy, the overlying epidermis shows variable appearances depending on the particular subtype ranging from normal to spongiosis to parakeratosis. The dermis shows tight perivascular infiltrate of lymphocytes in all the subtypes.

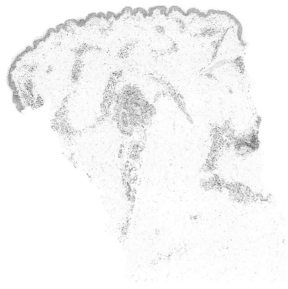

FIGURE 9.105   Gyrate Erythema

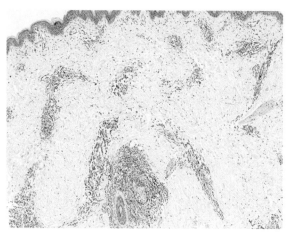

FIGURE 9.106   Gyrate Erythema-High Power

JESSNER'S LYMPHOCYTIC INFILTRATE

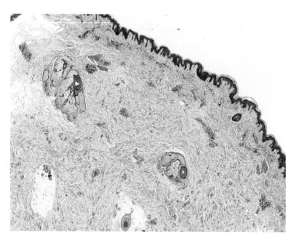

FIGURE 9.107   Jessner's Lymphocytic Infiltrate-Low Power

Jessner's lymphocytic infiltrate is a disorder of unknown etiology in which there is infiltration of lymphocytes in the dermis. They are usually seen on sun-exposed sites as brownish papules and plaques and are known not to evolve into lupus erythematosus.

On microscopy, there is no involvement of the epidermis, in particular there is no follicular plugging or hyperkeratosis as seen in lupus erythematosus. The dermis shows edema and perifollicular and perivascular infiltrate of lymphocytes, which are of the helper type. Lymphoid follicles are not seen. Occasionally plasma cells and histiocytes may be seen.

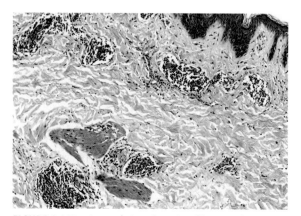

FIGURE 9.108   Jessner's Lymphocytic Infiltrate-High Power

REACTIVE ANGIOENDOTHELIOMATOSIS

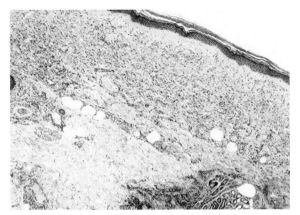

FIGURE 9.109   Reactive Angioendotheliomatosis-Low Power

Reactive angioendotheliomatosis is an uncommon condition presenting as plaques and macules. This may be associated with peripheral vascular disease, amyloidosis, antiphospholipid syndrome, and rheumatoid arthritis.

On microscopy, this is a dermal lesion with occasional extension into the subcutaneous fat. Multiple lobules of closely packed capillaries lined by plump endothelial cells are seen in the dermis. Occasionally the lumen is obliterated by plump endothelial cells.

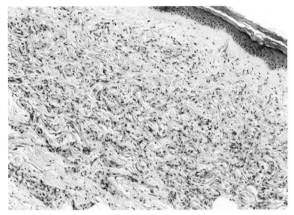

FIGURE 9.110   Reactive Angioendotheliomatosis-High Power

WARFARIN NECROSIS

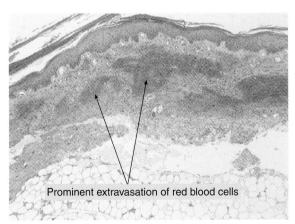

Prominent extravasation of red blood cells

FIGURE 9.111   Warfarin Necrosis

Warfarin necrosis usually develops between the third and the sixth day of warfarin therapy. Usually presents as painful well-circumscribed erythematous plaques. As the lesion progresses, large blood-filled blisters that breakdown accompanied by necrosis of the tissue are seen. Congenital deficiency of protein C and acquired or congenital deficiency of protein S may also be present.

On microscopy, the epidermal changes depend on the stage of the lesion. In majority of the cases, there is widespread extravasation of red blood cells. In advanced lesions subepidermal blistering is seen.

Adnexal Structures—Inflammatory and Neoplastic Diseases

INTRODUCTION

The adnexal or appendageal structures of skin include the folliculosebaceous apparatus, apocrine glands, and eccrine glands. The pathological entities involving hair follicles are dealt with in Chapter 13. The tumors of the adnexal structures far out number the inflammatory conditions, which is being described in this chapter.

COMEDONES

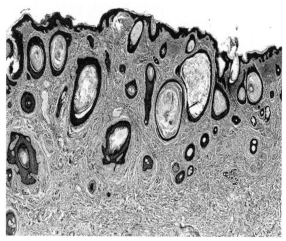

FIGURE 10.1   Comedones-Low Power

Comedonal nevus is an uncommon condition of pilosebaceous development and manifests as multiple comedones usually along the lines of Blaschko. Generally, they are arranged in a linear pattern unilaterally on the face and upper trunk. Association with other adnexal tumors such as hidradenoma papilliferum, syringocystadenoma papilliferum, and trichilemmal cysts has been documented.

On microscopy, the epidermis may be mildly acanthotic. Multiple cystically dilated hair follicles containing keratinous material are seen. Some of them open to the epidermal surface, but some are closed. The sebaceous glands may be normal or slightly reduced in number.

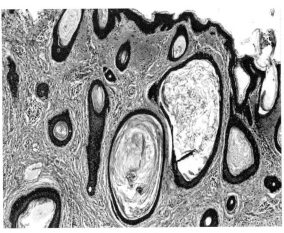

FIGURE 10.2   Comedones-High Power

DILATED PORE OF WINER

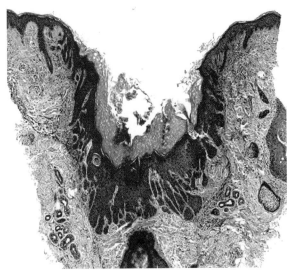

FIGURE 10.3   Dilated Pore of Winer

The dilated pore is a common lesion occurring in the head and neck area.

On microscopy, a cystically dilated follicle plugged with keratin is seen. The follicle is lined by acanthotic-stratified squamous epithelium. Numerous irregular projections of the squamous epithelium are seen extending to the adjacent dermis.

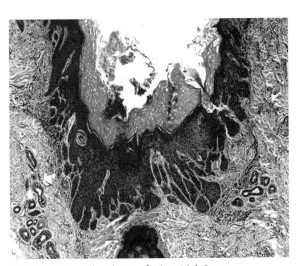

FIGURE 10.4   Dilated Pore of Winer-High Power

PILAR SHEATH ACANTHOMA

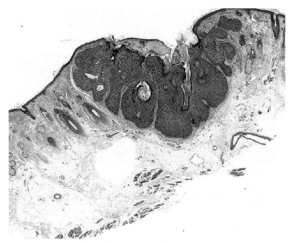

FIGURE 10.5   Pilar Sheath Acanthoma-Scanning View

Pilar sheath acanthoma is a benign nodule seen most commonly on the upper lip.

On microscopy, the typical appearance is that of cystic invagination of the epidermis into the underlying dermis, subcutaneous fat, or skeletal muscle. The involved epidermis is acanthotic and contains a granular layer. Many protrusions of the epidermis are seen extending to the periphery. The keratinization is that of infundibular type and keratocyst formation may be seen.

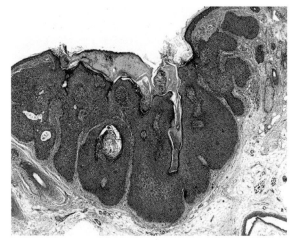

FIGURE 10.6   Pilar Sheath Acanthoma-Low Power

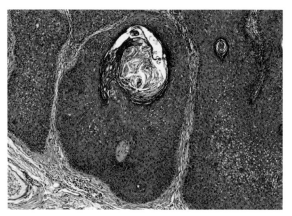

FIGURE 10.7   Pilar Sheath Acanthoma-High Power

TRICHOADENOMA

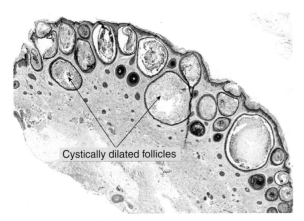

Cystically dilated follicles

FIGURE 10.8   Trichoadenoma-Low Power

Trichoadenoma is a benign tumor seen in the head and neck, upper extremities, and thighs as solitary firm or soft nodules. The tumor is considered to show differentiation toward infundibular part of the pilosebaceous unit.

On microscopy, the epidermis is normal. There are several dilated follicular infundibular structures containing keratinous material within the dermis. Some of them may be seen opening into the overlying epidermis. Mature hairs are not seen although very rarely vellus hairs may be seen. The stroma is fibrotic with scanty infiltration of lymphocytes.

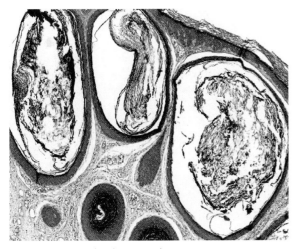

FIGURE 10.9   Trichoadenoma-High Power

TRICHILEMMOMA

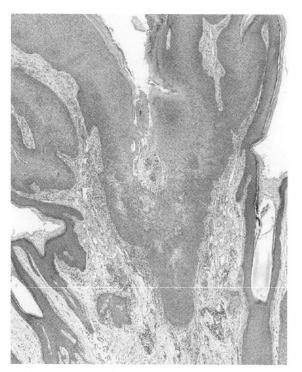

FIGURE 10.10   Tricholemmoma-Low Power

Trichilemmoma is a benign tumor, clinically presenting as solitary nodules on the face of elderly individuals. Uncommonly trichilemmomas present as multiple nodules when they are associated with Cowden's syndrome. The facial lesions are seen around the nose, mouth, and ears, and they may also be seen on the neck. Punctate and scaly keratoses of the palms and soles may also be seen. Cowden's syndrome is associated with carcinoma of the breast, thyroid, and endometrium and multiple gingival oral fibromas on the tongue and elsewhere in the oral cavity.

On microscopy, solitary trichilemmomas show proliferation of the outer root sheath. The tumor is seen in an endoexophytic pattern. The follicular epithelium grows down into the dermis as multiple lobules. The lobules show intensely eosinophilic hyaline material at the periphery. The cells exhibit peripheral nuclear palisading. The large part of the lobule is formed of cells with pale or clear cytoplasm and rounded or oval nuclei. Nuclear pleomorphism and mitotic activity are not seen. Duct formation is not a feature in this tumor, which is a helpful diagnostic clue in differentiating other adnexal tumors that may enter the differential diagnosis. The adjacent epidermis at the surface may show hyperkeratosis and focal parakeratosis.

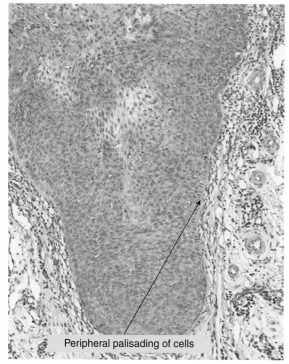

Peripheral palisading of cells

FIGURE 10.11   Tricholemmoma—The Base

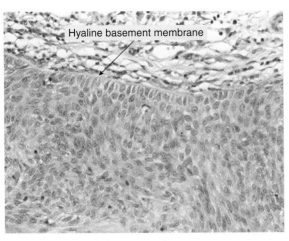

FIGURE 10.12   Tricholemmoma-High Power

DESMOPLASTIC TRICHILEMMOMA

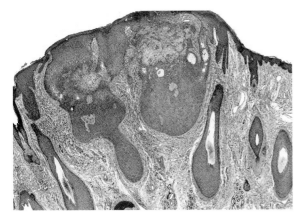

FIGURE 10.13   Desmoplastic Tricholemmoma-Low Power

Desmoplastic trichilemmoma is a variant of trichilemmoma seen more commonly in males. The lesions present as skin-colored nodules, and there is no association with Cowden's syndrome.

On microscopy, majority of the features are those of conventional trichilemmoma. However, the center of the tumor exhibits strands of follicular epithelial cells set in a fibrotic or desmoplastic stroma. This appearance can be easily confused with morpheic basal cell carcinoma or squamous cell carcinoma.

The conventional and desmoplastic trichilemmoma stain with cytokeratin and CD34. They do not stain with EMA (epithelial membrane antigen) or CEA (carcinoembryonic antigen).

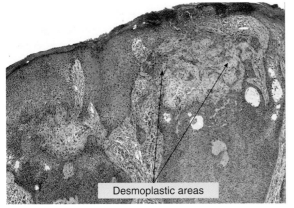

FIGURE 10.14   Desmoplastic Tricholemmoma-High Power

PROLIFERATING TRICHILEMMAL CYST

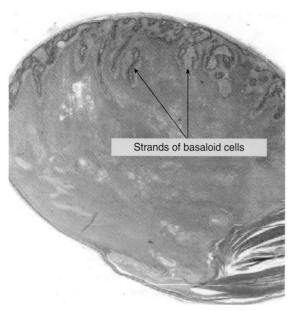

FIGURE 10.15 Proliferating Trichilemmal Cyst-Low Power

Proliferating trichilemmal cyst is a rare tumor seen on the scalp. They behave in a benign fashion in majority of the cases. Very rarely, these tumors are seen on other sites such as extremities and face. They are seen to develop within the wall of preexistent trichilemmal cyst. Clinically, they present as a multinodular tumor on the scalp, and they are usually multiple accompanied by usual trichilemmal cysts. They may invade the deeper structures and produce locally destructive symptoms.

On microscopy, proliferation of trichilemmal type of epithelium is seen. This is usually seen into the preexisting cyst. The proliferating strands lack a granular layer, and they exhibit peripheral palisading of the cells. Nuclear pleomorphism and mitotic activity are not seen. Squamous eddies may be seen. The cells may appear to be clear due to glycogen accumulation.

Malignant proliferating trichilemmal tumor shows frank features of malignancy such as nuclear pleomorphism, mitotic activity, and infiltration into the adjacent dermis. Reported cases are rare. These tumors tend to show loss of CD34 staining.

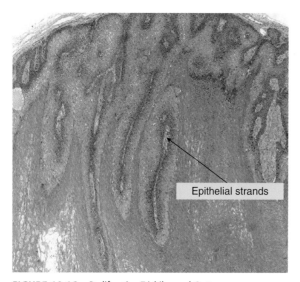

FIGURE 10.16 Proliferating Trichilemmal Cyst

PILOMATRIXOMA

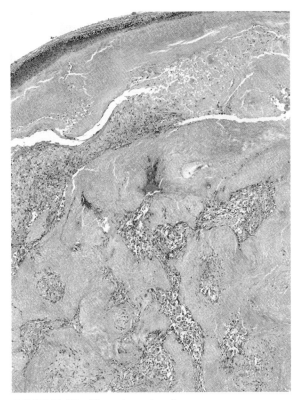

FIGURE 10.17   Pilomatrixoma-Low Power

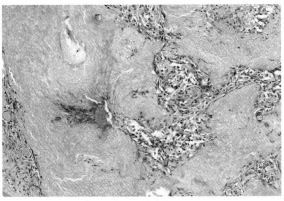

FIGURE 10.18   Pilomatrixoma-High Power

Pilomatrixoma also known as calcifying epithelioma of Malherbe is a benign tumor of follicular derivation. Clinically, they present as slow-growing firm nodules on various parts of the body with a predilection for the head and neck, trunk, and extremities. Calcification can be evident. Pilomatrixomas are commonly seen in young females. Beta-catenin and the Wnt-signaling pathway are said to be involved in the pathogenesis of pilomatrixoma.

On microscopy, pilomatrixoma exhibits features of hair matrix. The overlying epidermis may exhibit mild acanthosis. The tumor is located in the dermis and may extend to the subcutaneous fat. The tumor itself is multilobulated, and the individual lobules are composed of variable mixtures of basaloid cells and ghost cells. The basaloid cells are a prominent component in the early lesions. The cells have scanty cytoplasm and rounded or oval nuclei and exhibit brisk mitotic activity indicating rapid growth of the tumor. As the tumor matures, the basaloid cells acquire more cytoplasm and the nuclei become small and pyknotic. As the tumor evolves, the basaloid cells ultimately loose their nuclei and become ghost cells. Ghost cells appear as sheets of intensely eosinophilic keratinous debris with outlines of cells. Multinucleated giant cells and multiple foci of calcification may be seen. The keratinization in pilomatrixoma is of the trichilemmal type. Rarely in older individuals, the tumor may show predominance and pleomorphism of the basaloid cells with atypical mitotic activity. This is referred to as proliferating trichilemmal cyst.

Malignant pilomatrixoma is rare but documented. The tumor shows male predominance and can occur in any part of the body. The features that raise the possibility of malignant pilomatrixoma include large size (>4 cm), predominance of basaloid cells with nuclear pleomorphism, atypical mitotic activity, necrosis, infiltrative borders, and lymphatic or vascular invasion.

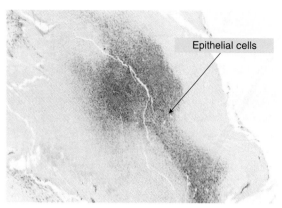

FIGURE 10.19   Pilomatrixoma—Epithelial Cells

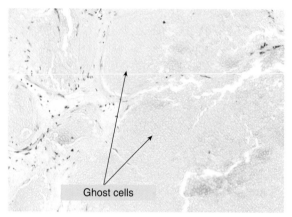

FIGURE 10.20   Ghost Cells in Pilomatrixoma

FOLLICULOCYSTIC SEBACEOUS HAMARTOMA

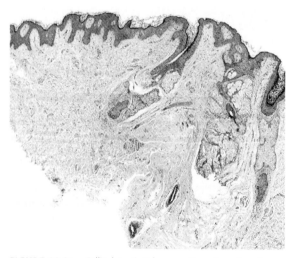

FIGURE 10.21   Folliculocystic Sebaceous Hamartoma-Low Power

Folliculocystic sebaceous hamartoma is a rare hamartomatous lesion formed of follicular, sebaceous, and mesenchymal elements. They are known to occur on the face, particularly around the nose.

On microscopy, the lesion is mainly dermal and very rarely an epidermal connection with a dilated follicular ostium is seen. Multiple small lobules of sebaceous glands are seen attached to the rudimentary follicles. Hair follicles in various stages of development are seen. The surrounding stroma may show fibroblastic proliferation. In addition, the stroma also shows variable prominence of collagen, elastic fibers, and adipose tissue and they form part of the tumor.

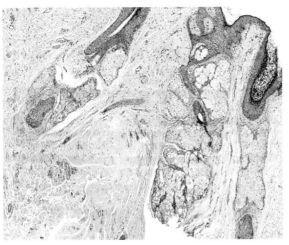

FIGURE 10.22   Folliculocystic Sebaceous Hamartoma-High Power

TRICHOEPITHELIOMA

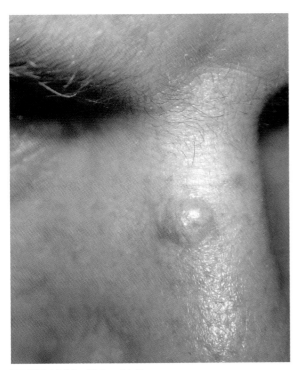

FIGURE 10.23   Trichoepithelioma

Trichoepithelioma may be solitary or multiple and may exhibit a familial tendency. Solitary trichoepitheliomas present as asymptomatic flesh-colored nodules on the face. Multiple trichoepitheliomas are seen in association with the autosomal dominant inherited Brooke-Spiegler syndrome (familial multiple cylindromatosis, spiradenomas, multiple trichoepitheliomas, and milia). The tumor suppressor gene *CYLD* has been identified as the candidate gene for Brooke-Spiegler syndrome, and the chromosomal abnormality has been identified to be the chromosome locus 16q12–13. The sonic hedgehog signaling pathway is known to be involved in the pathogenesis of solitary trichoepitheliomas. Similar to basal cell carcinomas, loss of heterozygosity of the patched gene (PTCH) has been documented in a small group of solitary trichoepitheliomas. The keratin expression of trichoepitheliomas is that of outer root sheath.

On microscopy, the epidermis may show mild hyperkeratosis. Majority of the tumors do not show any connection to the overlying epidermis and is strictly a dermal tumor. Lobules of basaloid cells of varying sizes are seen embedded in a fibroblastic stroma. The connective tissue around the primitive follicular structures condense giving rise to the papillary mesenchymal bodies. The cells have scanty cytoplasm and rounded or oval nuclei. They exhibit peripheral palisading and exhibit no nuclear pleomorphism. Occasional mitotic figures may be seen. Calcification and keratocyst formation are seen frequently.

The histological appearances raise the differential diagnosis of a basal cell carcinoma. The absence of connection to the overlying epidermis, absence of perilobular clefting, and absence of mucinous degeneration of the stroma are features that favor the diagnosis of trichoepithelioma. The presence of papillary mesenchymal bodies and keratocysts are additional features that support the diagnosis of trichoepithelioma. Immunohistochemical

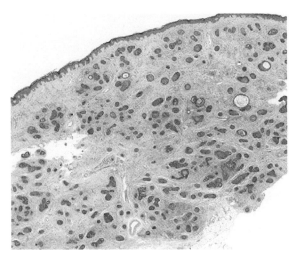

FIGURE 10.24   Trichoepithelioma-Low Power

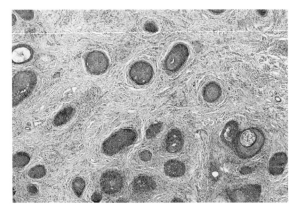

FIGURE 10.25   Trichoepithelioma-High Power

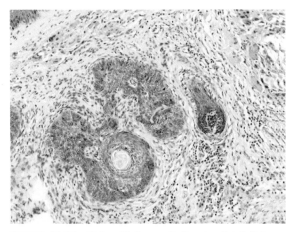

FIGURE 10.26   Trichoepithelioma—Rudimentary Hair Follicle

stains have only a very limited role in differentiating the two entities. CD34 stains the stromal cells in trichoepitheliomas but not in basal cell carcinomas. Bcl2 shows a peripheral pattern of staining in trichoepitheliomas, but diffusely throughout the lobule in basal cell carcinoma. CD15 decorates most of the lobules of trichoepitheliomas, but shows absent staining in basal cell carcinomas.

The clinical appearances are of paramount importance in deciding the final diagnosis. If the lesion is solitary and the patient is of older age group, it is best to treat the lesion as a basal cell carcinoma as none of the above mentioned features are helpful in the final diagnosis.

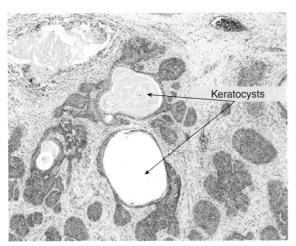

FIGURE 10.27   Trichoepithelioma—Keratocysts

DESMOPLASTIC TRICHOEPITHELIOMA

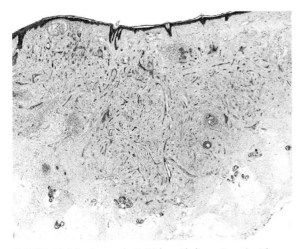

FIGURE 10.28   Desmoplastic Trichoepithelioma-Scanning View

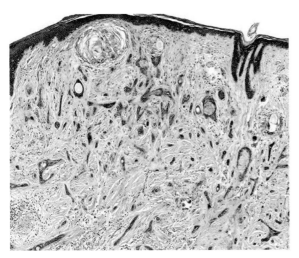

FIGURE 10.29   Desmoplastic Trichoepithelioma—Keratocysts

Desmoplastic trichoepithelioma presents as solitary slowly growing, firm 3–8 mm skin-colored to white annular lesion with a raised edge on the face or neck of young adults. Milia may be present on the raised edge of the lesion. It tends to show a predilection for females. Rarely multiple desmoplastic trichoepitheliomas may occur.

On microscopy, unlike conventional trichoepitheliomas, desmoplastic trichoepitheliomas show strands of basaloid cells in a fibroblastic stroma accompanied by keratocysts. The epidermis is generally uninvolved. The tumor involves the dermis and superficial subcutaneous fat. The tumor is composed of thin strands of small cuboidal cells. Nuclear pleomorphism and mitotic activity are not seen. The cells do not exhibit peripheral palisading. Keratocysts lined by similar cuboidal cells is a constant feature. Occasionally, the keratocysts may be lined by squamous epithelial cells. The stroma also shows many Merkel cells. Perineural invasion is never seen in desmoplastic trichoepithelioma.

The morphological appearances raise the differential diagnosis of morphoeic basal cell carcinoma, microcystic adnexal carcinoma, and syringoma. Keratocysts are absent in morphoeic basal cell carcinoma. This feature together with the absence of nuclear palisading and mitotic activity helps to differentiate between the two entities. Merkel cells in the stroma are an additional supporting feature in favor of desmoplastic trichoepitheliomas. Microcystic adnexal carcinoma and syringoma can be confirmed by the presence of duct formation, which is absent in follicular-derived desmoplastic trichoepithelioma. The duct formation can be demonstrated by immunohistochemical stains such as EMA and CEA.

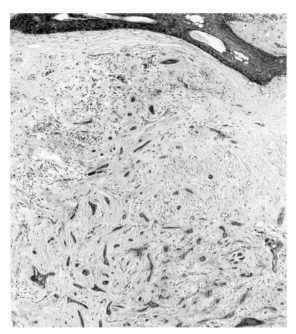

FIGURE 10.30   Desmoplastic Trichoepithelioma—Periphery

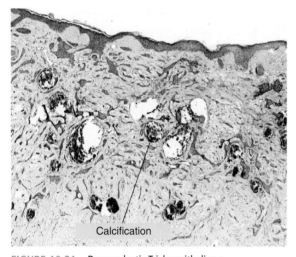

FIGURE 10.31   Desmoplastic Trichoepithelioma

GIANT SOLITARY TRICHOBLASTOMA

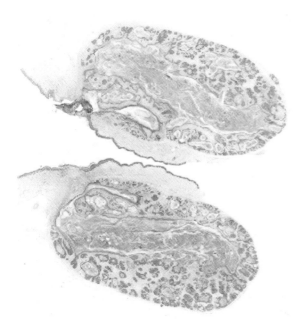

FIGURE 10.32   Giant Solitary Trichoblastoma

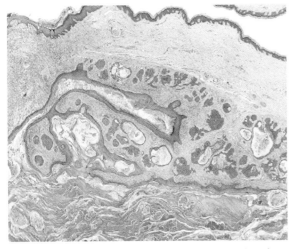

FIGURE 10.33   Giant Solitary Trichoblastoma-Scanning View

Trichoblastomas are benign tumors originating from the germinative cells of the hair bulb. Clinically, they present as solitary slowly growing nodules that can acquire size up to 10 cm, hence the designation giant trichoblastoma. Trichoblastomas have a predilection for the head and neck area, but they are seen also in the perianal region and the buttock, particularly the giant variant.

On microscopy, the tumor is entirely dermal and usually well circumscribed and is composed of lobules of basaloid cells exhibiting peripheral palisading. Unlike basal cell carcinoma, perilobular clefting is not a feature. The stroma surrounding the lobules is very fibrotic and it tends to show perilobular condensation. The cells have scanty cytoplasm and rounded or oval nuclei with brisk mitotic activity. Atypical mitoses are not a feature. Clear cell change may be seen.

Basal cell carcinoma and conventional trichoepithelioma are the two entities that enter the differential diagnosis. The dermal location of the tumor and the absence of myxoid stroma should favor trichoblastoma over basal cell carcinoma. It can be difficult to differentiate trichoblastoma from conventional trichoepithelioma, particularly on a small biopsy. Wide excision of the lesion is the safest option from the treatment point of view.

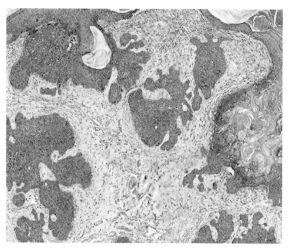

FIGURE 10.34   Giant Solitary Trichoblastoma-High Power

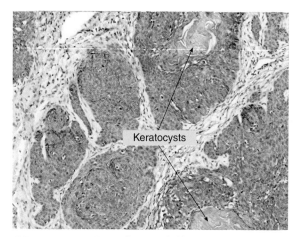

FIGURE 10.35   Giant Solitary Trichoblastoma—Keratocysts

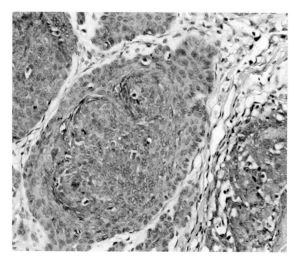

FIGURE 10.36   Giant Solitary Trichoblastoma

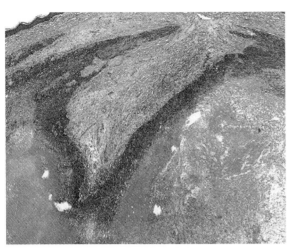

FIGURE 10.37   Trichoblastoma-Low Power

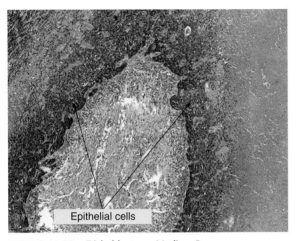

Epithelial cells

FIGURE 10.38   Trichoblastoma-Medium Power

CUTANEOUS LYMPHADENOMA

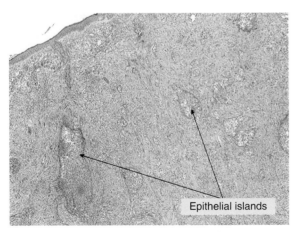

Epithelial islands

FIGURE 10.39   Cutaneous Lymphadenoma-Low Power

Cutaneous lymphadenoma is also known as lymphoepithelial tumor of skin. Clinically, it presents as a slow-growing skin-colored nodule most commonly on the head and neck area. It clinically resembles nodular basal cell carcinoma. The histogenesis of cutaneous lymphadenoma is controversial with views that this could be a variant of trichoblastoma with adenomatoid differentiation.

On microscopy, cutaneous lymphadenoma is a primarily dermal tumor that may extend into the subcutaneous fat. The tumor itself is composed of islands of epithelial cells embedded in a fibroblastic stroma containing large numbers of small mature lymphocytes. The epithelial islands show peripheral rimming by one or more layers of basaloid cells. The islands are formed of cells with clear glycogen-rich cytoplasm and central nuclei. Mitotic activity is not seen. Merkel cells positive for CK20 and S100 positive dendritic cells are seen within the stroma and within the islands.

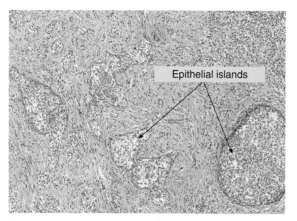

FIGURE 10.40   Cutaneous Lymphadenoma-High Power

SEBACEOUS HYPERPLASIA

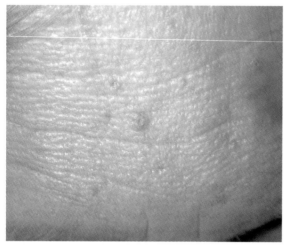

FIGURE 10.41   Sebaceous Hyperplasia

Sebaceous hyperplasia is a very common condition seen on the face and cheek of elderly men. Less commonly, it may occur at other sites and in females and children. Clinically, they are seen as small 1–2 mm dome-shaped, umbilicated, yellowish papules often on the background of chronically sun damaged skin.

On microscopy, there is proliferation of sebaceous glands draining by a single duct to a dilated follicle. The intervening dermis may show some solar elastosis.

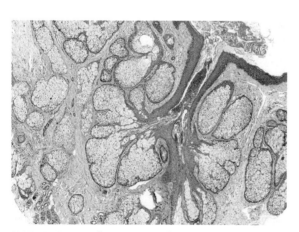

FIGURE 10.42   Sebaceous Hyperplasia-Low Power

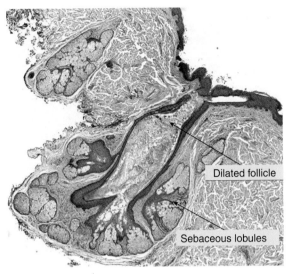

FIGURE 10.43   Sebaceous Hyperplasia-Low Power

BASAL CELL CARCINOMA ARISING IN THE BACKGROUND OF SEBACEOUS NEVUS

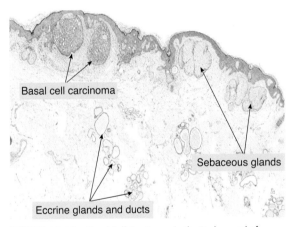

FIGURE 10.44   Basal Cell Carcinoma in the Background of Sebaceous Nevus

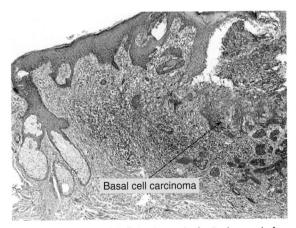

FIGURE 10.45   Basal Cell Carcinoma in the Background of Sebaceous Nevus

Sebaceous nevus (nevus sebaceous of Jadassohn or organoid nevus) is not an uncommon lesion. It is usually present at birth but can manifest at a later age. Clinically, it presents as a well-circumscribed rounded lesion. Some of them may have a yellow cerebriform appearance. Alopecia is known to develop secondary to sebaceous nevus. The lesions are commonly seen in the head and neck area especially the scalp. Very rarely, oral cavity and peri-anal area may be involved. Sebaceous nevus is associated with many other syndromes and extracutaneous manifestations (sebaceous nevus syndrome). There is possibly 5% risk of malignant transformation in adulthood to basal carcinoma but various other appendageal tumors including syringocystadenoma papilliferum and trichoblastoma may develop.

On microscopy, the epidermis is acanthotic or papillomatous. Many primitive hair follicles are seen attached to the epidermis. The sebaceous glands may show hyperplastic changes or may be abortive. They are seen to drain to the infundibular part of the follicle, high up in the dermis, some of them draining directly into the epidermis. Sebaceous glands are increased in number. Marked reduction in the number of hair follicles is noted and some of the follicles may be atrophic. The eccrine glands and ducts are also increased in number and seen higher up in the papillary dermis. Sebaceous nevus is seen in association with many other benign and malignant tumors particularly basal cell carcinoma, which is the commonest malignant tumor arising in the background of nevus sebaceous.

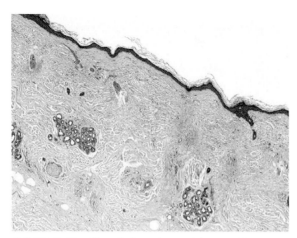

FIGURE 10.46   Alopecia Secondary to Sebaceous Nevus

SEBACEOUS ADENOMA

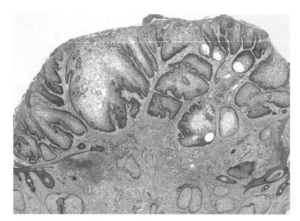

FIGURE 10.47   Sebaceous Adenoma

Sebaceous adenoma represents the benign end of the spectrum of neoplastic changes in sebaceous glands. Clinically, it presents as a yellow-red dome-shaped nodule in the head and neck area preferentially. They are most often misdiagnosed clinically as basal cell carcinomas. Sebaceous adenomas are associated with Muir-Torre syndrome. A variety of changes are seen in sebaceous glands ranging from benign to malignant sebaceous tumors in Muir-Torre syndrome.

On microscopy, the tumor is multilobulated and shows proliferation of lobules of sebaceous glands in a haphazard pattern. The lobules are separated by a thin fibrous capsule. The basaloid germinative cells are seen at the periphery and are more than one to two layers thick but do not occupy the majority of the lobule.

SEBACEOMA

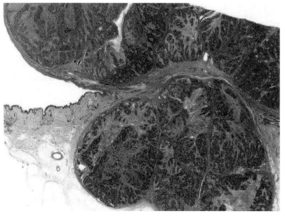

FIGURE 10.48   Sebaceoma-Scanning View

Clinically, sebaceoma has a predilection for females and presents as skin-colored papules on the head and neck area. It is also seen in association with Muir-Torre syndrome.

On microscopy, the tumor is predominantly dermal with epidermal attachment seen in a small number of cases. The tumor itself is composed of lobules of sebocytes but with marked predominance of basaloid cells, almost occupying the entire lobule in some cases. The lobules merge with one another, but the periphery is well preserved with no infiltration into the adjacent dermis. There is no peripheral palisading of cells. The basaloid cells are small with scanty cytoplasm and vesicular nuclei. Mitotic figures are rarely seen and nuclear pleomorphism is not a feature.

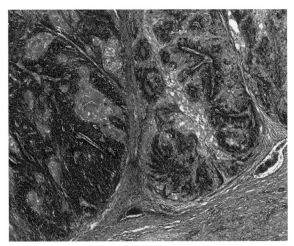

FIGURE 10.49   Sebaceoma-Medium Power

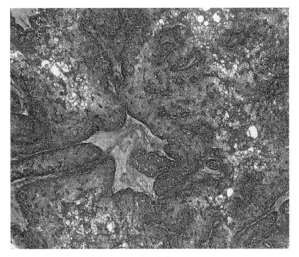

FIGURE 10.50   Sebaceoma-High Power

SEBACEOUS CARCINOMA

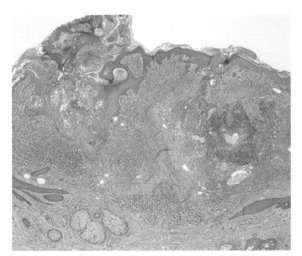

FIGURE 10.51   Sebaceous Carcinoma-Low Power

Sebaceous adenoma enters the differential diagnosis but can be distinguished by the well-maintained lobular architecture and lack of predominance of basaloid cells in sebaceous adenoma. Sebaceous carcinoma can be differentiated by the infiltrative nature and necrosis seen in sebaceous carcinoma. Basal cell carcinoma with sebaceous differentiation can be differentiated by the presence of cleft formation and mucinous stroma in basal cell carcinoma.

Sebaceous carcinoma is a very rare tumor. There are two variants described. The more aggressive form occurs in a periocular location. Tumors in the extraocular location are also known to recur and metastasize. The periocular sebaceous carcinoma is known to arise from the adnexal glands within and around the eyelids such as meibomian glands and the glands of Zeiss. Clinically, sebaceous carcinoma is commonly mistaken for basal cell carcinoma or squamous cell carcinoma. The periocular tumors invade locally and intracranial extension has been reported. Metastasis to regional lymph nodes and to visceral organs such as lung, bone, brain, and liver has been documented.

On microscopy, the tumor cells are arranged in sheets and large islands with focal attachment to the overlying epidermis. In the periocular variant, the cells might even exhibit Pagetoid spread into the overlying epidermis. The tumor cells loose the lobular architecture. Basaloid cells predominate and the cells exhibit marked nuclear atypia. Many mitotic figures including

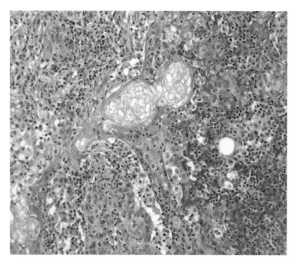

atypical mitoses are seen. Foci of necrosis are identified. Lymphovascular and perineural invasion is documented. Sebaceous differentiation is not readily identified but could be demonstrated by staining with epithelial membrane antigen (EMA).

Sebaceous carcinoma is a very aggressive tumor, and the indicators of poor prognosis include size larger than 1 cm, vascular or lymphatic involvement, periocular location, and poor differentiation of the tumor with nearly absent clear cell change.

FIGURE 10.52   Sebaceous Carcinoma-High Power

APOCRINE HIDROCYSTOMA

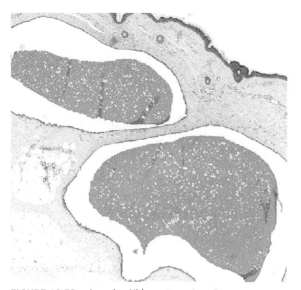

Apocrine hidrocystoma is an uncommon cystic lesion found in the head and neck area of middle-aged and elderly females. It also occurs in areas where apocrine glands are normally seen such as axilla and the genital area. Clinically, it presents as a dome-shaped translucent nodule. Some of them can attain big size up to 5 cm.

On microscopy, apocrine hidrocystoma shows unilocular or multilocular cystic spaces within the dermis. The cysts are lined by double layer of cells. The outer layer is composed of flattened myoepithelial cells and an inner layer of columnar cells with abundant eosinophilic cytoplasm and a nucleus located at the base. Projections of the secretions into the luminal surface of the cells referred to as apocrine snouts are commonly seen. These cells eliminate the apocrine decapitation secretions into the lumen of the cysts. The apocrine cells express specific keratins on immunohistochemical staining. The apocrine keratins are K7, K8, and K18.

FIGURE 10.53   Apocrine Hidrocystoma-Low Power

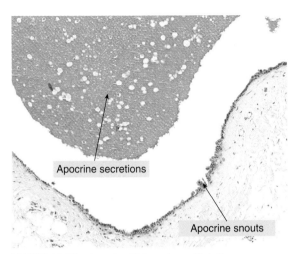

FIGURE 10.54   Apocrine Hidrocystoma-High Power

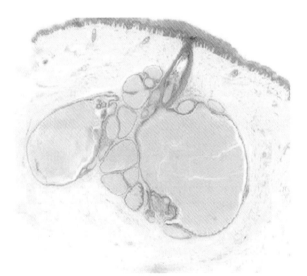

FIGURE 10.55   Apocrine Hidrocystoma-Scanning View

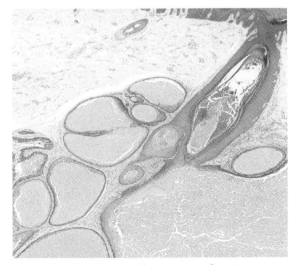

FIGURE 10.56   Apocrine Hidrocystoma-Medium Power

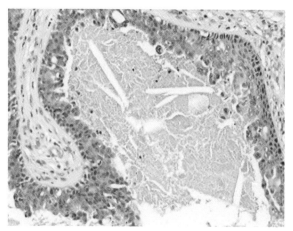

FIGURE 10.57 Apocrine Hidrocystoma-Closer View

TUBULAR APOCRINE ADENOMA

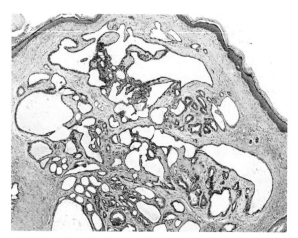

FIGURE 10.58 Tubular Apocrine Adenoma-Scanning View

Tubular apocrine adenoma, also known as apocrine adenoma and tubulopapillary hidradenoma is a rare benign tumor of the apocrine glands. The tumor is most commonly seen on the scalp, although other sites such as face, axillae, and the genitalia could be involved. The tumor presents as a dome-shaped nodule and could be longstanding particularly in the ones associated with nevus sebaceous.

On microscopy, the tumor is circumscribed and purely dermal in majority of the cases. Very rarely, subcutaneous fat may be involved. The tumor is composed of papillary or tubular structures lined by double layer of cells. The outer layer is composed of flattened cuboidal cells, and the inner layer is columnar cells exhibiting the apocrine secretions. The cells may show mild nuclear pleomorphism. Mitotic activity is very scanty. The luminal cells of apocrine adenoma shows positive staining with EMA and CEA. The myoepithelial cells are positive for smooth muscle actin and S100. The surrounding dermis and subcutaneous fat may show features of mild chronic inflammation.

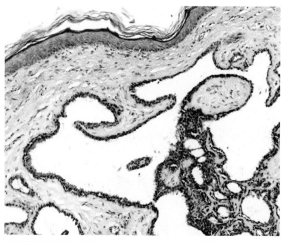

FIGURE 10.59 Tubular Apocrine Adenoma-High Power

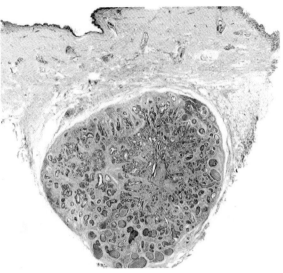

FIGURE 10.60   Tubular Apocrine Adenoma-Scanning View

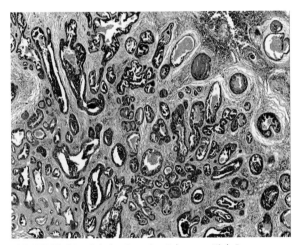

FIGURE 10.61   Tubular Apocrine Adenoma-High Power

APOCRINE CARCINOMA

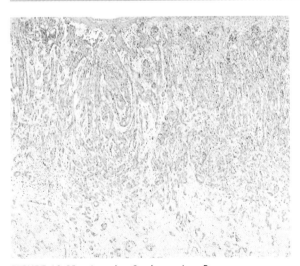

FIGURE 10.62   Apocrine Carcinoma-Low Power

Apocrine carcinoma is a rare malignant tumor of the apocrine glands. The tumor is most commonly seen in the axilla. Occasionally, they may be seen on the scalp, eyelid, ear, and anogenital region. Clinically, the tumor presents as single or multiple small cysts or nodules and would have been present for a long time. Very rarely, they are ulcerated.

On microscopy, apocrine carcinomas show a dermal tumor diffusely infiltrating into the subcutaneous fat. The tumor cells are arranged as strands and in an adenomatous pattern. The cells have abundant eosinophilic cytoplasm and rounded and vesicular nuclei. The cells exhibit nuclear pleomorphism, and mitotic activity is frequently seen. Apocrine secretions are seen in the tumor cells, and normal and hyperplastic apocrine glands are usually seen in the vicinity of the tumor. The tumor cells are positive for cytokeratins. The myoepithelial cells are lost and hence the tumor lobules show negative staining with smooth muscle actin.

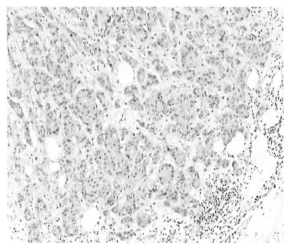

Metastatic apocrine carcinoma from the breast is the closest differential diagnosis, which is impossible to differentiate on histological grounds alone. Clinical and radiological examination of the breast is indicated to exclude this possibility.

FIGURE 10.63   Apocrine Carcinoma-High Power

ECCRINE HIDROCYSTOMA

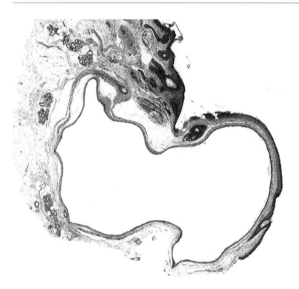

Eccrine hidrocystoma is a common tumor seen in adults. Clinically, they present as tense cystic structures on the face particularly in a periocular location. They may also be seen in the axilla and the anogenital region. Large majority of the lesions are solitary, but they may occasionally be multiple.

On microscopy, eccrine hidrocystoma is dermal and is composed of a cystic structure lined by double layer of cuboidal cells. A hyalinized band composed of basement membrane substance is seen beneath the lining cells. Most often a connection with the neighboring eccrine duct can be established.

FIGURE 10.64   Eccrine Hidrocystoma-Low Power

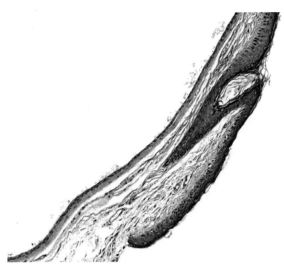

FIGURE 10.65   Eccrine Hidrocystoma-High Power—Flattened
Eccrine Lining

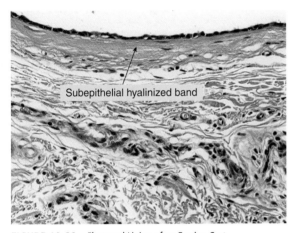

Subepithelial hyalinized band

FIGURE 10.66   Flattened Lining of an Eccrine Cyst

ECCRINE POROMA

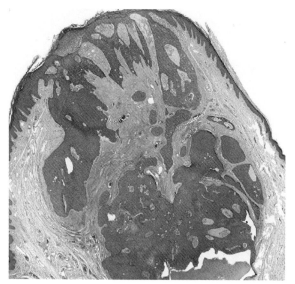

FIGURE 10.67 Eccrine Poroma-Low Power

Eccrine poroma is a benign adnexal tumor. They present as pink- to red-colored nodules most commonly on the sole or sides of the feet.

On microscopy, the tumor is considered to arise from the outer layer of the acrosyringeal part of the eccrine duct. The tumor grows down from the epidermis as broad bands into the underlying dermis. The cells forming the tumor are cuboidal and smaller than the keratinocytes of the adjacent epidermis. Duct formation is a conspicuous diagnostic feature. There is no nuclear pleomorphism, mitotic activity, or peripheral palisading of cells.

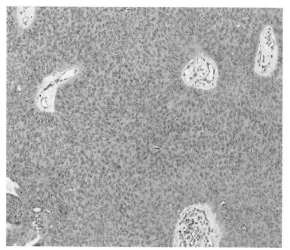

FIGURE 10.68 Eccrine Poroma-Medium Power

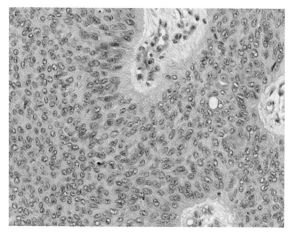

FIGURE 10.69 Eccrine Poroma-High Power

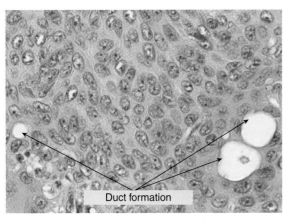

FIGURE 10.70   Eccrine Poroma—Duct Formation

DERMAL DUCT TUMOR

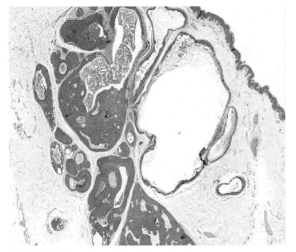

FIGURE 10.71   Dermal Duct Tumor-Low Power

Dermal duct tumor presents as skin-colored nodules on the head and neck and lower extremities with an elderly female predominance.

On microscopy, the tumor is entirely dermal and arises from the dermal part of the eccrine duct. The pattern of arrangement and the cells forming the tumor are exactly the same as eccrine poroma. Nuclear pleomorphism and mitotic activity are not seen. Duct formation is readily identified.

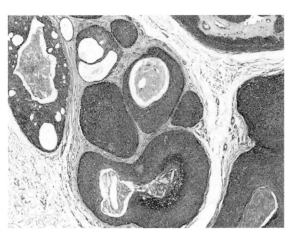

FIGURE 10.72   Dermal Duct Tumor-Medium Power

ECCRINE POROCARCINOMA

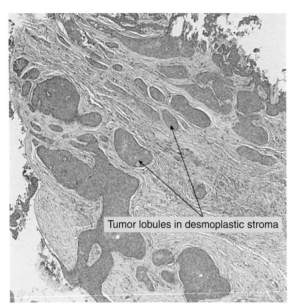

FIGURE 10.73 Eccrine Porocarcinoma-Low Power

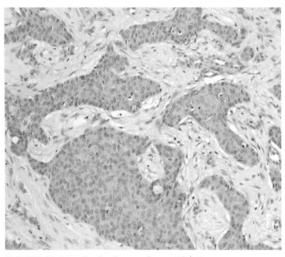

FIGURE 10.74 Eccrine Porocarcinoma-High Power

Eccrine porocarcinoma or malignant eccrine poroma is the commonest malignant adnexal tumor. Clinically, it is more commonly seen in elderly females and presents as polypoid or verrucous nodules and plaques. Ulceration may be seen. The tumor can present on any cutaneous site, but there is a predilection for lower extremities. Usually, there is a history of longstanding nodule, suggesting malignant transformation in a benign poroma.

On microscopy, a benign poroma is identified in only a very small percentage of tumors. There may be an in situ component with the malignant poroma cells amongst the keratinocytes of the epidermis. Duct formation is identified in the in situ component. The invasive part of the tumor may show a broad pushing margin or an infiltrative pattern where thin strands and lobules of tumor are seen in a desmoplastic stroma. There are two histological patterns of eccrine porocarcinoma. In one of the variants, the tumor is arranged in strands and as small islands infiltrating the surrounding desmoplastic stroma. Nuclear pleomorphism and mitotic activity are not conspicuously seen. The infiltrative nature of the tumor is the diagnostic clue. In the second variant, in addition to the infiltrative pattern, there is marked nuclear pleomorphism and mitotic activity. Tumor necrosis is seen. The presence of duct formation helps in confirming the diagnosis of a porocarcinoma. Ductal differentiation can be confirmed by the Periodic acid Schiff (PAS) stain or immunohistochemical markers such as EMA and CEA. Other histological variants such as eccrine porocarcinoma with clear cell change and squamous differentiation have also been reported.

SYRINGOMA

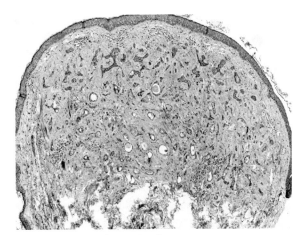

FIGURE 10.75   Syringoma-Low Power

Syringoma is a common benign tumor of eccrine derivation. Syringomas usually present as multiple firm skin-colored papules. They occur in a variety of cutaneous sites in the body, but most characteristically occur on the lower eyelids and cheeks, often in a symmetrical distribution. They occur more commonly in Asian races.

On microscopy, syringomas are located in the upper dermis and are formed of interconnecting strands of double-layered cuboidal cells set in a fibrous stroma. The cells are also arranged in a tadpole configuration around a cuticle. Some of these epithelial lined structures have a lumina containing keratinous debris. Clear cell change of the epithelial cells is seen in the variant described as clear cell syringoma.

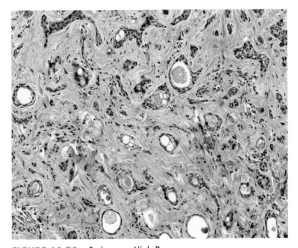

FIGURE 10.76   Syringoma-High Power

HIDRADENOMA PAPILLIFERUM

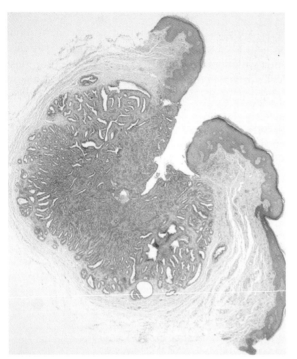

FIGURE 10.77   Hidradenoma Papilliferum-Low Power

Hidradenoma papilliferum is a benign adnexal tumor exclusive to young and middle-aged females. Clinically, the tumor presents as dome-shaped papules in the vulval region (usually the labia majora) and perianal areas. Very rarely, the papules may be umbilicated or ulcerated.

On microscopy, hidradenoma papilliferum is known to arise from the eccrine glands, apocrine glands, or anogenital mammary-like glands. The epidermis may be ulcerated or acanthotic. The tumor may show continuation with the overlying epidermis, but in majority of the cases it is a well-demarcated dermal nodule. This is lined by a fibrous capsule. The cells are lined along papillary structures, and they project cystic spaces. The papillae are lined by double layers of cells. The inner layer is the flattened cuboidal myoepithelial cells. The luminal cells are either of the apocrine type with decapitation secretions or the eccrine type with rounded or oval nuclei and scanty cytoplasm. Malignant change in a hidradenoma papilliferum is extremely rare.

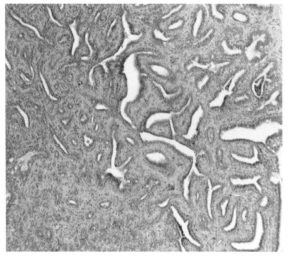

FIGURE 10.78   Hidradenoma Papilliferum-Medium Power

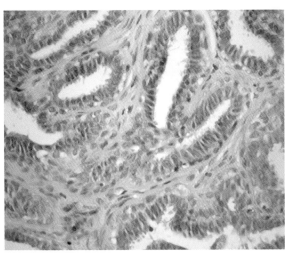

FIGURE 10.79   Hidradenoma Papilliferum-High Power

SYRINGOCYSTADENOMA PAPILLIFERUM

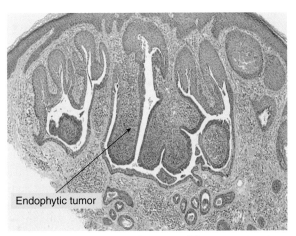

Endophytic tumor

FIGURE 10.80   Syringocystadenoma Papilliferum-Scanning View

Syringocystadenoma papilliferum is a benign tumor most commonly seen on the head and neck area. Less than one third of the cases are associated with an organoid (sebaceous) nevus, and 10% are associated with a basal cell carcinoma. Clinically, the tumor presents as raised warty nodule or plaque.

On microscopy, there are duct-like structures seen growing down from the surface epithelium. In the dermal part of the tumor, they are lined by double-layered columnar and cuboidal epithelium. The superficial part of the tumor may be lined by squamous epithelium. The ductular proliferations may lead to cystic structures lined by double-layered epithelium. The surrounding stroma may contain numerous plasma cells and some lymphocytes. CEA is present in these cells. Published literature suggests origin from eccrine and apocrine cells. Malignant variant called syringocystadenocarcinoma papilliferum has been reported.

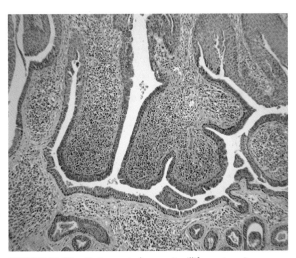

FIGURE 10.81   Syringocystadenoma Papilliferum-Low Power

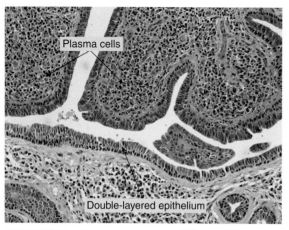

FIGURE 10.82   Syringocystadenoma Papilliferum-High Power

AGGRESSIVE DIGITAL PAPILLARY ADENOCARCINOMA

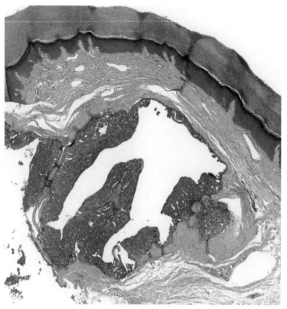

FIGURE 10.83   Aggressive Digital Papillary Adenocarcinoma-
Scanning View

Aggressive digital papillary adenocarcinoma is the preferred term for this locally aggressive, rarely metastasizing tumor. They are rare tumors and exhibit a range of clinical and histological features. Clinically, they present as painful nodules and masses on the digits or the volar aspect of the fingertip. They are also seen on the palms and soles. Very commonly the tumor is painful.

On microscopy, aggressive digital papillary adenocarcinoma is located in the deep dermis and subcutaneous fat and may invade the muscle, tendon, and bone. The tumor characteristically is composed of papillary and adenomatous structures. They are lined by columnar cells with eosinophilic cytoplasm and in places by apocrine type cells with decapitation secretions. The epithelial cell show staining with cytokeratin and S100 protein.

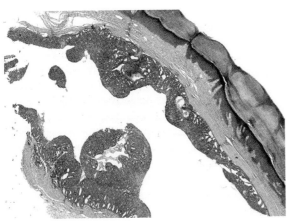

FIGURE 10.84   Aggressive Digital Papillary Adenocarcinoma-Low Power

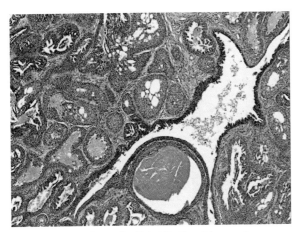

FIGURE 10.85   Aggressive Digital Papillary Adenocarcinoma-Closer View

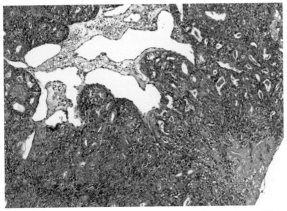

FIGURE 10.86   Aggressive Digital Papillary Adenocarcinoma-High Power

CYSTIC ECCRINE CLEAR CELL HIDRADENOMA

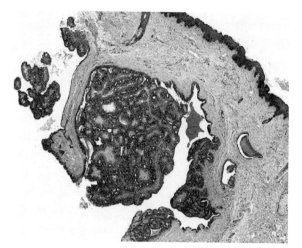

FIGURE 10.87   Cystic Eccrine Clear Cell Hidradenoma-Low Power

Clear cell hidradenoma presents as a slow-growing painless flesh-colored nodule that can occur on almost any part of the body.

On microscopy, solid and cystic variants are identified. The tumor has mixed apocrine and eccrine derivation. It is a circumscribed but nonencapsulated tumor. Two types of cells are identified in hidradenomas. A large majority of the tumors have cells with rounded or oval nuclei and scanty cytoplasm. The second population of cells have pale or clear cytoplasm and vesicular nuclei. The proportion of the two cell types can vary in individual tumors. Nuclear pleomorphism, mitotic activity, and tumor necrosis are not seen. Duct formation within the tumor is readily identified. Squamous metaplasia and areas of mucin-rich goblet cells are seen. Nuclear pleomorphism, macronucleoli, and mitotic activity more than 2 per 10 high-power fields are features of atypical behavior.

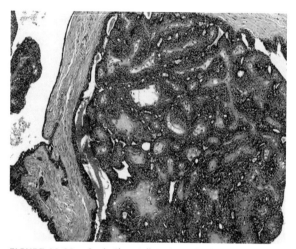

FIGURE 10.88   Cystic Clear Cell Eccrine Hidradenoma-High Power

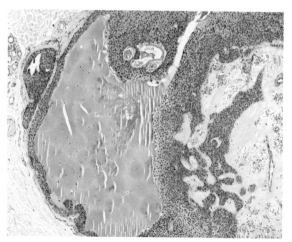

FIGURE 10.89   Clear Cell Hidradenoma-Low Power

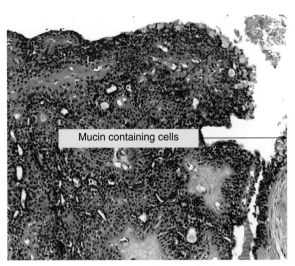

FIGURE 10.90   Mucinous Metaplasia in Hidradenoma

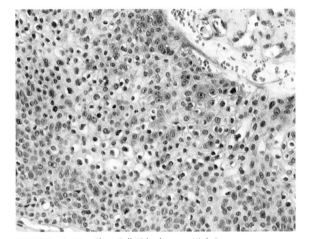

FIGURE 10.91   Clear Cell Hidradenoma-High Power

HIDRADENOCARCINOMA

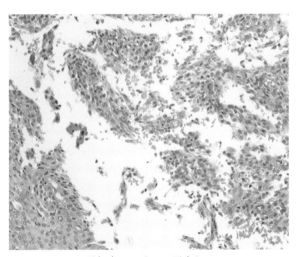

FIGURE 10.92   Hidradenocarcinoma-High Power

Hidradenocarcinoma is a very rare tumor occurring over a wide variety of cutaneous sites.

On microscopy, the tumor is purely dermal and infiltration into the adjacent stroma is easily identified. The cells may exhibit clear cell change and squamous differentiation is noted. There is brisk mitotic activity and atypical mitoses are seen. Foci of necrosis are identified. Ductal differentiation is an important diagnostic clue as many other malignant tumors with clear cell differentiation enter the differential diagnosis such as clear cell squamous carcinoma, clear cell melanoma, and metastatic clear cell carcinoma from other locations. Immunohistochemical stains, detailed clinical history, and other investigations may be needed to confirm the diagnosis.

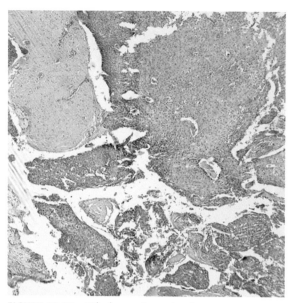

FIGURE 10.93   Hidradenocarcinoma-Low Power

BROOKE-SPIEGLER SYNDROME

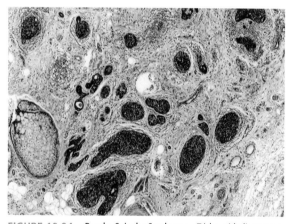

FIGURE 10.94   Brooke-Spiegler Syndrome—Trichoepitheliomatous Areas

Brooke-Spiegler is an autosomal dominant syndrome characterized by multiple trichoepitheliomas, multiple cylindromas, eccrine spiradenomas, and milia. These tumors may occur in isolation or in various different combinations. The syndrome has a predilection for females and the penetrance is high.

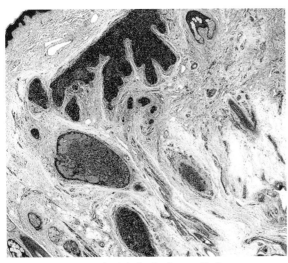

FIGURE 10.95   Brooke-Spiegler Syndrome—Rudimentary
Cylindroma

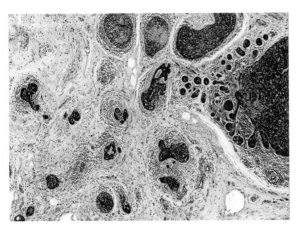

FIGURE 10.96   Brooke-Spiegler Syndrome—Multiple
Cylindromatous Foci

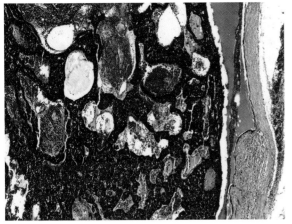

FIGURE 10.97   Brooke-Spiegler Syndrome—Eccrine Spiradenoma

CYLINDROMA

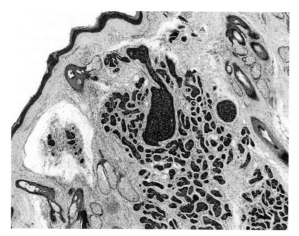

FIGURE 10.98   Cylindroma-Low Power

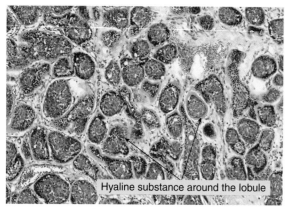

Hyaline substance around the lobule

FIGURE 10.99   Cylindroma-Medium Power

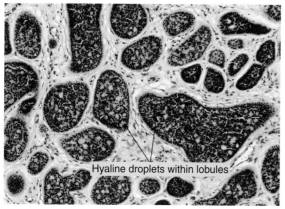

Hyaline droplets within lobules

FIGURE 10.100   Cylindroma-High Power

Cylindroma is a relatively common benign adnexal tumor that occurs in the head and neck area predominantly. Other unusual sites include abdomen and breast. Clinically, cylindromas present as flesh-colored or pink nodules. Multiple cylindromas are seen in Brooke-Spiegler syndrome, which is also referred to as turban tumor syndrome. Rare associations of the tumor include basal cell adenomas of the parotid gland.

On microscopy, cylindromas are dermal tumors. They characteristically show irregular lobules of basaloid cells arranged in a jigsaw pattern. The lobules are formed of small cells with scanty cytoplasm at the periphery and larger cells with pale cytoplasm in the center. The periphery of the lobules shows eosinophilic hyaline substance, which is PAS positive. Such hyaline droplets are also seen within the lobules in varying numbers. The lobules stain positive for CEA. Occasionally, cylindromas are seen in combination with eccrine spiradenomas, and they are then referred to as spiradenocylindromas. Cylindromas have been genetically linked to *CYLD* gene, which is a tumor suppressor gene. Malignant change in a cylindroma is extremely rare. The diagnosis can be made only when a transition from a benign cylindroma can be identified. There is loss of the jigsaw architecture, the hyaline droplets. The cells exhibit marked nuclear pleomorphism with prominent mitotic activity.

GIANT ECCRINE SPIRADENOMA

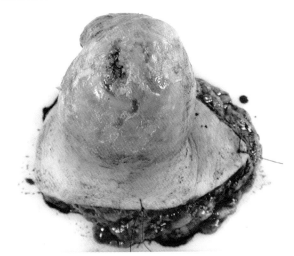

FIGURE 10.101   Giant Eccrine Spiradenoma-Macroscopic View

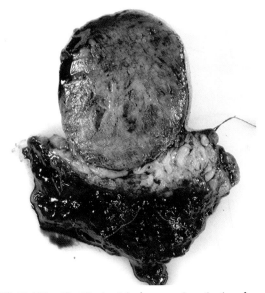

FIGURE 10.102   Giant Eccrine Spiradenoma—Cross Section of the Tumor

Eccrine spiradenoma is a benign adnexal tumor of the eccrine glands. Clinically, it is characteristically painful or tender small solitary nodule with bluish overlying skin. Eccrine spiradenoma can present on any anatomical site, the commonest being the head and neck. Giant and multiple forms have also been documented.

On microscopy, eccrine spiradenoma is a well-circumscribed and encapsulated dermal tumor extending into the subcutaneous fat. The overlying epidermis is uninvolved and normal. The tumor is composed of lobules of small basaloid cells. The cells are of two distinct types with the small cells at the periphery and the larger cells with pale cytoplasm and vesicular nuclei toward the center. Ductal differentiation is notably seen. Eccrine spiradenoma characteristically shows proliferation of large numbers of blood vessels of varying sizes. Conspicuous presence of pink hyaline basement membrane is noted. Sprinkling of lymphocytes and lymphedema is also a notable feature. Features of cylindroma can be seen, which may or may not be associated with Brooke-Spiegler syndrome. The tumor cells stain with cytokeratin 7, 8, and 18 and EMA and CEA.

Malignant eccrine spiradenoma is extremely rare. A benign counterpart within the tumor is a requirement for confirming the diagnosis. The malignant changes include loss of dual cell population, marked nuclear pleomorphism, necrosis, and prominent mitotic activity including the atypical forms. Low-grade and high-grade forms have been recognized. The low-grade form is very difficult to recognize as the changes are very subtle. There is loss of dual cell population with mild nuclear pleomorphism and scanty mitotic activity. These tumors may recur locally, but metastasis is not reported. The high-grade form shows prominent carcinomatous changes such as marked nuclear pleomorphism and increased mitotic activity. Adenocarcinomatous, squamous, and sarcomatous differentiation in the form of leiomyosarcoma and rhabdomyosarcoma has been documented.

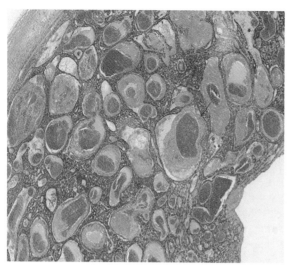

FIGURE 10.103 Eccrine Spiradenoma-Low Power

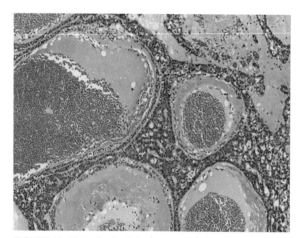

FIGURE 10.104 Eccrine Spiradenoma-High Power

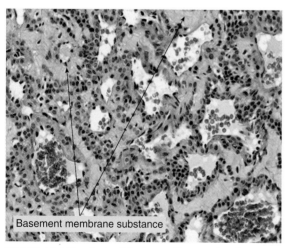

FIGURE 10.105 Eccrine Spiradenoma-Basement Membrane Substance

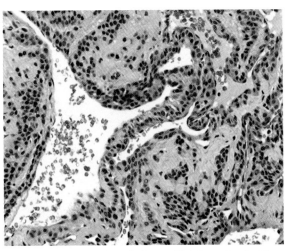

FIGURE 10.106   Eccrine Spiradenoma-High Power-Another View

SYRINGOID ECCRINE CARCINOMA

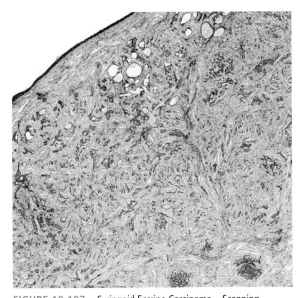

FIGURE 10.107   Syringoid Eccrine Carcinoma—Scanning

Syringoid eccrine carcinoma is a very rare tumor clinically manifesting as painful plaque or ulcerated non healing lesion. This is a longstanding tumor and local recurrences are very common. Syringoid eccrine carcinomas rarely metastasize to the regional lymph nodes.

On microscopy, the tumor is dermal and infiltrates into the subcutaneous fat or underlying muscle. It is composed of basaloid cells set in a sclerotic and hyalinized stroma. The tumor cells are arranged as narrow strands and sometimes lining cystic spaces. The cells have scanty cytoplasm and rounded or oval nuclei. Nuclear pleomorphism and mitotic activity are rarely seen. Duct formation is identified. Keratocysts are conspicuously absent. Perineural infiltration is frequently seen. The tumor cells stain strongly for MNF116, AE1/AE3, and Cam 5.2. The ductular differentiation is highlighted by EMA and CEA.

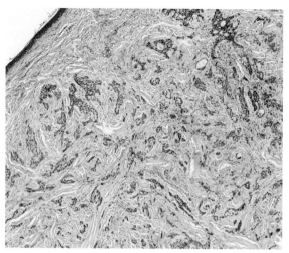

FIGURE 10.108   Syringoid Eccrine Carcinoma-Low Power View

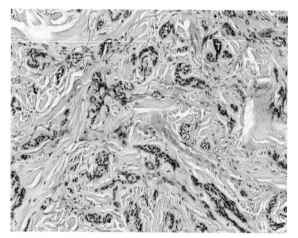

FIGURE 10.109   Syringoid Eccrine Carcinoma-High Power

MICROCYSTIC ADNEXAL CARCINOMA

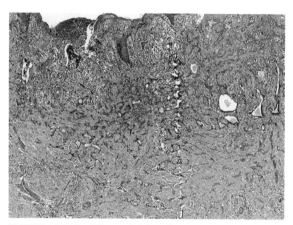

FIGURE 10.110   Microcystic Adnexal Carcinoma-Low Power

Microcystic adnexal carcinoma is a rare eccrine tumor presenting predominantly in the perinasal and periorbital areas. It is also known by other names such as sclerosing sweat duct carcinoma and malignant syringoma. Clinically, the tumor presents as slow-growing hard nodule or as a plaque of longstanding duration.

On microscopy, it is a poorly circumscribed tumor localized in the dermis but deeply infiltrating into the subcutaneous fat and even underlying muscle. Very rarely, they show connection to the overlying epidermis or follicle. The cells forming the tumor are arranged as strands and small cysts. A tadpole-like morphology is often seen. Keratocysts are frequently identified. The cells may exhibit mild nuclear pleomorphism or occasional mitotic activity. Ductular differentiation is frequently seen.

The tumor cells stain with AE1/AE3. Duct formation is highlighted by CEA and EMA. The morphological appearances raise the differential diagnosis of desmoplastic trichoepithelioma, morphoeic basal cell carcinoma, and syringoma. Desmoplastic trichoepithelioma and syringoma are located in the superficial dermis and show no ductal differentiation or perineural invasion. Morphoeic basal cell carcinoma again shows no ductal differentiation. A definitive diagnosis can be very difficult on punch or shave biopsies and hence a wider excision is always indicated.

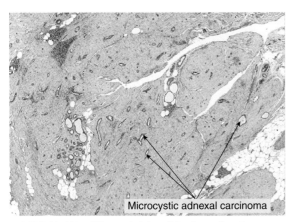

FIGURE 10.111   Microcystic Adnexal Carcinoma-Low Power

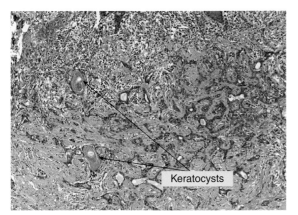

FIGURE 10.112   Microcystic Adnexal Carcinoma with Keratocysts

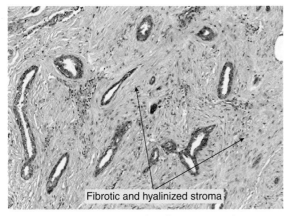

FIGURE 10.113   Microcystic Adnexal Carcinoma-High Power

PRIMARY CUTANEOUS ADENOID CYSTIC CARCINOMA

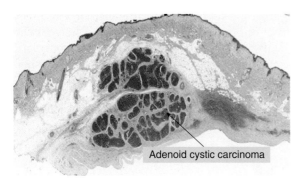

Adenoid cystic carcinoma

FIGURE 10.114   Primary Cutaneous Adenoid Cystic Carcinoma

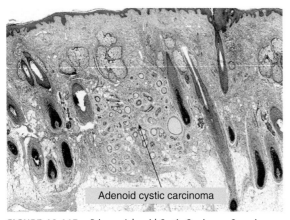

Adenoid cystic carcinoma

FIGURE 10.115   Primary Adenoid Cystic Carcinoma-Scanning View

Primary cutaneous adenoid cystic carcinoma is a rare neoplasm occurring in the head (usually the scalp) and neck area. Less common sites include abdomen breast and back. Clinically, the tumor presents as a very slow-growing plaque or nodule. Local recurrence is often seen, but metastasis is uncommon.

On microscopy, the tumor shows eccrine differentiation in majority of the cases, but apocrine differentiation has also been documented. The tumor is located in the mid and deep dermis and may extend into the subcutaneous fat. The tumor cells are characteristically arranged in a cribriform pattern in a loose myxoid background. The tumor cells are small and uniform with scanty cytoplasm and rounded nuclei. Very rarely, tubular and sheet-like patterns are also identified. Duct formation is identified. PAS-positive, diastase-resistant hyaline basement membrane material is seen amongst the tumor cells or in between the lobules. Immunohistochemically, the basement membrane substance is identified to be collagen IV, V, and laminin. Abundant Alcian blue positive mucinous material is seen within and in between the lobules. The tumor cells stain strongly with high- and low–molecular-weight cytokeratins. The ductal differentiation can be highlighted with EMA and CEA.

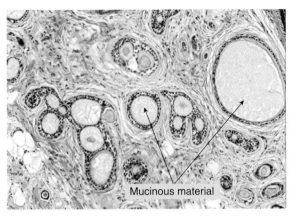

FIGURE 10.116   Primary Adenoid Cystic Carcinoma-High Power

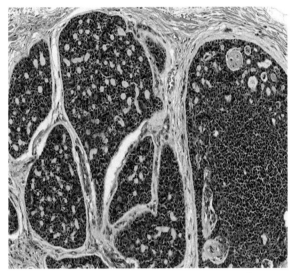

FIGURE 10.117   Primary Adenoid Cystic Carcinoma-High Power

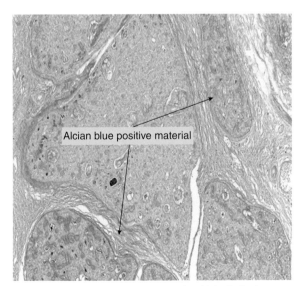

FIGURE 10.118   Primary Cutaneous Adenoid Cystic Carcinoma—
Alcian Blue Stain

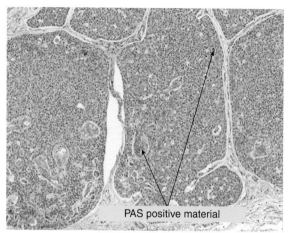

FIGURE 10.119   Primary Cutaneous Adenoid Cystic Carcinoma—Periodic Acid-Schiff with Diastase Stain

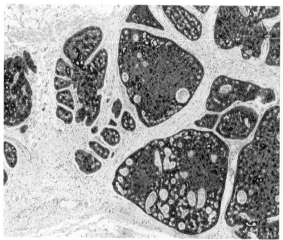

FIGURE 10.120   Primary Cutaneous Adenoid Cystic Carcinoma—MNF116

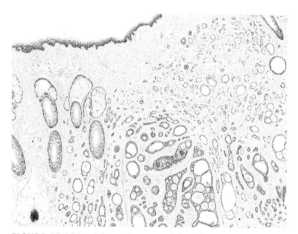

FIGURE 10.121   Primary Cutaneous Adenoid Cystic Carcinoma 63

PRIMARY CUTANEOUS MUCINOUS CARCINOMA

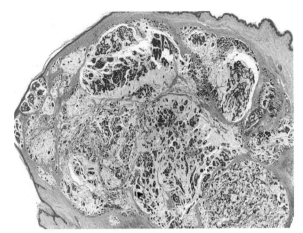

FIGURE 10.122   Primary Cutaneous Mucinous Carcinoma-Low Power

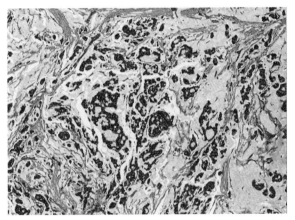

FIGURE 10.123   Primary Cutaneous Mucinous Carcinoma-High Power

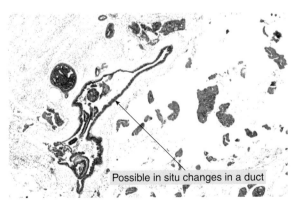

Possible in situ changes in a duct

FIGURE 10.124   Primary Cutaneous Mucinous Carcinoma—MNF 116

Primary cutaneous mucinous carcinoma is a rare tumor, primarily affecting the head and neck area. It occurs on other sites less commonly. Clinically, they present as slow-growing flesh-colored, erythematous or blue nodules. After removal, local occurrence in regional lymph nodes may occur but distant metastasis occurs rarely.

On microscopy, the tumor cells are set in a markedly myxoid stroma. The cells are arranged in groups of varying sizes, in a papillary, adenomatous, or glandular pattern. The tumor cells have scanty cytoplasm and rounded or oval nuclei. Nuclear pleomorphism and mitotic activity are not seen significantly. The myxoid or mucinous material is diastase resistant, PAS positive, and Alcian blue positive. The tumor cells stain strongly for broad spectrum cytokeratins such as AE1/AE3, MNF116, and specialized cytokeratin CK7. The cells are also positive for estrogen and progesterone receptors (ER and PR).

It is almost impossible to differentiate primary cutaneous mucinous carcinoma from a mucinous metastatic tumor from the breast, gastrointestinal tract, and genitourinary tract. Immunohistochemical staining for CK20 may possibly exclude a lower gastrointestinal primary, but clinical history and investigation are of paramount importance in confirming the diagnosis. The possibility of identifying in situ component in the tumor supporting the diagnosis of a primary mucinous carcinoma has been suggested by some authors but needs larger studies to validate it.

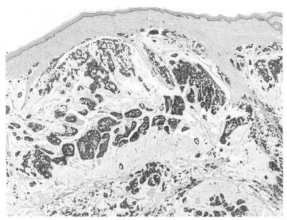

FIGURE 10.125   Primary Cutaneous Mucinous Carcinoma—
Cytokeratin 7

CHONDROID SYRINGOMA

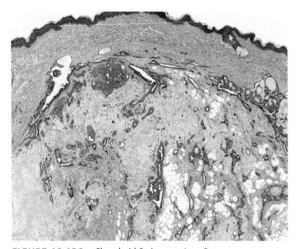

FIGURE 10.126   Chondroid Syringoma-Low Power

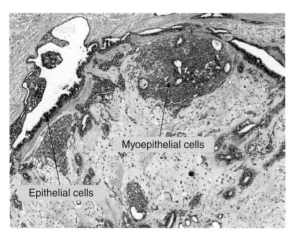

Myoepithelial cells

Epithelial cells

FIGURE 10.127   Chondroid Syringoma-High Power

Chondroid syringoma or cutaneous mixed tumor is a relatively common tumor occurring in the head and neck area and face. Clinically, they present as small firm to hard nodules. Very rarely giant forms have been described.

On microscopy, the tumor is dermal and well circumscribed with no involvement of the epidermis. The epithelial component is arranged as strands, cords, and glandular pattern of cells with eosinophilic cytoplasm and rounded nuclei. Decapitation secretions are identified within the lumina of the glands. In most instances, the lining is composed of double layers of cells. Aggregates of spindle-shaped and plasmacytoid myoepithelial cells are seen. Other features of note are squamous differentiation and clear cell change. The stroma has a bluish background with cartilage being the prominent component. Hyaline mucinous material, mucin, and adipose tissue are also identified. The eccrine variant of chondroid syringoma shows small strands and glandular pattern of eccrine cells in a significant proportion. Malignant change is rare in a chondroid syringoma.

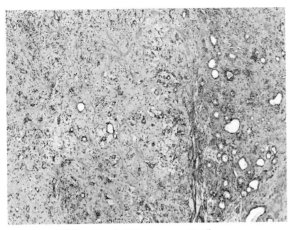

FIGURE 10.128   Chondroid Syringoma—Cartilage

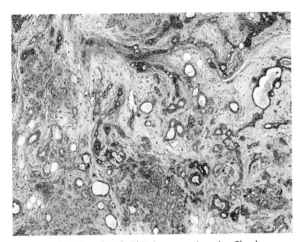

FIGURE 10.129   Chondroid Syringoma—Apocrine Glands

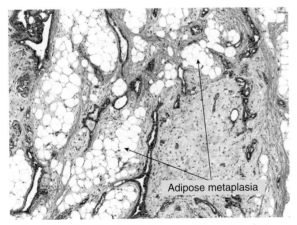

Adipose metaplasia

FIGURE 10.130   Chondroid Syringoma—Adipose Metaplasia

MALIGNANT CHONDROID SYRINGOMA

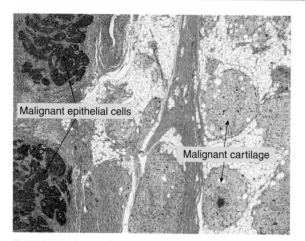

FIGURE 10.131   Malignant Chondroid Syringoma-Low Power

Malignant chondroid syringoma is an extremely rare tumor affecting the hands or feet of mainly elderly females. The tumor behaves in an aggressive fashion with frequent metastasis to regional lymph nodes and lung.

On microscopy, in a large majority of cases the epithelial component show malignant features in addition to malignant cartilage. There is marked nuclear pleomorphism of the epithelial component with brisk mitotic activity. Malignant cartilage shows increased cellularity and nuclear pleomorphism. Areas of necrosis and lymphovascular permeation are seen. Satellite nodules are a conspicuous feature of this tumor. The epithelial component of the tumor stains with cytokeratin.

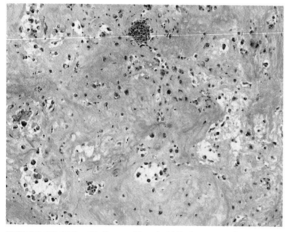

FIGURE 10.132   Malignant Chondroid Syringoma—Showing Malignant Cartilage

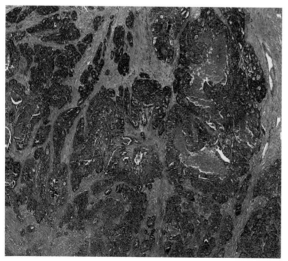

FIGURE 10.133   Malignant Chondroid Syringoma-Epithelium-Carcinoma

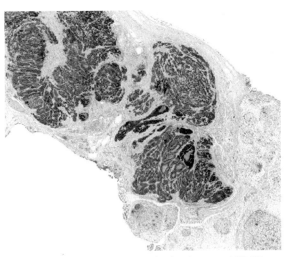

FIGURE 10.134   Malignant Chondroid Syringoma—MNF116

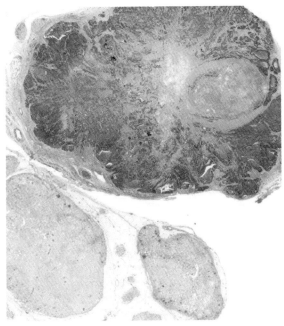

FIGURE 10.135   Malignant Chondroid Syringoma—Satellite Nodules

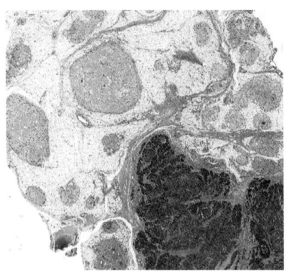

FIGURE 10.136   Malignant Chondroid Syringoma—Satellite Nodules-A Different View

CUTANEOUS MYOEPITHELIOMA

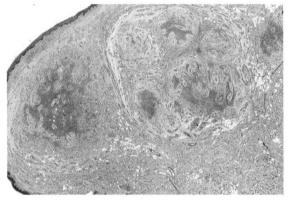

FIGURE 10.137   Cutaneous Myoepithelioma-Scanning View

Cutaneous myoepitheliomas are rare benign tumors that can occur in any layer of the skin except the epidermis. They can also occur in the deep soft tissues. Clinically, they present as flesh-colored or violaceous nodules in a variety of sites.

On microscopy, the tumor is dome shaped and nonencapsulated. The overlying epidermis is uninvolved. The cells are arranged as whorls, sheets, or scattered in the dermal collagen. The cells may be spindle shaped, plasmacytoid, or epithelioid. Nuclear pleomorphism, mitotic activity, and necrosis are not seen. The tumor cells stain positively for cytokeratins, S100, calponin, and smooth muscle myosin. Malignant change is extremely rare but can occur.

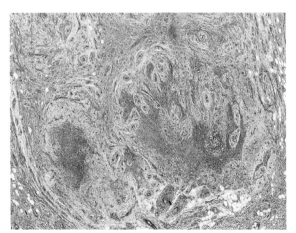

FIGURE 10.138   Cutaneous Myoepithelioma-Medium Power

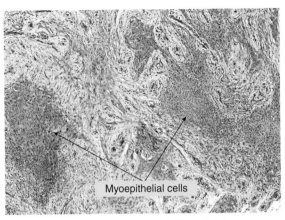

FIGURE 10.139   Cutaneous Myoepithelioma-High Power

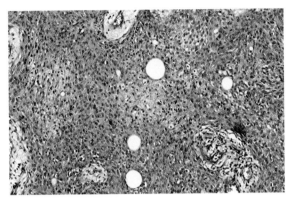

FIGURE 10.140   Cutaneous Myoepithelioma—Bland
Myoepithelial Cells

BIBLIOGRAPHY

McKee PH. Pathology of the Skin, 3rd Ed. Mosby, Elsevier, 2005.
Weedon D. Skin Pathology, 4th Ed. Churchill Livingstone, 2009.

Subcutaneous Fat—Inflammatory and Neoplastic Diseases

INTRODUCTION

The subcutaneous fat is seen beneath the reticular dermis. It is composed of lobules of mature adipocytes separated by fibrous septae. Small arteries, nerves, lymphatics, and venules are seen within the fibrous septae. The inflammatory diseases involving subcutaneous fat are called panniculitis. There are three categories of panniculitis:

1. Septal panniculitis

2. Lobular panniculitis

3. Panniculitis associated with vasculitis.

The histological appearances of panniculitis depend to a large extent on the stage at which the lesion is biopsied. The early stages show acute inflammatory cells, whereas the later stages may show fibrosis, chronic inflammatory, and granulomas. There is lot of overlap of features between septal and lobular panniculitis, so much so that the terms predominantly septal and predominantly lobular panniculitis are universally accepted. Clinical correlations with ancillary laboratory techniques are useful in arriving at a diagnosis.

The neoplastic diseases of fat are variants of lipomas and liposarcomas.

ERYTHEMA NODOSUM

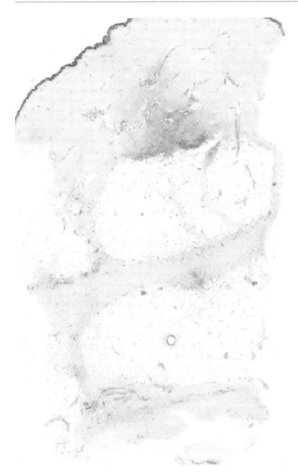

FIGURE 11.1   Erythema Nodosum-Scanning View

Erythema nodosum is the classical example of predominantly septal panniculitis. Clinically, it presents as painful nodules on the anterior aspect of the lower extremities. Other sites such as arms and trunk are less often involved. The lesions are associated with a wide variety of clinical conditions and could also occur following an infection or could be drug induced. It is basically considered an allergic reaction.

On microscopy, the changes are seen predominantly in the subcutaneous fat. The inflammation primarily affects the septae with variable spill over into the lobules. In the early stages, neutrophils predominate the inflammatory component. In the later stages, there is fibrosis and marked thickening of the septae with infiltration of lymphocytes and histiocytes and the formation of giant cells and granulomas. Frank vasculitis is not identified although there may be swelling of the endothelial cells.

Septal panniculitis can also be seen in factitial panniculitis, necrobiosis lipoidica, and scleroderma.

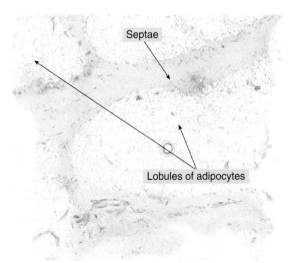

FIGURE 11.2   Erythema Nodosum-Low Power

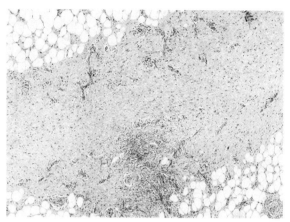

FIGURE 11.3   Erythema Nodosum-Medium Power

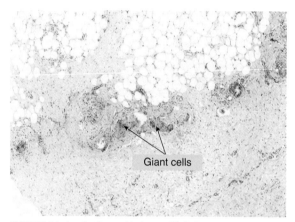

Giant cells

FIGURE 11.4   Erythema Nodosum-High Power

ERYTHEMA INDURATUM

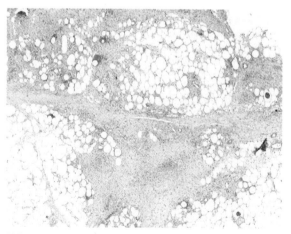

FIGURE 11.5   Erythema Induratum-Low Power

Erythema induratum is a rare inflammatory disorder characterized by painful nodules on the lower legs. Erythema induratum is considered a tuberculid, with circumstantial evidence to support this. In other situations, the lesion is designated nodular vasculitis.

On microscopy, the features of predominant lobular panniculitis are seen. Granulomatous reaction pattern is a notable feature accompanied by vasculitis.

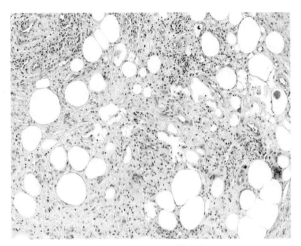

FIGURE 11.6   Erythema Induratum-High Power

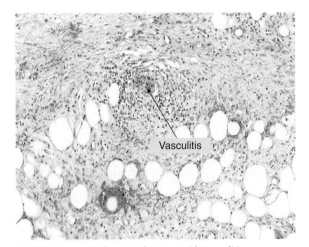

FIGURE 11.7   Erythema Induratum with Vasculitis

CYTOPHAGIC HISTIOCYTIC PANNICULITIS

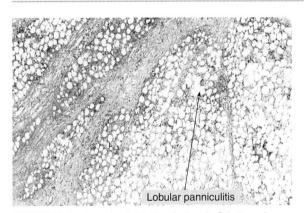

FIGURE 11.8   Cytophagic Histiocytic Panniculitis-Scanning View

Cytophagic histiocytic panniculitis belongs to the spectrum of diseases of the hemophagocytic syndrome. The disease is characterized by recurring panniculitis with infiltration of phagocytic histiocytes into the subcutaneous fat. The disease eventually becomes a multisystem disorder that terminates in hemorrhagic diathesis. Very rarely, this is a self-limiting disorder confined to the cutaneous location. This is a predominantly lobular panniculitis with minimal septal involvement.

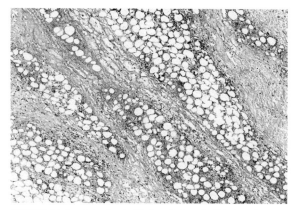

FIGURE 11.9   Cytophagic Histiocytic Panniculitis-Low Power

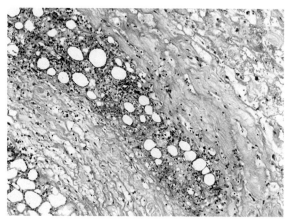

FIGURE 11.10   Cytophagic Histiocytic Panniculitis-High Power

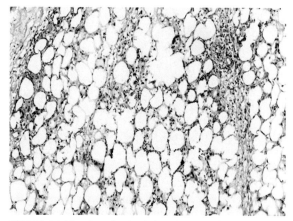

FIGURE 11.11   Cytophagic Histiocytic Panniculitis-High Power-Another View

LOBULAR PANNICULITIS IN LUPUS PROFUNDUS

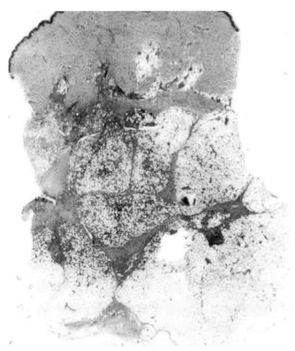

Involvement of subcutaneous fat in lupus erythematosus is designated lupus profundus. This is a chronic recurring disorder affecting 1 to 4% of patients with lupus erythematosus. The lesions are commonly seen on the upper extremities and trunk. Clinically, the lesions precede or follow the onset of lupus erythematosus. They are seen as painful nodules and plaques.

On microscopy, the epidermal and dermal changes of lupus erythematosus are seen in most cases. The notable feature is a predominantly lobular panniculitis with a dense infiltration of lymphocytes. The lymphocytes do not exhibit cytological atypia or rimming around the adipocytes. Lymphoid follicles with germinal centers are a prominent feature.

FIGURE 11.12   Lobular Panniculitis in Lupus Profundus-Scanning View

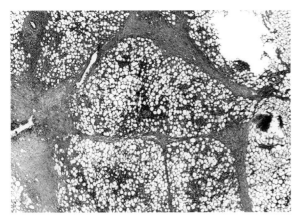

FIGURE 11.13   Lobular Panniculitis in Lupus Profundus-High Power

NEUTROPHILIC PANNICULITIS

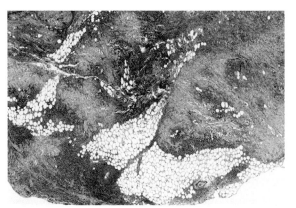

FIGURE 11.14   Neutrophilic Panniculitis-Scanning View

Neutrophilic panniculitis is a histological reaction pattern seen in conditions where the etiological factor is an infective agent. A wide variety of fungal, mycobacterial, and helminthic infections have been implicated as the cause for this condition. Clinically, the lesions occur on multiple sites of the body as painful subcutaneous nodules. The overlying skin may be erythematous or ulcerated.

On microscopy, the histological changes are seen as predominantly lobular panniculitis. There is extension of the inflammation into the subcutaneous fat. A large majority of cells are neutrophils with granulomatous inflammation in some of the cases depending on the etiology. Fibrinoid necrosis in the stroma and secondary vasculitis may be seen. In a large number of cases, the inflammation is also seen in the reticular dermis.

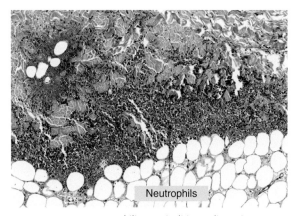

FIGURE 11.15   Neutrophilic Panniculitis-Medium View

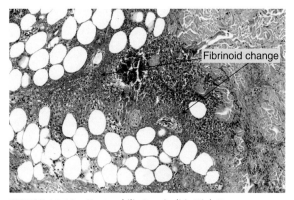

FIGURE 11.16   Neutrophilic Panniculitis-High Power

POLYARTERITIS NODOSA

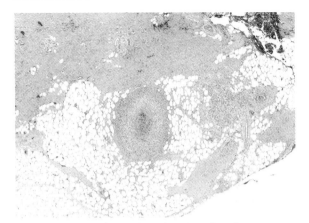

FIGURE 11.17   Polyarteritis Nodosa-Scanning View

Polyarteritis nodosa is a multisystem disorder. The cutaneous manifestations are mainly due to the involvement of the small- and medium-sized vessels. Purely cutaneous form of the disease has also been reported. Clinically, the lesions present as painful nodules and ulcerated plaques in the lower limbs.

On microscopy, the cutaneous lesions involve the small- and medium-sized blood vessels in the deep dermis and subcutaneous fat. In the early stages, the vessels are infiltrated by neutrophils and lymphocytes with the occasional eosinophils. Fibrinoid necrosis of the vessels is seen. Luminal thrombi may also be seen. Leukocytoclasia is also identified.

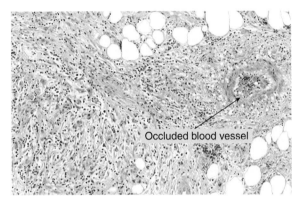

FIGURE 11.18   Polyarteritis Nodosa-Medium Power

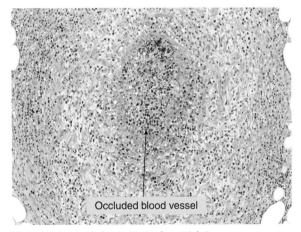

FIGURE 11.19   Polyarteritis Nodosa-High Power

CALCIPHYLAXIS

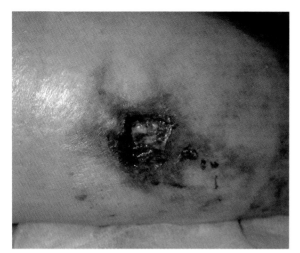

FIGURE 11.20   Calciphylaxis

Calciphylaxis clinically presents as bilateral painful and tender eruptions on the lower limbs. Lesions are rarely identified on other sites of the body. Ulceration and bulla formation are typically seen. The lesions are seen in patients with renal impairment and subsequent altered calcium/phosphorous metabolism and hyperparathyroidism.

On microscopy, the overlying epidermis is ulcerated. The small- and medium-sized blood vessels of the subcutaneous fat show deposition of calcium in the lumina of the blood vessels. Quite often, the vessels are thrombosed.

Calciphylaxis is a fatal condition in almost 60% of patients.

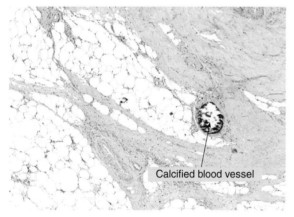

Calcified blood vessel

FIGURE 11.21   Calciphylaxis

LIPOMA

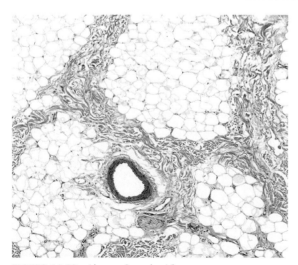

FIGURE 11.22   Lipoma-Scanning View

Lipomas are the most common benign tumors of adipose tissue. They are seen on all parts of the body, particularly the extremities and the trunk. They are broadly classified into solitary and multiple lipomas. The solitary variants are of the superficial and deep types. Superficial lipomas are either dermal or subcutaneous in location. Multiple lipomas are also commonly encountered. These tumors are usually associated with several syndromes, the notable ones being Cowden syndrome, where multiple lipomas are associated with hemangiomas, lichenoid, and papular lesions of skin and goiter. Frohlich syndrome, also known as prune- belly syndrome, and Bannayan-Zonana syndrome are associated with multiple lipomas.

On microscopy, they are encapsulated tumors composed of mature univacuolated adipocytes separated by fibrous septae. Several histological variants of lipoma where the tumor is infiltrated by different components of the mesenchymal tissue have been described. They include fibrolipoma, myxolipoma,

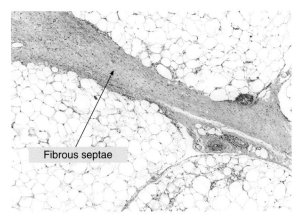

FIGURE 11.23   Lipoma

angiomyxolipoma, and myolipoma. Secondary changes are commonly seen in lipomas. This is the result of either secondary inflammation or impaired blood supply. Inflammatory changes are usually manifested as fat necrosis where aggregates of foamy histiocytes are seen within lipoma. Long-standing ischemia can result in infarction within a lipoma, which leads to secondary calcification. Cytogenetic examinations of lipomas show karyotypic abnormalities involving 12q, 6p, and 13q.

ANGIOLIPOMA

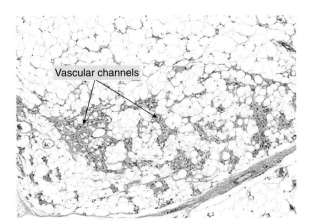

FIGURE 11.24   Angiolipoma-Low Power

Angiolipomas are benign variants of lipoma. Clinically, they are tender and present as bluish nodules preferably on the upper half of the body. Multiple angiolipomas have been associated with diabetes mellitus.

On microscopy, the lesions are encapsulated and are composed of mature adult-type adipocytes. Varying proportions of vascular channels are identified, and most of them contain fibrin thrombi in the lumen. Mast cells are commonly seen. Cellular angiolipomas show markedly increased numbers of vascular channels in a closely packed pattern. Cellular angiolipomas can be confused with a vascular tumor if the adipocytic differentiation is not identified. Cytogenetic examination has not revealed any karyotypic abnormality within the tumor.

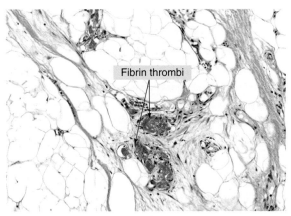

FIGURE 11.25   Angiolipoma-Fibrin Thrombi

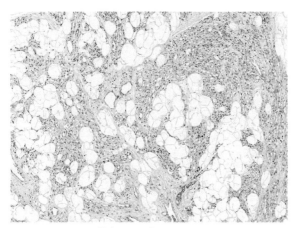

FIGURE 11.26   Cellular Angiolipoma-Low Power

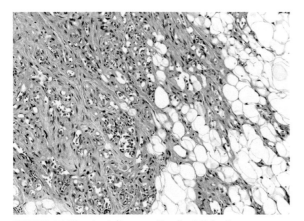

FIGURE 11.27   Angiolipoma—Focally Cellular Area

INTRADERMAL SPINDLE CELL LIPOMA

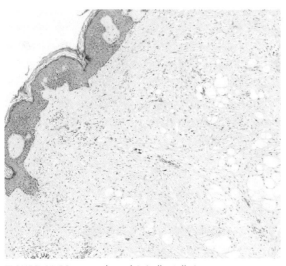

FIGURE 11.28   Intradermal Spindle Cell Lipoma-Low Power

Spindle cell lipoma is an uncommon variant of lipoma occurring on the back of neck and shoulder region of middle-aged and elderly men.

On microscopy, spindle cell lipomas are in dermal and subcutaneous locations. They are generally encapsulated tumors. The tumors are composed of mature adipocytes diffusely infiltrated by short spindly cells in a myxoid background. The collagen within the tumor is increased compared with an ordinary lipoma and shows a ropey appearance. Scattered mast cells are seen within the tumor. Slight variation in the size of the adipocytes is readily seen, but atypical hyperchromatic nuclei are not seen. The vascularity within the tumor is variable, and focally, hemangiopericytomatous vessels are also seen. The amount of adipocytes can vary markedly, and some tumors are completely devoid of adipose tissue. Such cases are quite challenging histologically.

The spindle cells are positive for CD34 and bcl2, and the adipocytes stain for S100 protein.

Spindle cell lipoma is entirely benign and local recurrence may occur. The tumor shows cytogenetic abnormalities, the notable ones being monosomy and partial loss of chromosome 13 and 16. This cytogenetic abnormality can be used to confirm the diagnosis.

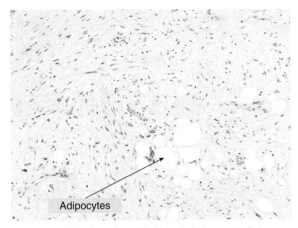

FIGURE 11.29   Intradermal Spindle Cell Lipoma-High Power

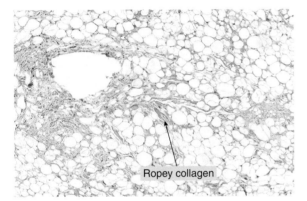

FIGURE 11.30   Spindle Cell Lipoma-Low Power View

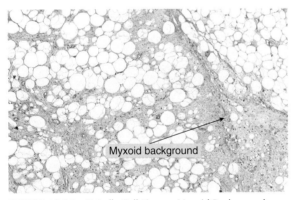

FIGURE 11.31   Spindle Cell Lipoma-Myxoid Background

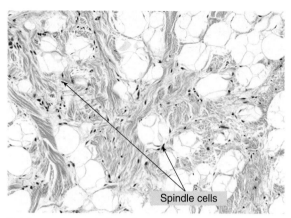

FIGURE 11.32   Spindle Cell Lipoma-High Power

PLEOMORPHIC LIPOMA

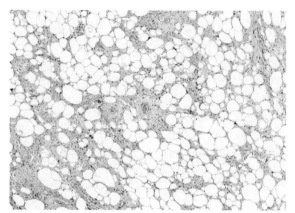

FIGURE 11.33   Pleomorphic Lipoma—Variation in Size of the Adipocytes

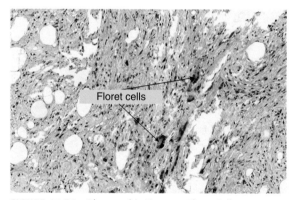

FIGURE 11.34   Pleomorphic Lipoma—Floret Cells

Pleomorphic lipoma is a variant of lipoma and belongs to the family of spindle cell lipoma. It occurs in the same clinical setting as spindle cell lipoma in the subcutaneous tissue of the back of neck and shoulder of elderly men. Very unusually, similar to spindle cell lipoma, they may arise in other parts of the body.

On microscopy, there is marked variation in histological appearance from an ordinary lipoma. There is a range of histological appearances. The amount of adipose tissue can vary markedly, similar to spindle cell lipoma. In addition to adipocytes, which may show variation in sizes, pleomorphic lipomas also show many giant cells formed of hyperchromatic nuclei. These are referred to as floret cells. Ropey collagen bundles and myxoid change are also notable features similar to spindle cell lipoma.

The spindle cells in pleomorphic lipoma are positive for CD34 and bcl2. Cytogenetic examination shows deletion of chromosome 13q and 16q.

The most important differential diagnosis to be considered is that of a well-differentiated liposarcoma. The identification of MDM2 (murine double minute 2) gene amplification in a liposarcoma is useful in differentiating the two entities.

CHONDROID LIPOMA

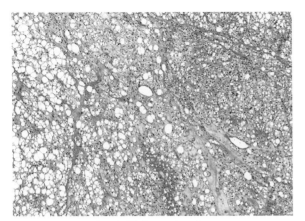

FIGURE 11.35   Chondroid Lipoma-Low Power

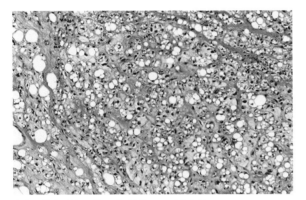

FIGURE 11.36   Chondroid Lipoma-High Power

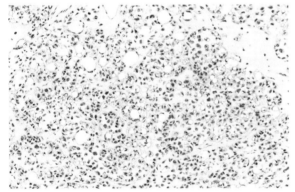

FIGURE 11.37   Chondroid Lipoma—CD68

Chondroid lipoma is a rare variant of lipoma seen mostly in the lower extremities of middle-aged individuals, predominantly women. Unusually, they occur in other anatomical locations. Chondroid lipomas are entirely benign tumors with no tendency to recur or metastasize.

On microscopy, chondroid lipomas show sheets of rounded cells in a myxoid or chondroid background. Most cells have eosinophilic cytoplasm, whereas others have multivacuolated cytoplasm. In most cases, the latter type of cells predominates. Stains for adipose tissue such as oil red O are positive in these cells, confirming adipocytic differentiation. Nuclear pleomorphism, necrosis, and mitotic activity are not seen. Focally, calcification and hemosiderin deposition may be seen.

The cells show focal staining for CD68 and occasionally with cytokeratins. Cytogenetic examination of the tumor shows balanced translocation t(11;16)(q13;p12–13), which is considered a characteristic finding.

HIBERNOMA

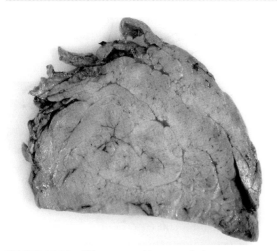

FIGURE 11.38   Hibernoma—Macroscopic Appearance

Hibernomas are tumors of brown fat and occur in a wide variety of anatomical locations in the body. They arise in young to middle-aged adults, and the commonest location is the scapular region and the thighs. Macroscopically, it has the characteristic yellowish matt appearance.

On microscopy, hibernomas are well-encapsulated tumors. Although four different morphological features have been described, the most common pattern is that of sheets of cells with uniform rounded nuclei and granular eosinophilic cytoplasm. The other less common appearances include the myxoid variant, spindle cell variant, and lipoma-like variant. Nuclear pleomorphism, necrosis, and mitotic activity are not seen in any of these tumors. Immunohistochemical staining shows the tumor cells to be positive for S100. Cytogenetic examination of the tumor shows structural rearrangements of 11q13–21, which is the most common finding identified.

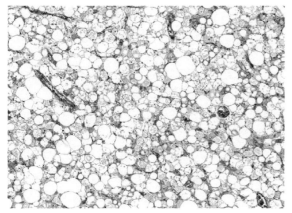

FIGURE 11.39   Hibernoma-Low Power

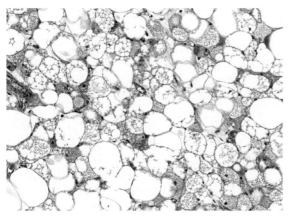

FIGURE 11.40   Hibernoma-High Power

LIPOSARCOMA AND CYTOGENETIC ABNORMALITIES

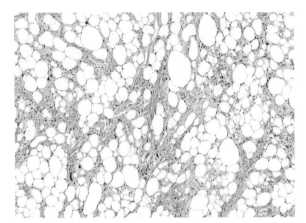

FIGURE 11.41   Well-Differentiated Liposarcoma—Atypical Hyperchromatic Cells

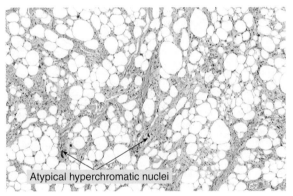

FIGURE 11.42   Well-Differentiated Liposarcoma

MDM2 amplification in WDLPS
Home-grown RP11-450G15 clone

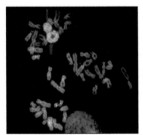
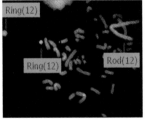

Ring (12)   Rods and rings

FIGURE 11.43   Well-Differentiated Liposarcoma, MDM-2 Amplification. Courtesy of Paul Roberts, St. James's University Hospital, Leeds, UK

Well-differentiated liposarcoma very rarely involve the subcutaneous fat. It is more commonly seen in the deep soft tissue. The subcutaneous variants present as ill-defined masses mostly on the extremities and back.

On microscopy, well-differentiated liposarcoma is nonencapsulated. The tumor predominantly shows mature adipocytes, which exhibit variation in sizes. Hyperchromatic spindle-shaped cells scattered among the adipocytes and/or in the fibrous septae is the most important diagnostic feature. Lipoblasts may or may not be seen and is a feature that should not be relied upon for the diagnosis of liposarcoma. Fat atrophy and fat necrosis may enter the differential diagnosis, due to the presence of variation of sizes of the adipocytes in these two conditions. The presence of atypical hyperchromatic nuclei can be quite sparse, which makes the confirmation of the diagnosis difficult at times. The identification of MDM2 gene amplification in liposarcomas is a useful test to confirm the diagnosis.

BIBLIOGRAPHY

Enzinger and Weiss's Soft Tissue Tumours, 5th Ed.
McKee PH. Pathology of the Skin, 3rd Ed. Mosby, Elsevier, 2005.

Infections and Infestations

INTRODUCTION

Cutaneous infections and infestations can occur de novo or in a setting where the patient is immunocompromised. The histopathological appearances of cutaneous infections are varied and present as granulomatous inflammation, neutrophilic infiltrates, and eosinophilic infiltrates. The parasitized organisms are identified within the histiocytes in a large number of cases.

BACTERIAL INFECTIONS

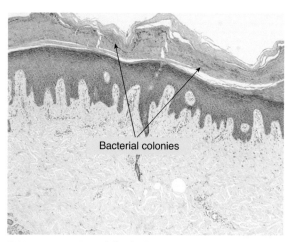

FIGURE 12.1   Bacterial Colonies-Low Power

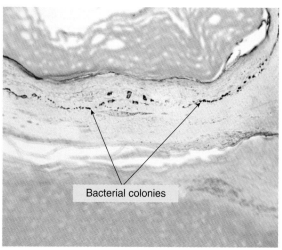

FIGURE 12.2   Bacterial Colonies-Gram Stain

Bacterial Colonies and Dermal Abscesses

Bacteria are either normal residents of the skin, or they could be pathogenic. Bacterial infections could be either superficial as in impetigo, Staphylococcal scalded skin syndrome, and ecthyma or deep, when it is termed cellulitis. Necrotizing fasciitis is also a manifestation of deep bacterial infection. The commonest bacterial infections are caused by pyogenic organisms such as *Staphylococcus aureus* and strains of Streptococci. Not uncommonly, mycobacterial infection is emerging as a significant cause of infections, particularly in the background of compromised immune status.

On microscopy, pyogenic infections generally presents as an abscess. An abscess is a collection of neutrophils. Mycobacterial and parasitic infections usually presents as dermal granulomas. Suppurative granulomas or caseating granulomas are seen in the dermis or subcutaneous fat.

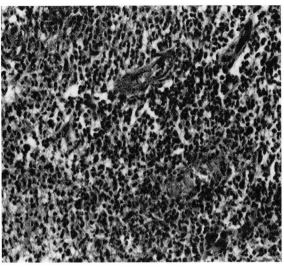

FIGURE 12.3   Dermal Abscess

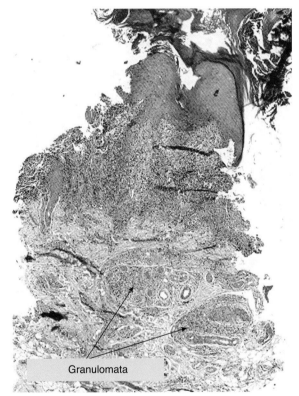

Granulomata

FIGURE 12.4   Tuberculosis Verrucosa Cutis-Scanning View.
Courtesy of Manoj Singh, AIIMS, India

Tuberculosis Verrucosa Cutis

Tuberculosis verrucosa cutis is a variant of lupus vulgaris and is an uncommon condition. It occurs by direct inoculation in individuals with good immunity. Clinically, the lesions show marked hyperkeratosis and verrucous appearance and are usually seen on acral skin.

On microscopy, there is marked hyperkeratosis and papillomatosis of the epidermis. The upper dermis shows a dense infiltrate composed of lymphocytes and histiocytes. Granulomas composed of epithelioid histiocytes, which are the diagnostic hallmark of tuberculosis verrucosa cutis, are seen in the deep dermis. This also highlights the importance of a deep biopsy in confirming the diagnosis.

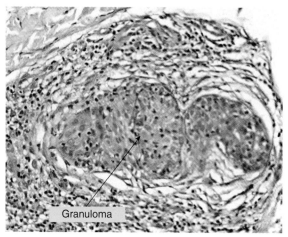

FIGURE 12.5 Tuberculosis Verrucosa Cutis—Deep Granuloma. Courtesy of Manoj Singh, AIIMS, India

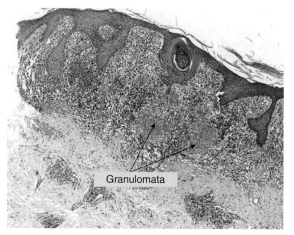

FIGURE 12.6 Lupus Vulgaris-Low Power. Courtesy of M Ramam, AIIMS, India.

Lupus Vulgaris

Lupus vulgaris is the commonest form of reinfection cutaneous tuberculosis. It is usually caused by *Mycobacterium tuberculosis*. The lesions are seen in the head and neck area and extremities as multiple erythematous papules–forming plaques.

On microscopy, the classical appearance is that of multiple granulomas that show a tendency to be confluent. Caseation necrosis may be seen, and there may be a cuff of lymphocytes in the periphery of the granulomas.

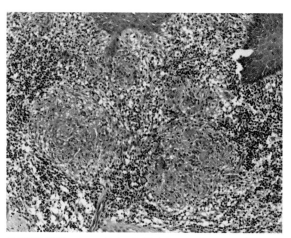

FIGURE 12.7 Lupus Vulgaris-High Power. Courtesy of M Ramam, AIIMS, India

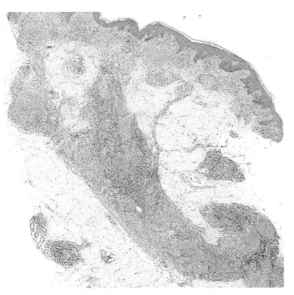

FIGURE 12.8   Tuberculoid Leprosy-Scanning View-Courtesy of Manoj Singh, AIIMS, India

Tuberculoid Leprosy

Tuberculoid leprosy is a localized form of leprosy. Clinically, the lesions are well defined and hypopigmented with a central anesthetic patch. A thickened and beaded nerve supplying the involved area is usually seen.

On microscopy, the striking appearance is that of caseating well-defined granulomatous inflammation. The granulomas may involve the appendageal structures. An important diagnostic clue is the absence of confluence of the granulomas. Acid-fast bacilli are not demonstrated in tuberculoid leprosy.

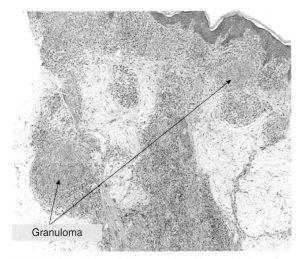

FIGURE 12.9   Tuberculoid Leprosy-Low Power. Courtesy of Manoj Singh, AIIMS, India

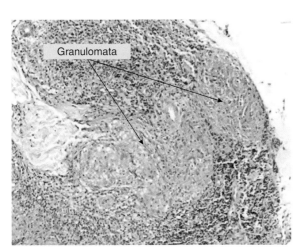

FIGURE 12.10   Tuberculoid Leprosy-High Power. Courtesy of Manoj Singh, AIIMS, India

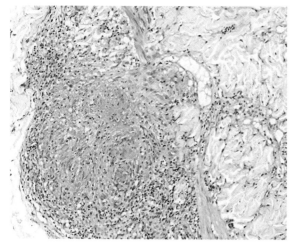

FIGURE 12.11   Granuloma in Tuberculoid Leprosy. Courtesy of Manoj Singh, AIIMS, India

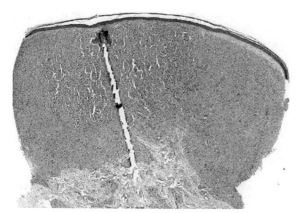

FIGURE 12.12   Lepromatous Leprosy-Scanning View. Courtesy of Manoj Singh, AIIMS, India

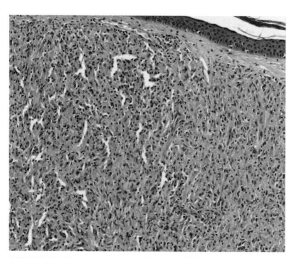

FIGURE 12.13   Lepromatous Leprosy-High Power. Courtesy of Manoj Singh, AIIMS, India

Lepromatous Leprosy

Lepromatous leprosy is a systemic disease with the prominent lesions occurring in the skin. The organism, *M. leprae* can be seen in almost all organs except brain and spinal cord. Mucosal involvement can be a notable clinical feature manifested as nasal stuffiness. Nodular thickening of the skin, which is classically manifested on the ear lobes, is a typical feature. The affected skin may show hypopigmented patches with little or no sensory loss in the early stages. In advanced stages, there is sensorimotor neuropathy of the "glove-and-stocking" type. Bone resorption in the late stage of the disease leads to damage in the nasal bone and long bones of hands and feet.

On microscopy, the density of the infiltration varies with the stage of the disease. The earlier stage of the disease shows sparse infiltrate of lymphocytes and histiocytes. The later stages show dense infiltrate of the same cells with a grenz zone at the dermoepidermal junction. The histiocytes appear foamy, termed as lepra cells or Virchow cells, and they are heavily parasitized. Acid-fast bacilli are easily demonstrated arranged as large masses called globi.

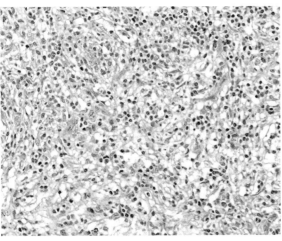

FIGURE 12.14   Lepromatous Leprosy-High Power. Courtesy of Manoj Singh, AIIMS, India

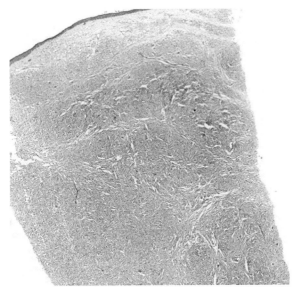

FIGURE 12.15   Histoid Leprosy-Low Power. Courtesy of M Ramam AIIMS, India

Histoid Leprosy

Histoid leprosy is a rare variant of leprosy, clinically presenting as multiple skin-colored nodules and papules. It was thought to be manifestation of drug resistance but has been reported in individuals who have received no treatment.

On microscopy, the infiltrate is seen in the dermis beneath the grenz zone. The cells are spindle shaped, and they are arranged in sheets. Foamy histiocytes containing the bacilli are seen admixed with the spindle cells. The acid-fast stain demonstrates the organisms as discrete bacilli. They tend to be longer than the usual *M. leprae* and are not arranged as globi.

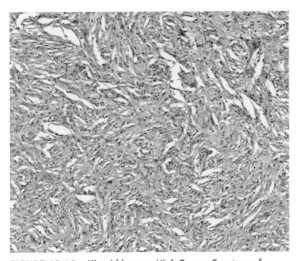

FIGURE 12.16   Histoid leprosy-High Power. Courtesy of M Ramam, AIIMS, India

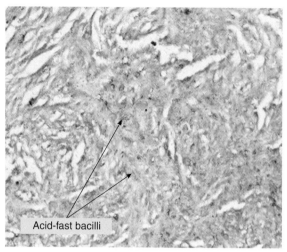

FIGURE 12.17 Histoid Leprosy—Acid-Fast Bacilli. Courtesy of M Ramam, AIIMS, India

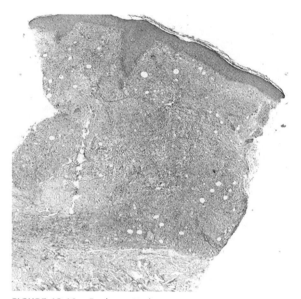

FIGURE 12.18 Erythema Nodosum Leprosum-Low Power. Courtesy of M Ramam, AIIMS, India

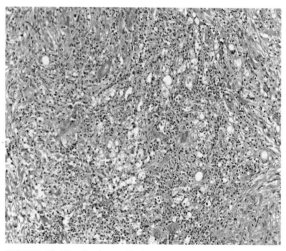

FIGURE 12.19 Erythema Nodosum Leprosum-High Power. Courtesy of M Ramam, AIIMS, India

Erythema Nodosum Leprosum

Erythema nodosum leprosum is a type of reaction at the lepromatous end of the spectrum. It is also known as type 2 reaction. It is similar to serum sickness and develops in patients who are already on treatment or have received no treatment for leprosy. Antileprosy treatment is considered a trigger for erythema nodosum leprosum. Patients develop systemic symptoms such as joint pains and fever. Multiple tender nodules are seen away from the original lesions, and the original lesions are unaffected. These nodules subside in 7 to 10 days.

On microscopy, features of lepromatous leprosy are seen, but the sharp circumscription of the granulomas seen in lepromatous leprosy is lost. The intervening dermis is infiltrated by foamy histiocytes and many neutrophils. The neutrophils are also seen around the appendageal structures and blood vessels. Occasional cases may show features of leukocytoclastic vasculitis. Acid-fast bacilli are seen but may be difficult to identify if the patient had been on long-term treatment.

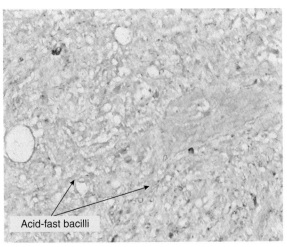

FIGURE 12.20   Erythema Nodosum Leprosum—Acid-Fast Bacilli. Courtesy of M Ramam, AIIMS, India

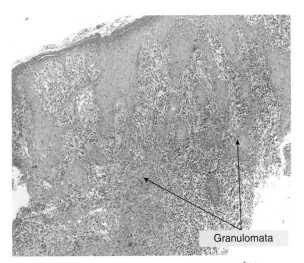

FIGURE 12.21   Tuberculids-Low Power. Courtesy of M Ramam, AIIMS, India

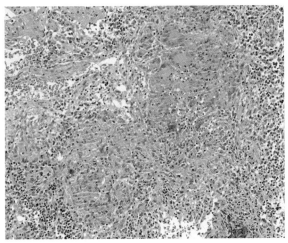

FIGURE 12.22   Tuberculids-High Power. Courtesy of M Ramam, AIIMS, India

Tuberculids

Tuberculids are cutaneous hypersensitivity lesions developing in individuals with a high degree of immunity or allergic sensitivity to the organism, who develop tuberculosis elsewhere in the body. The criteria to diagnose tuberculids are as follows:

a. Skin lesions should show features of tuberculosis.

b. Acid-fast bacilli should not be demonstrable on the skin lesion.

c. Tuberculin test must be strongly positive.

d. Treatment of the underlying tuberculosis should result in the resolution of the skin lesion.

Lichen scrofulosorum is the commonest type of tuberculid. It is clinically manifested as crops of lesions with a predilection for the trunk. Individual lesions may heal leaving areas of hyperpigmentation, but the crops may continue to be present for several months.

On microscopy, lichen scrofulosorum shows multiple granulomas composed of lymphocytes, histiocytes, and Langhan type of giant cells. The granulomas are centered on appendageal structures. Clinically and histologically, lichen scrofulosorum may be confused with lichen nitidus.

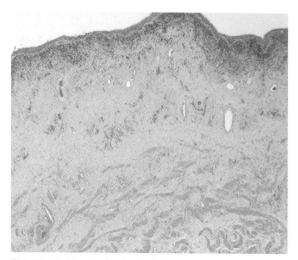

FIGURE 12.23   Penile Skin Syphilis-Low Power

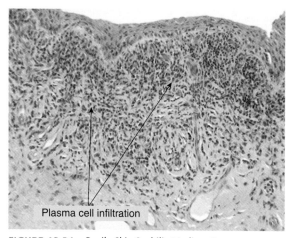

Plasma cell infiltration

FIGURE 12.24   Penile Skin Syphilis-Medium Power

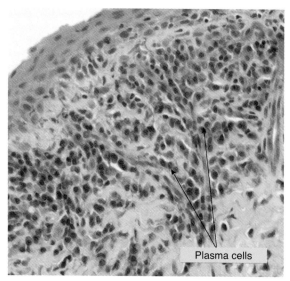

Plasma cells

FIGURE 12.25   Penile Skin Syphilis-High Power

Syphilis

Syphilis is caused by the spirochete *Treponema pallidum*. The infection is acquired by sexual contact. Acquired syphilis is manifested in different stages such as primary, secondary and latent, and tertiary syphilis. The earliest stage, which is primary syphilis, presents as painless ulcer with well-defined edges in genital or perianal skin. These lesions are referred to as chancre. Approximately 4 to 8 weeks after the development of the chancre, in untreated cases, constitutional symptoms such as fever, lymphadenitis, and hepatitis develop. The cutaneous lesions do not have any specific appearance and can vary from condyloma acuminata to alopecia syphilitica. Latent syphilis is a manifestation of secondary syphilis when the cutaneous lesions may relapse but the systemic symptoms subside. The serology remains positive in latent syphilis. Tertiary syphilis involves the cardiovascular and nervous systems and appears many years after secondary syphilis. The testes, lymph nodes, and skin may be involved. The cutaneous lesions in tertiary syphilis may be an ulcerated nodule or a gummatous ulcer.

On microscopy, the characteristic feature of primary syphilis is the presence of sheets of plasma cells in the subepithelial region. The overlying epidermis may be acanthotic initially but may be thinned out in later stages. The blood vessels show prominent endothelial swelling. *T. pallidum* can be demonstrated by silver stains, such as Warthin-Starry or Levaditi, or immunohistochemical methods. Secondary syphilis may show a granulomatous reaction pattern in addition to mixed inflammatory cell infiltration, which includes lymphocytes, histiocytes, and plasma cells. Tertiary syphilis typically shows prominent endothelial swelling and infiltration of lymphocytes, histiocytes, and fibroblasts. *T. pallidum* is hard to identify in the tissue sections.

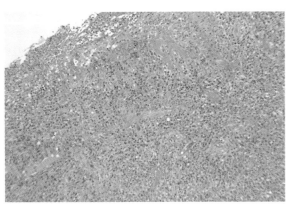

FIGURE 12.26   Penile Skin Syphilis-Low Power

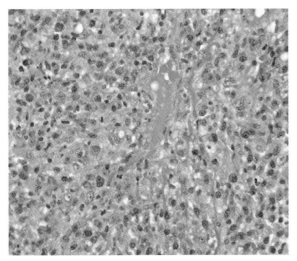

FIGURE 12.27   Penile Skin Syphilis-High Power

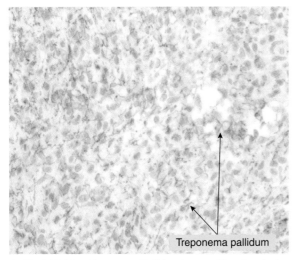

Treponema pallidum

FIGURE 12.28   *Treponema Pallidum*-Immunohistochemical Stain

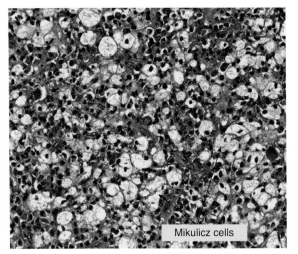

FIGURE 12.29   Rhinoscleroma

Rhinoscleroma

Rhinoscleroma is a chronic inflammatory disease affecting the nasal and oral mucosa caused by *Klebsiella rhinoscleromatis*. It is an opportunistic infection and affects immunocompromised individuals.

On microscopy, the lesions usually demonstrate a mixture of lymphocytes and plasma cells with prominent Russell bodies. Several macrophages with vacuolated cytoplasm containing the organism are seen. They are called Mikulicz cells. The organisms can be demonstrated by periodic acid-Schiff (PAS) stain, Gram stain, or Warthin-Starry stain. The overlying mucosa could be hyperplastic or atrophic.

FUNGAL INFECTIONS

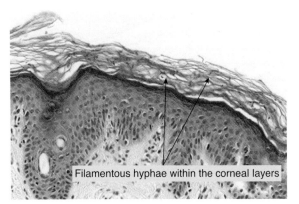

FIGURE 12.30   Superficial Dermatophytoses

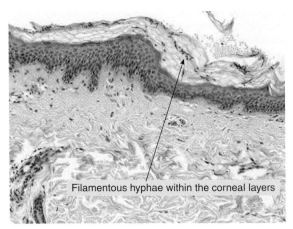

FIGURE 12.31   Superficial Dermatophytoses—Periodic Acid-Schiff Stain

Tinea Corporis

Fungal infections have clinical appearances varying from hypopigmented patches to ulcerated nodules. Direct examination of tissue scrapings in 10% potassium hydroxide clears the tissue, allowing direct visualization of the fungi. The special stains used are PAS, Grocott methenamine silver, and mucicarmine stains. Immunohistochemical antibodies are also available to identify fungal organisms.

Tinea corporis belongs to the superficial filamentous fungal infection called dermatophytosis. The clinical appearances usually are those of an annular centrifugal lesion with central clearing and peripheral desquamation. Chronic infections may occur in immunocompromised individuals.

On microscopy, filamentous hyphae are seen in the corneal layer, sandwiched between the different layers of the corneal layer. Ackerman designated this feature as the "sandwich sign." The epidermis may show spongiosis and vesiculation. The underlying dermis shows mixed inflammatory cell infiltration or sometimes granulomatous inflammation.

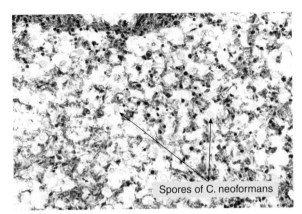

FIGURE 12.32   Cryptococcus Neoformans

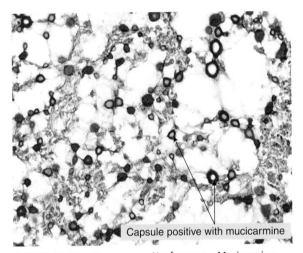

FIGURE 12.33   Cryptococcus Neoformans—Mucicarmine Stain

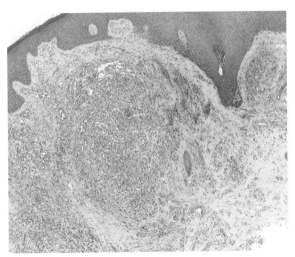

FIGURE 12.34   Histoplasmosis H&E Section-Low Power

Cryptococcosis

The causative organism of cryptococcosis is *Cryptococcus neoformans*, which is a yeast-like fungus. Most lesions present as nodules ulcers and pustules and are commonly seen in immunocompromised patients. Primary cutaneous cryptococcosis is rare, the cutaneous lesions being manifestations of occult systemic infection. Face, neck, and the upper arms are the favored sites. The most common mode of entry is through the respiratory tract, and the lesions manifest as pulmonary granulomas.

On microscopy, tuberculoid type of granulomas in the dermis or dense mixed inflammatory infiltrate mixed with large numbers of organisms can be seen. The overlying epidermis may show pseudoepitheliomatous hyperplasia. The organisms are rounded yeast-like forms with refractile walls. The capsule of *C. neoformans* stains with mucicarmine.

Histoplasmosis

Histoplasmosis is caused by *Histoplasma capsulatum*. The cutaneous lesions presents as ulcerated nodules or cellulites-like areas at the site of inoculation. Most lesions occur in immunocompromised individuals, and lung appears to be the commonest site of primary infection. The laboratory diagnosis of histoplasmosis is made by serological testing, histological evaluation of the affected tissue, and culture.

On microscopy, the overlying epidermis may be ulcerated or acanthotic. The dermis shows granulomatous inflammation or mixed inflammatory cell infiltration. The yeast-like organisms surrounded by a clear halo are seen within macrophages. Extracellular organisms can also be seen. The organisms stain positive with the PAS stain.

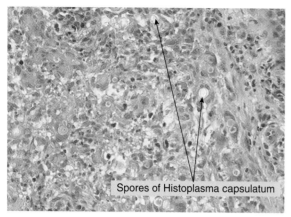

FIGURE 12.35 Histoplasmosis H&E Sections-High Power

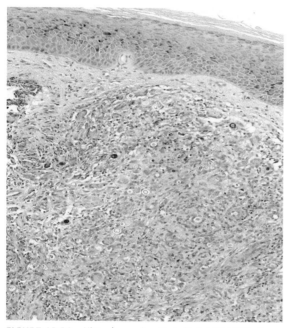

FIGURE 12.36 Histoplasmosis—Periodic Acid-Schiff Stain

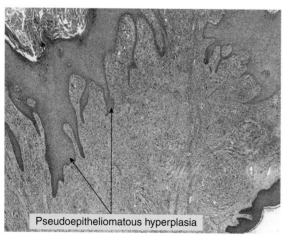

FIGURE 12.37 Chromoblastomycosis-H&E Section-Low Power

Chromoblastomycosis

Chromoblastomycosis is a chronic infection caused by a group of dematiaceous (pigmented fungi). The brown pigment in the fungi is melanin. Lower extremities are most commonly affected. The lesions usually follow superficial trauma, and the lesions develop into verrucous nodules or plaques.

On microscopy, the overlying epidermis exhibits pseudoepitheliomatous hyperplasia. The dermis shows granulomatous inflammation. Suppurative granulomas are not seen, and caseating necrosis is not a feature. Thick-walled, rounded, golden-brown forms of fungi are seen within the histiocytes or lying free in the interstitium. These rounded structures are called sclerotic bodies, muriform cells, or medlar bodies. These are considered to be the intermediate vegetative forms arrested between the yeast and hyphal stages. The fungal forms can be highlighted by the PAS and Grocott methenamine silver stains.

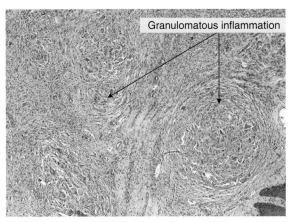

FIGURE 12.38   Chromoblastomycosis-H&E Sections-Medium Power

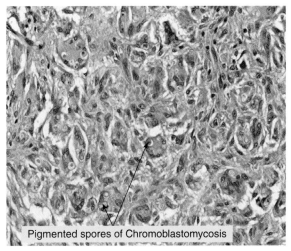

FIGURE 12.39   Chromoblastomycosis-H&E Section-High Power

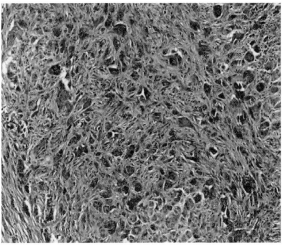

FIGURE 12.40   Chromoblastomycosis—Periodic Acid-Schiff Stain

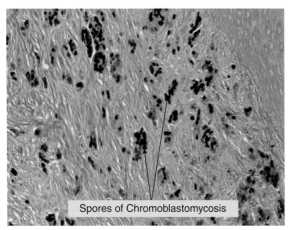

FIGURE 12.41 Chromoblastomycosis—Grocott's Methenamine Silver Stain

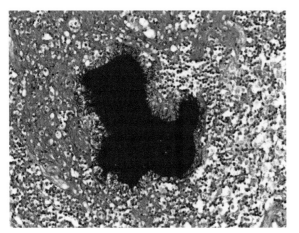

FIGURE 12.42 Actinomycotic Colony—Periodic Acid-Schiff Stain

Actinomycosis

The causative organism of actinomycosis is *Actinomyces israelii*. It is a chronic fatal infection, which could involve any part of the body. The cutaneous manifestations include fluctuant swellings in the cervicofacial, thoracic, and abdominal regions. Underlying visceral involvement or a history of previous surgery is usually elicited. *A. israelii* are filamentous organisms that form soft sulfur granules detected in the pus.

On microscopy, the lesions are usually located in the deep dermis or subcutaneous fat. The commonest presentation is that of an abscess at the center of which is located a colony of granules. The granules exhibit numerous slender beaded filaments radiating in a parallel fashion from the border. The granules stain with PAS and with methenamine silver stain, they appear black.

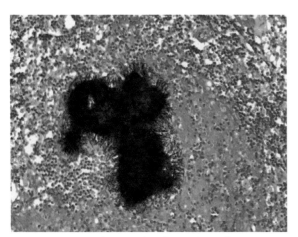

FIGURE 12.43 Actinomycotic Colony—Grocott's Methenamine Silver

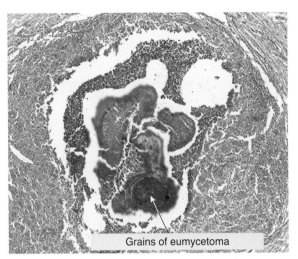

Grains of eumycetoma

FIGURE 12.44   Madurella Mycetoma. Courtesy of Manoj Singh, AIIMS, India

Madurella Mycetoma

The causative organism is *Madurella mycetomatis*. Mycetoma is a chronic fungal infection characterized by swelling, draining sinuses, and discharging granules. The lower extremities, particularly the feet, are commonly affected, hence the term Madura foot. Repeated minor trauma is thought to be the portal of entry for the organism. The sinuses develop in few weeks, and involvement of the underlying fascia, muscle, and bone is a frequent feature. The grains discharged from the sinuses have different colors and are a useful clue to the identification of the organism.

On microscopy, the colored grains and the organism are seen surrounded by Splendore-Hoeppli phenomenon. This is seen in the middle of a suppurative granuloma. The grains are formed of brown cement substance in which septate filamentous hyphae of *M. mycetomatis* are embedded.

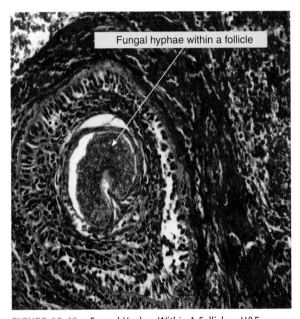

Fungal hyphae within a follicle

FIGURE 12.45   Fungal Hyphae Within A Follicle—H&E Section

Pityrosporum Folliculitis

The causative organism is *Malassezia furfur*. Clinically, the lesions are erythematous follicular papules, which could be intensely itchy. Follicular occlusion is the primary event, followed by plugging of the follicle by the organism.

On microscopy, the involved follicles are dilated and plugged with keratin. The intervening dermis may show moderate to severe inflammatory cell infiltration. Foreign body giant cell reaction due to the released keratin from the follicle may be seen. The follicles on deeper sections show plugging by oval yeast-like organisms. The organisms stain positive with PAS and methenamine silver stains.

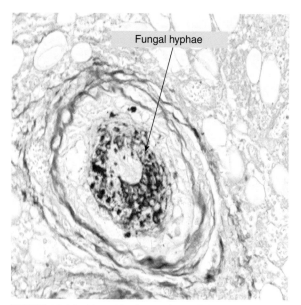

FIGURE 12.46   Fungal hyphae Within Follicle—Grocott's Methenamine Silver Stain

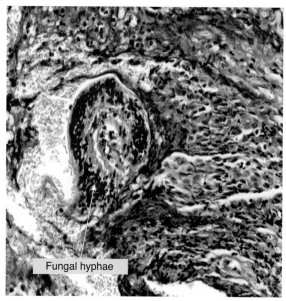

FIGURE 12.47   Fungal Hyphae Within Follicle—Periodic Acid-Schiff Stain

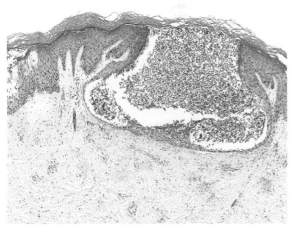

FIGURE 12.48   Phaeohyphomycosis-Low Power

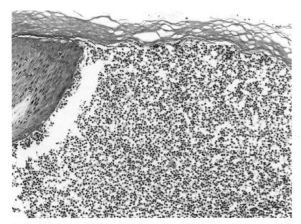

FIGURE 12.49   Phaeohyphomycosis-High Power

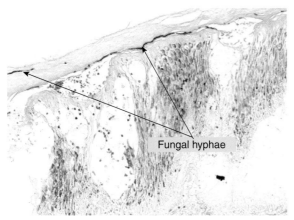

Fungal hyphae

FIGURE 12.50   Phaeohyphomycosis—Grocott's
Methenamine Silver Stain

Phaeohyphomycosis

The causative organisms are a diverse group of fungi that are pigmented in most cases. Clinically, the lesions are nodular or cystic.

On microscopy, the typical lesion is a cyst or an abscess. Granulomatous reaction can also be seen. The hyphal forms of the organism are seen on the surface or within the abscess or in the giant cells.

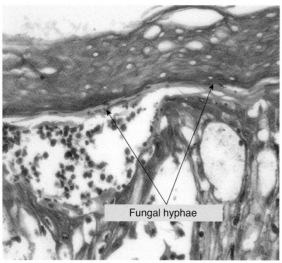

FIGURE 12.51 Phaeohyphomycosis—Periodic Acid-Schiff Stain

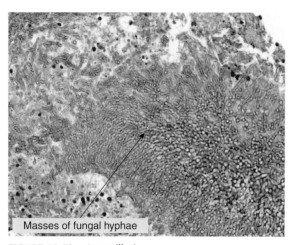

FIGURE 12.52 Aspergillosis

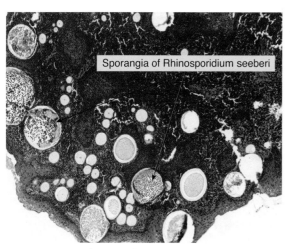

FIGURE 12.53 Rhinosporidiosis-Low Power

Aspergillosis

The causative organism is *Aspergillus flavus*. Aspergillosis is an opportunistic fungal infection seen more commonly in immuno-compromised patients. Cutaneous involvement is very rare, and it involves the lung primarily. Cutaneous involvement commonly is seen in patients with previous malignancies, and the lesions develop at the site of intravenous cannulae.

On microscopy, the appearances can vary from granulomas to abscess formation. Masses of septate hyphae are seen among the inflammatory cells.

Rhinosporidiosis

The causative organism is *Rhinosporidium seeberi*. Rhinosporidiosis is primarily a mucosal lesion. Cutaneous involvement is by contiguous spread from the mucosal lesion.

On microscopy, the diagnostic feature is the presence of sporangia containing many spores. A mixed inflammatory cell infiltrate is seen, which may or may not form granulomas.

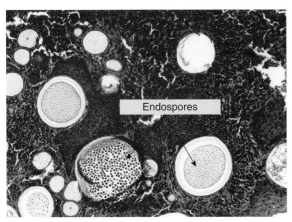

FIGURE 12.54   Rhinosporidiosis-High Power

VIRAL INFECTIONS

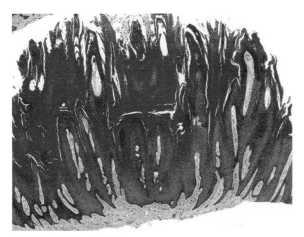

FIGURE 12.55   Viral Wart

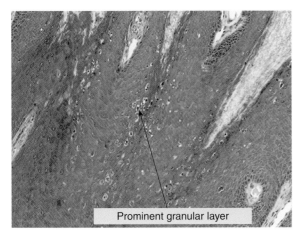

FIGURE 12.56   Viral Wart-High Power

Viral Infections

Viral diseases clinically manifest as erythematous maculopapular rash or urticarial lesions. Viruses are divided into separate families on the basis of the presence of RNA or DNA particles within them. The laboratory methods used to detect suspected viral diseases include light and electron microscopy, serology, viral culture, and immunomorphological methods. The development of monoclonal antibodies to various viruses to be used with fluorescent, immunoperoxidase, and ELISA (enzyme-linked immunosorbent assay) techniques has tremendously helped the rapid diagnosis of viral diseases.

Human papillomavirus (HPV) produces various types of warts on different parts of the body. HPV belongs to the family of papovavirus, which is a DNA virus. Modern techniques of viral DNA isolation have helped in the identification of 70 different types of HPV.

Viral warts or verrucae have been classified into the following:

- Verruca vulgaris or common warts
- Palmoplantar warts including superficial or deep types
- Verruca plana
- Epidermodysplasia verruciformis
- Condyloma acuminatum.

Verruca vulgaris is associated with Human papillomaviruses-1, 2, 4, and 7. They are commonly seen in children and young adults.

On microscopy, there is marked acanthosis, hyperkeratosis, and papillomatosis. Tiers of parakeratosis are seen overlying the parakeratotic columns. The granular layer is markedly prominent. The diagnostic feature is the presence of koilocytes, which have pyknotic or "raisinoid" nuclei and perinuclear halo. Occasional dyskeratotic cells may be seen. The dermal changes are minimal and consist of perivascular lymphocytic infiltration. The papillomavirus antigen can be detected by immunoperoxidase methods or polymerase chain reaction (PCR).

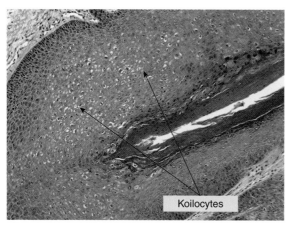

FIGURE 12.57   Koilocytes

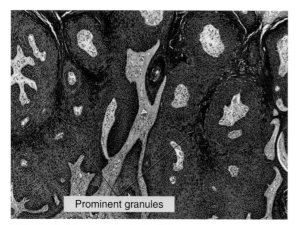

FIGURE 12.58   Granules in Viral Wart

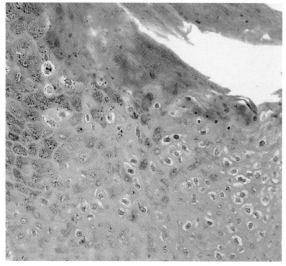

FIGURE 12.59   Koilocytosis and Hypergranulosis

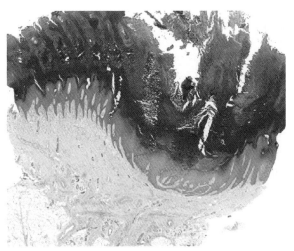

FIGURE 12.60   Palmoplantar Wart-Scanning View

Palmoplantar Wart

As the name implies, palmoplantar warts are seen on the palms and soles. They are painful lesions and occur beneath pressure points and could be confused with callosities. The causative organisms are HPV-1 and HPV-4. The traditionally described variants are the superficial or mosaic type and the deep type also known as myrmecia. Unusual forms such as a nodular or ridged variant, a pigmented verrucous variant, and a whitish punctuate keratotic variant have also been described.

On microscopy, the acanthotic epidermis is seen to grow well into the underlying dermis. There is marked hyperkeratosis. There is prominence of keratohyaline granules, and they are seen as characteristic eosinophilic granules, particularly in HPV-1 infections. The underlying dermis may show mild perivascular lymphocytic infiltration.

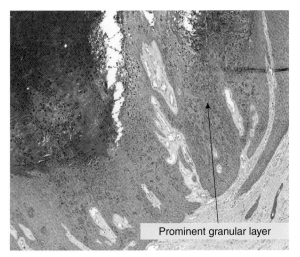

FIGURE 12.61   Palmoplantar Wart-Low Power

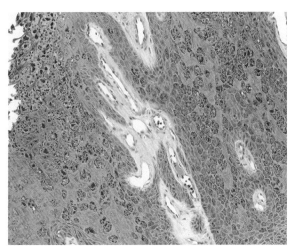

FIGURE 12.62   Palmoplantar Wart-Pink Granules

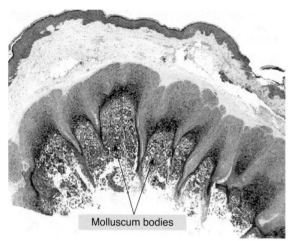

FIGURE 12.63   Molluscum Contagiosum-Scanning View

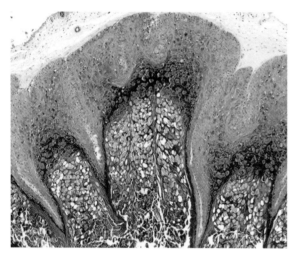

FIGURE 12.64   Molluscum Bodies

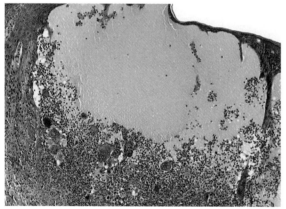

FIGURE 12.65   Herpes Simplex-Low Power

Molluscum Contagiosum

The causative organism is a DNA pox virus. Clinically, molluscum contagiosum presents as solitary or crops of umbilicated waxy papules on the flexural areas or genitalia of young adults and children.

On microscopy, the striking feature is the presence of lobules of hyperplastic epidermis that invaginate into the underlying dermis. The cytoplasm of the keratinocytes lodges the eosinophilic inclusion bodies. At the level of the granular layer, the inclusion bodies become basophilic, and they are finally extruded to the surface through the follicular ostia. A variable number of lymphocytic infiltrations may be seen within the dermis.

Herpes Simplex Infection

The herpes simplex virus (HSV) has two types: HSV-1 and HSV-2. The commonest infection is seen in children with HSV-1. Recurrent lesions occurring around the lip are called cold sores or herpes labialis. HSV-2 infections are seen in the genital areas, and it is sexually transmitted. Clinically, they present as a group of clear vesicles, and they heal without scarring. The viral antigens can be detected on tissue sections by using immunoperoxidase and immunofluorescence techniques or PCR.

On microscopy, both types of herpes viruses show similar features. The earliest change is the characteristic peripheral clumping of the keratinocyte nuclei with the formation of the ground glass appearance. The cytoplasmic vacuolization is also noted. These changes gradually involve the entire epidermis. This results in an intraepidermal vesicle. The keratinocytes undergo two types of degeneration, namely ballooning degeneration or reticular degeneration. Ballooning degeneration is more common, where the affected cells are swollen and the cytoplasm of the cells become intensely eosinophilic and swollen. These cells also become multinucleate and are referred to as Tzanck cells.

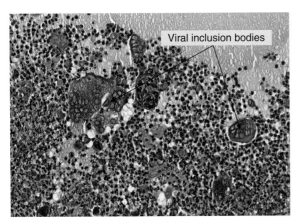

FIGURE 12.66   Herpes Simplex-High Power

The intraepidermal vesicles extend further down to become subepidermal vesicles due to the reticular degeneration of the epidermal keratinocytes. The vesicles are surrounded by a mixed inflammatory cell infiltrate, which also includes a significant number of neutrophils. The underlying dermis shows extension of the inflammatory cell infiltration from the vesicle.

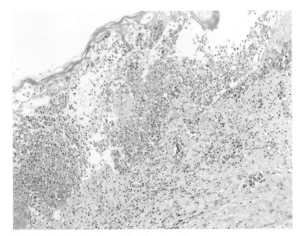

FIGURE 12.67   Herpes Simplex-Low Power

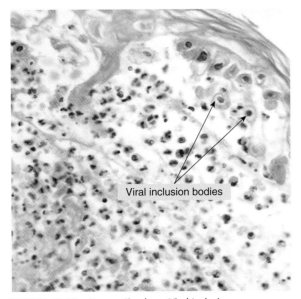

FIGURE 12.68   Herpes Simplex—Viral Inclusions

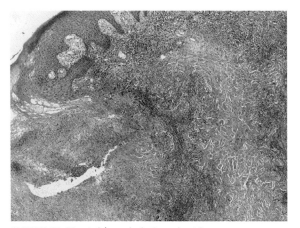

FIGURE 12.69   Leishmaniasis-Scanning View

Leishmaniasis

Cutaneous leishmaniasis is caused by protozoon called *Leishmania tropica* in Asia and Africa and *Leishmania mexicana* in Central and South America. The vector for the disease is a sandfly belonging to the family of Phlebotomus. Clinically, acute, chronic, and disseminated forms have been recognized. The lesions start as ulcerated nodules, which later heal, leaving scars.

On microscopy, the epidermis may be mildly acanthotic. The changes are seen in the dermis with a dense infiltrate of lymphocytes, plasma cells, histiocytes, and some neutrophils. The histiocytes contain the amastigote form of the parasites, which is better seen on Giemsa stain.

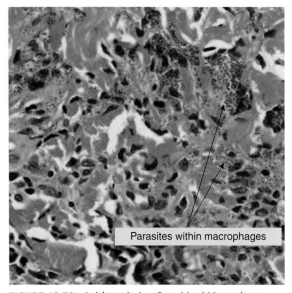

FIGURE 12.70   Leishmaniasis—Parasitized Macrophages

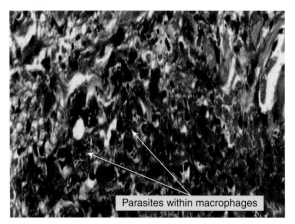

FIGURE 12.71   Leishmaniasis—Giemsa Stain

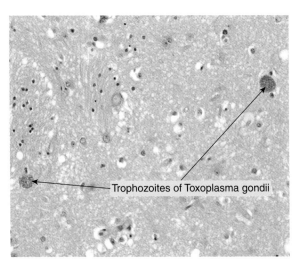

FIGURE 12.72   Toxoplasmosis

Toxoplasmosis

The causative organism is called *Toxoplasma gondii*. Congenital and acquired forms have been described. Cutaneous involvement of both forms is very rare. The changes in the acquired form, which are slightly more common, have been described as maculopapular–, lichenoid–, and erythema multiforme–like changes.

On microscopy, the epidermis may show pseudoepitheliomatous hyperplasia. The dermis shows an infiltrate of lymphocytes, and the parasites in the form of trophozoites may be seen lying free in the dermis or in the form of a pseudocyst.

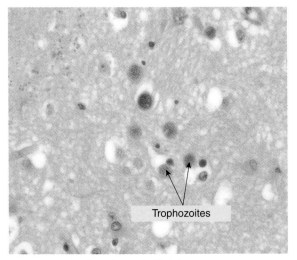

FIGURE 12.73   Toxoplasmosis-High Power

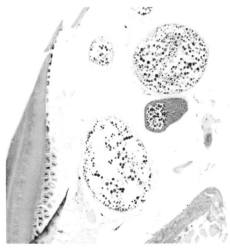

FIGURE 12.74   Jigger Flea *Tunga Penetrans*

Tungiasis

The causative organism is the pregnant female sand flea *Tunga penetrans*, commonly seen in Africa, Central and South America, and Pakistan. Clinically, the lesions have a predilection for the feet and are seen as papules and nodules with a central black dot and erythematous base.

On microscopy, the diagnostic feature is the identification of the exoskeleton and the internal parts of the flea in the dermis or epidermis. This is usually surrounded by mixed inflammatory cell infiltration.

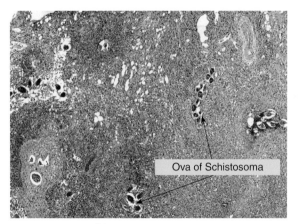

FIGURE 12.75   Schistosomiasis-Low Power

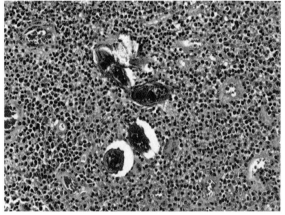

FIGURE 12.76   Schistosomiasis-High Power

Schistosomiasis

The causative organism is the trematode belonging to the family of Schistosoma. The different species identified are *Schistosoma japonicum, S. haematobium*, and *S. mansoni*. The cutaneous manifestations described have a variety of appearances, and they include pruritic erythematous lesions to granulomatous warty lesions. Squamous cell carcinoma has been described to develop as a late complication of some cases of warty genital lesions.

On microscopy, the epidermis may show marked spongiosis and intraepidermal vesicles, pseudoepitheliomatous hyperplasia, or microabscesses. The dermis contains dense infiltrate of mixed inflammatory cells, which includes many eosinophils and many ova. The ova of each species have characteristic features. *S. haematobium* have an apical spine, *S. mansoni* have a lateral spine, and *S. japonicum* have no spine.

BIBLIOGRAPHY

McKee PH. Pathology of the Skin, 3rd Ed. Mosby, Elsevier, 2005.
Weedon D. Skin Pathology, 4th Ed. Churchill Livingstone, 2009.

Diseases of Hair and Nail

BIOPSIES OF CONDITIONS AFFECTING THE SCALP

Assessment of scalp disorders can be difficult clinically and histologically. Selection of the appropriate area for biopsy and subsequent histological examination is crucial. Interpretation of biopsy specimens requires clinicopathological correlation. In most cases, scalp biopsies are performed for evaluating alopecia and its causes.

In selecting the site for biopsy, the optimum site should be at sites of early clinical disease:

- In the center of the lesion in a representative area
- At the "active" edge of the scalp condition in a representative area.

SELECTION OF BIOPSY SITES

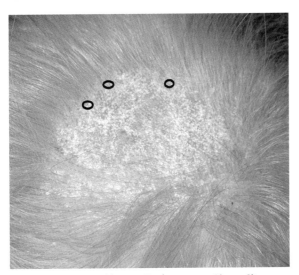

FIGURE 13.1   Discoid Lupus Erythematosus-Biopsy Sites Selection at Presumed Active Edge

In some cases, early disease may not be easily appreciated clinically. Sites of end-stage disease (e.g., sites where there are no hair follicles or extensive scarring is present) are of very limited use. Sites of marked inflammation with pustules sometimes do not provide sufficient diagnostic information. In areas of pustule formation, microbiological swabs and pulled hair samples of hair bulbs and roots may be obtained to be examined by microscopy and microbiological evaluation for fungal organisms if a fungal kerion (an area of markedly inflamed fungal infection affecting hair follicles and skin) is suspected.

Multiple biopsies (sampling) from the early affected areas generally improve the diagnostic yield by reducing sampling error. A biopsy of normal unaffected scalp skin can provide a useful normal internal control to compare with the affected scalp skin.

All scalp biopsies are taken under local anesthetic cover. Biopsy sites should be marked up with a surgical marker prior to infiltration of the local anesthetic. Biopsies may be obtained by punch biopsy or alternatively as a small thin incisional biopsy. When obtaining a punch biopsy, the trajectory of the punch biopsy as it is twisted into the scalp skin should be parallel to the trajectory of the hair shafts as they enter the skin. Punch biopsy specimens are traditionally sectioned along the vertical axis of the specimen; however, when evaluating alopecia, vertical and transverse sectioning yield more diagnostic information.

When evaluating scalp biopsies for alopecia, a minimum of three samples of tissue are required for:

1. Traditional vertical axis sectioning,

2. Transverse sectioning, and

3. Tissue for direct immunofluorescence for evaluation of presence or absence of immune deposits (complement and immunoglobulin) in early alopecia areata, autoimmune blistering conditions, and suspected cutaneous lupus erythematosus.

An additional sample of normal unaffected scalp hair may be useful in some settings, for example, evaluation of male-type androgenetic alopecia. If other conditions are suspected clinically, a single punch biopsy for hematoxylin and eosin examination in 10% formalin and a separate biopsy in Michel medium for immunofluorescence study are submitted.

VERTICAL SECTION OF A PUNCH BIOPSY OF THE SCALP

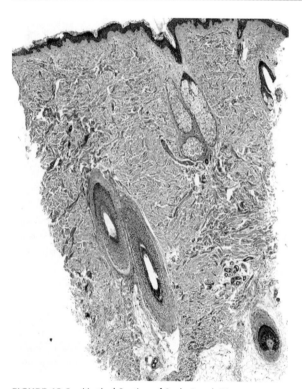

FIGURE 13.2   Vertical Section of Scalp Punch Biopsy

This specimen is useful for assessing the epidermal changes, particularly when discoid lupus erythematosus or other variants of lupus erythematosus are suspected, for assessment of the hair bulb architecture and the level(s) at which inflammation may be present. Traditional vertical sectioning does not give sufficient information about hair density and often may not contain sufficient hair follicles to examine.

TRANSVERSE SECTION AT THE LEVEL OF UPPER DERMIS, UPPER SUBCUTIS, DEEP SUBCUTIS

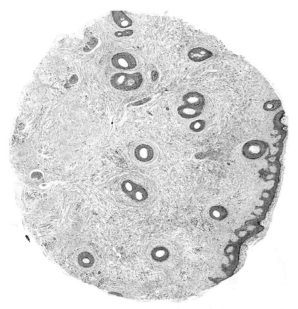

Transverse sections are used for assessment of hair density, anagen:telogen ratio, and hair shaft diameters. Serial transverse sections also may give an indication of the level(s) where the pathological process affects the follicles that are not apparent with examination of vertical sections as more section of hair follicles are easily seen with this type of sectioning compared with vertical axis sectioning.

FIGURE 13.3   Transverse Section at the Level of Upper Dermis

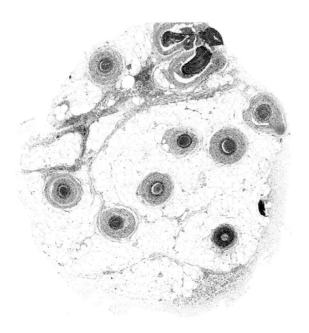

FIGURE 13.4   Transverse Section at the Level of Upper Subcutis

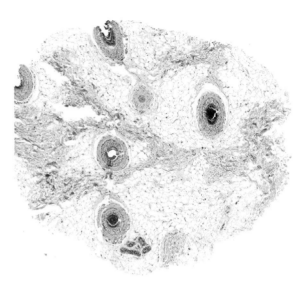

FIGURE 13.5   Transverse Section at the Level of Deep Subcutis

IMMUNOFLUORESCENCE STAINING

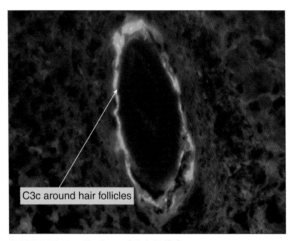

C3c around hair follicles

FIGURE 13.6   C3c Around Hair Follicles

Immunofluorescence staining of skin biopsies is useful in confirming the diagnosis of bullous disorders, alopecia areata, and lupus erythematosus.

In cases where a single punch biopsy is submitted, the specimen may be sectioned in the normal vertical axis, if scarring alopecia is suspected or in transverse sections if nonscarring alopecia is suspected.

STRUCTURE OF NORMAL HAIR

Hairs can be broadly divided into long thick terminal hairs and short hypopigmented vellus hairs. In transverse sections of scalp biopsies, terminal and vellus hairs can be identified by measuring their transverse diameters. Terminal hairs have diameters greater than 0.06 mm and vellus hairs have diameters less than 0.03 mm.

The terminal hair follicle undergoes three different phases in the hair cycle. The anagen phase, which is the longest and active phase, on an average, lasts for 3 years; the catagen or the regressing phase lasts for approximately 3 weeks; and the telogen or the resting phase lasts for approximately 3 months on an average.

SEGMENTS OF HAIR FOLLICLE

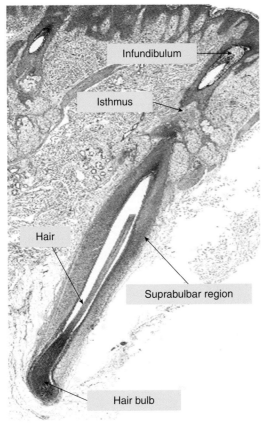

FIGURE 13.7   Segments of Hair Follicle

An anagen hair can be described to have four segments. Beginning from the surface is the infundibulum, which is a continuation of the epidermis into the follicular epithelium. The outer root sheath of the follicular epithelium of the infundibulum is cornified and has a granular layer similar to the epidermis. The infundibulum opens to the epidermal surface through the follicular ostium. The lower limit of the infundibulum is the entrance of the sebaceous ducts. The region in between the entrance of the sebaceous duct and the arrector pili muscle is the isthmus. The cells of the outer root sheath of the isthmus begin to cornify without forming the granular layer and results in trichilemmal type of keratinization. The region below the attachment of the arrector pili muscle is the suprabulbar zone. The hair bulb is normally located in the subcutaneous fat.

SEBACEOUS GLAND AND ARRECTOR PILI MUSCLE

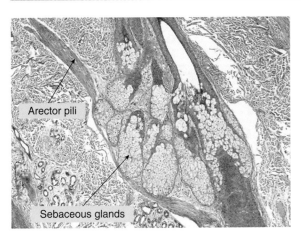

FIGURE 13.8   Sebaceous Gland and Arrector Pili Muscle

The region between the entrance of the sebaceous duct and the arrector pili muscle is called the isthmus. This is an important region of the follicle due to the formation of tricholemmal type of keratinization by the absence of the granular layer. Common scalp tumors such as tricholemmal cysts, proliferating tricholemmal cysts, and tricholemmal carcinomas arise from this region of the hair follicle.

The bulge region containing the stem cells are located in the region just above the attachment of the arrector pili muscle. The stem cells are known to stain positive for Cytokeratin 15.

HAIR BULB IN THE SUBCUTANEOUS FAT

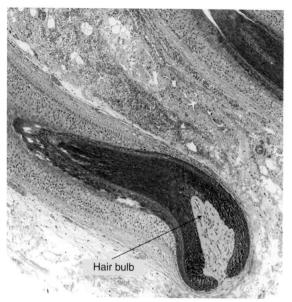

FIGURE 13.9   Hair Bulb in the Subcutaneous Fat

The hair bulb is normally located in the subcutaneous fat. It is mainly composed of the hair papilla surrounded by the hair matrix, which is formed of the pigmented germinative cells. The papilla continues with the outer fibrous sheath through the stalk. The hair and the inner root sheath are formed from the pluripotential cells present in the matrix. The melanin present in the cells of the hair matrix is transferred to the future cells of the hair in varying quantities by the process of phagocytosis. As the cells mature toward the surface, different layers of the follicle, the hair cortex, and the medulla are formed.

ANAGEN HAIR-LAYERS

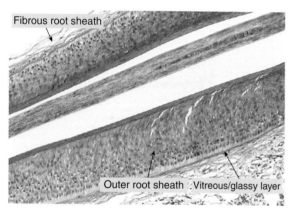

FIGURE 13.10   Anagen Hair-Layers of the Follicle-Suprabulbar Region

The suprabulbar region exhibits the different layers of the anagen hair. The outermost layer of the follicle is the fibrous root sheath. Inner to this is the thin well defined glassy (vitreous) layer. The outer root sheath is the thick cellular layer seen inside the vitreous layer. The cells of the outer root sheath cornifies without forming the granular layer at the level of isthmus. This results in tricholemmal type of keratinization.

CORTEX AND MEDULLA OF THE FOLLICLE

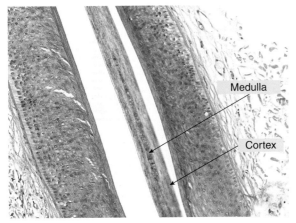

FIGURE 13.11   Cortex and Medulla of the Follicle

The cortex and the medulla of the follicle are formed from the pluripotential cells of the hair matrix.

LAYERS OF THE FOLLICLE-BULBAR REGION

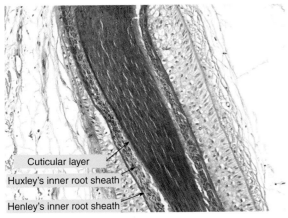

FIGURE 13.12   Layers of the Follicle-Bulbar Region

The cuticular layer, Huxley inner root sheath, and Henley inner root sheath are essentially formed from the pluripotential cells of the hair matrix.

HAIR BULB-HIGH POWER

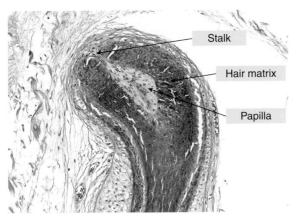

FIGURE 13.13   Hair Bulb-High Power

The hair bulb is located in the subcutaneous fat. The dermal papilla of the bulb is continuous with the fibrous root sheath through the stalk. The papilla and the stalk are surrounded by the hair matrix, which contains the germinative or pluripotential cells. A considerable numbers of melanocytes are also seen admixed with the germinative cells. The hair and the layers of the follicular epithelium are formed from the pluripotential cells. The melanocytes transfer the pigment to the primitive hair cells as required.

INFLAMMATORY DISEASES OF THE FOLLICLES

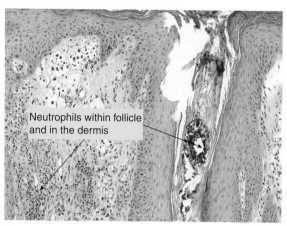

FIGURE 13.14   Suppurative Folliculitis-High Power

Inflammatory conditions affecting the follicular units are common. A large majority of cases are acneiform lesions, superficial folliculitis, deep folliculitis, and the diseases constituting the follicular occlusion triad.

SUPPURATIVE FOLLICULITIS

Suppurative folliculitis occurs in a number of clinical settings. It could be superficial folliculitis or deep folliculitis as in furuncle, pseudomonas folliculitis or other bacterial folliculitis caused by *Klebsiella* sp. or *Escherichia coli*.

Deep folliculitis may also be caused by dermatophytes such as *Microsporum canis* or *Malassezia* sp., which causes Pityrosporum.

On microscopy, the organisms are identified very rarely on routine microscopy. There is dense collection of neutrophils forming abscesses within the follicle or surrounding it. Microbiological culture of the tissue is the most helpful diagnostic tool.

ACNE KELOIDALIS

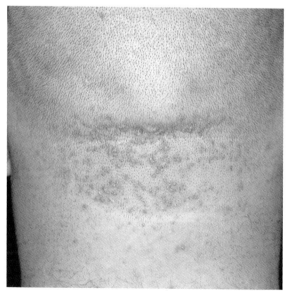

FIGURE 13.15   Acne Keloidalis Nuchae

Acne keloidalis is also known as folliculitis keloidalis nuchae, which is an uncommon inflammatory condition occurring on the nape of the neck in adult men. Clinically, there are plaques and pustules, which are follicular based.

On microscopy, there is rupture and destruction of the follicle with liberation of the hair shaft into the dermis. The inflammatory response varies with the stage of the disease. The early stages show abscess formation and infiltration of neutrophils into the follicles. As the lesion progresses, or in recurrent lesions, there is extensive scarring and chronic inflammatory response. Granulomas may be seen surrounding the released keratin.

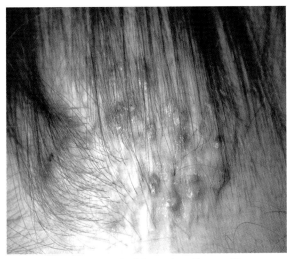

FIGURE 13.16   Acne Keloidalis Nuchae-Close-up View

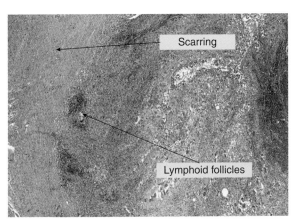

FIGURE 13.17   Acne Keloidalis Nuchae-Low Power

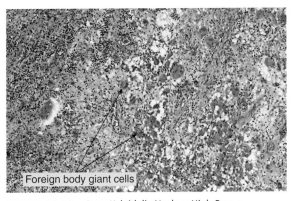

FIGURE 13.18   Acne Keloidalis Nuchae-High Power

HIDRADENITIS SUPPURATIVA

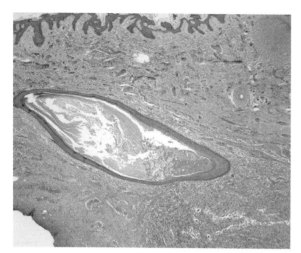

FIGURE 13.19   Hidradenitis Suppurativa-Low Power

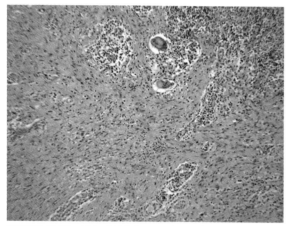

FIGURE 13.20   Hidradenitis Suppurativa-High Power-Giant Cells

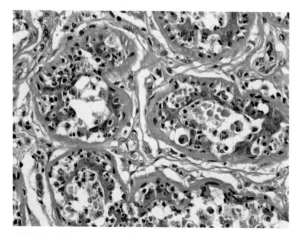

FIGURE 13.21   Hidradenitis Suppurativa-High Power

Hidradenitis is a chronic recurring inflammatory disease and is one of the follicular occlusion triads. The disease involves the axilla, groin, and the pubic regions most commonly. Clinically, the disease is characterized by recurring pustules, which gets complicated by scarring. It is thought to be an androgen-dependent disorder. Very rarely, squamous cell carcinoma develops at the sites of long-standing hidradenitis suppurativa.

On microscopy, the overlying epidermis may show acanthosis and pseudoepitheliomatous hyperplasia. The histological changes reflect the stage of the disease. In the early acute stages, there is dense infiltrate of neutrophils forming abscesses. Sinus tracts may form, leading up to the skin surface. The sinuses are lined by stratified squamous epithelium and may well represent residual follicular epithelium. In the chronic stage, granulation tissue composed of foreign body giant cells and chronic inflammatory cells such as lymphocytes are seen. Extensive areas of scarring are also seen, particularly in the recurrent cases. The adnexal glands particularly apocrine gland in the axilla could be involved in a large number of cases. Hidradenitis is still considered a follicular disease due to the involvement of the follicles in the large majority of cases.

FOLLICULITIS DECALVANS

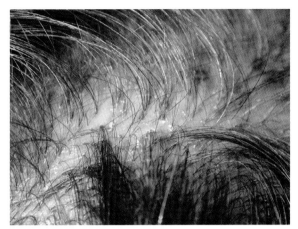

FIGURE 13.22   Folliculitis Decalvans-Close-up View

Folliculitis decalvans is a chronic disease affecting the deep follicles. Clinically, it is known to affect any hair-bearing part of the body and presents as alopecia.

On microscopy, follicular destruction by infiltrating neutrophils is the earliest change. The release of hair and keratin into the adjacent dermis results in granuloma formation with foreign body giant cell reaction and scarring.

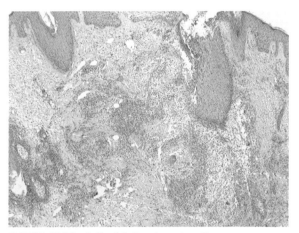

FIGURE 13.23   Folliculitis Decalvans-Low Power

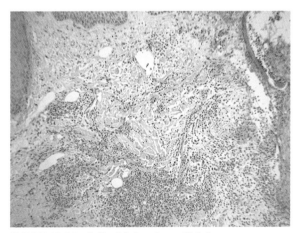

FIGURE 13.24   Folliculitis Decalvans-High Power

EROSIVE PUSTULAR DERMATOSIS

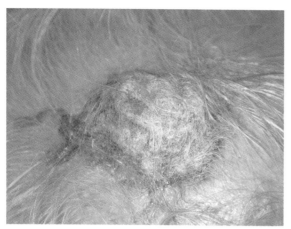

FIGURE 13.25   Erosive Pustular Dermatosis

Erosive pustular dermatosis of the scalp is a very uncommon condition resulting in scarring alopecia.

On microscopy, there is ulceration of the epidermis. The dermis shows diffuse infiltration of neutrophils with involvement of the follicles and the eccrine glands and ducts. *Staphylococcus aureus* has been implicated as the causative organism in some of the cases.

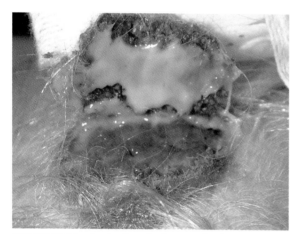

FIGURE 13.26   Erosive Pustular Dermatosis-Close-up View

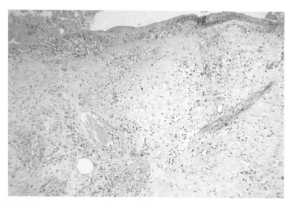

FIGURE 13.27   Erosive Pustular Dermatosis-Scanning View

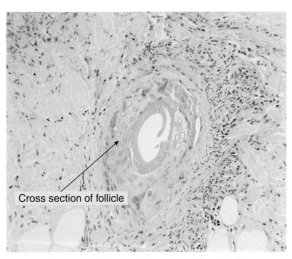

FIGURE 13.28   Erosive Pustular Dermatosis-Follicular Involvement

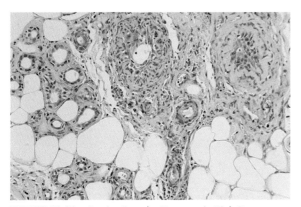

FIGURE 13.29   Erosive Pustular Dermatosis-High Power

ALOPECIA

Alopecia is broadly divided into scarring and nonscarring types. The commonest causes of scarring alopecia are lichen planopilaris and its subtypes and lupus erythematosus. Scarring alopecia can also be due to a number of uncommon conditions such as nevus sebaceous. The commonest type of nonscarring alopecia is alopecia areata and androgenetic alopecia.

LICHEN PLANOPILARIS

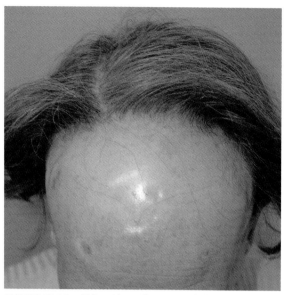

FIGURE 13.30   Lichen Planopilaris-Frontal Fibrosing Type

Lichen planopilaris is also known as follicular lichen planus. Clinically, it manifests as scarring alopecia with erythema and scarring.

On microscopy, the changes are seen mainly in the perifollicular area. There is lichenoid infiltration of the follicular epithelium, which results in the destruction of the follicles, and at a later stage, there is fibrosis and perifollicular scarring.

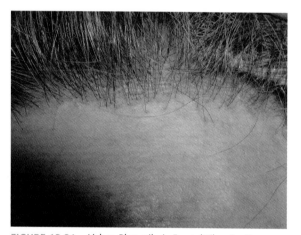

FIGURE 13.31   Lichen Planopilaris-Frontal Fibrosing Type-Follicular Plugging and Erythema

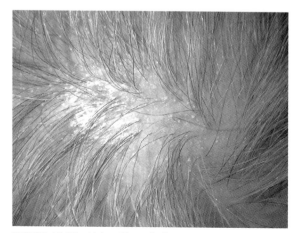

FIGURE 13.32   Lichen Planopilaris

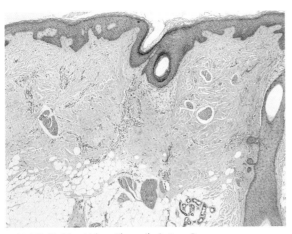

FIGURE 13.33   Lichen Planopilaris-Low Power

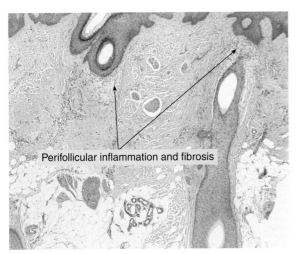

Perifollicular inflammation and fibrosis

FIGURE 13.34   Lichen Planopilaris-High Power

SCARRING ALOPECIA

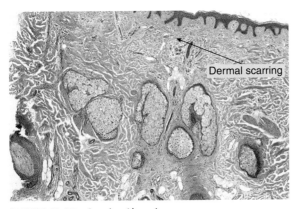

Dermal scarring

FIGURE 13.35   Scarring Alopecia

Scarring alopecia is one of the commonest types of alopecia. The lesions are represented by lichen planopilaris and lupus erythematosus.

On microscopy, the characteristic change identified is interfollicular scarring. The changes of lichen planopilaris and lupus erythematosus will be seen as the case may be.

LUPUS ERYTHEMATOSUS

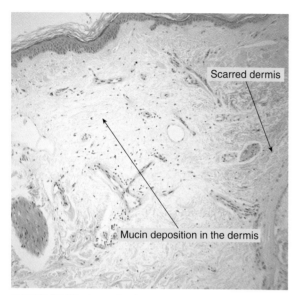

FIGURE 13.36 Lupus Erythematosus-Low Power

Lupus erythematosus is one of the commonest causes of scarring alopecia. Different clinical forms have been described. Discoid lupus erythematosus is the commonest type involving the scalp and resulting in scarring alopecia.

On microscopy, the classical features of discoid lupus erythematosus such as basal cell vacuolation, basement membrane thickening, and lichenoid infiltration of lymphocytes in the papillary dermis. The infiltrate may also involve the follicular epithelium and result in the destruction of the follicles. In addition, separation of the dermal collagen may be the only diagnostic feature seen in some cases of lupus erythematosus. This finding is due to the deposition of dermal mucin. The presence of dermal mucin can be confirmed by the Alcian blue stain.

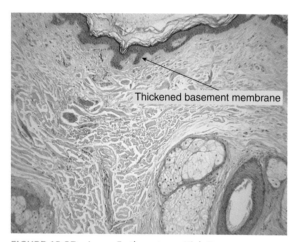

FIGURE 13.37 Lupus Erythematosus-High Power

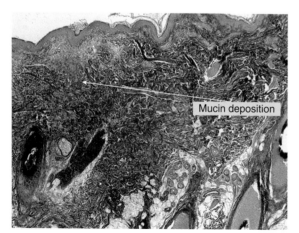

FIGURE 13.38 Lupus Erythematosus-Alcian Blue

ALOPECIA AREATA

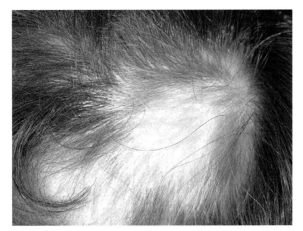

FIGURE 13.39   Alopecia Areata-Regrowth

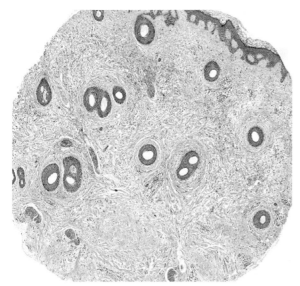

FIGURE 13.40   Transverse Section of Scalp Skin-Alopecia Areata

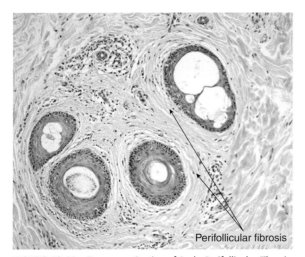

Perifollicular fibrosis

FIGURE 13.41   Transverse Section of Scalp-Perifollicular Fibrosis

Alopecia areata is one of the commonest causes of nonscarring alopecia. The disease can affect any part of the body. Clinically, it presents as circumscribed patches on the scalp or total body hair loss.

On microscopy, the changes are seen in three different stages. The earliest is the acute stage when the total numbers of the follicles may appear normal. Many of the follicles enter the telogen phase. There is peribulbar inflammation, which may be subtle in some cases. Vacuolization and necrosis of the matrix cells are a characteristic features of alopecia areata and may be found in some of the cells. Clumps of pigment may be found in the epithelium of the catagen follicles.

The second phase, is the most common phase encountered by the pathologists. The catagen/telogen numbers are increased. The peribulbar inflammation tends to subside, and the hair bulbs are generally free of inflammation. The third phase, also known as the chronic phase, is seen in well-established cases. The follicles get miniaturized, but the total numbers of follicles may remain normal. Nanogen hairs, which are abnormally formed, are a distinctive feature of alopecia areata. Nanogen hairs are identified in transverse sections by the absence of the hair shaft and incompletely cornified hair shaft. In addition, they have thin outer and inner root sheaths. Mitotic activity, which is a feature of active growth and apoptosis, indicating cell death, is simultaneously seen in alopecia areata. Few stelae, which are composed of numerous capillaries, inflammatory cells, and clumps of melanin are also identified.

MALE PATTERN ALOPECIA

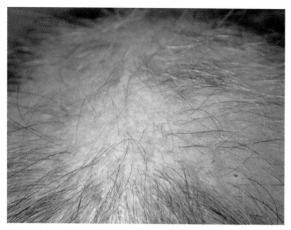

FIGURE 13.42   Male Pattern Alopecia

Androgenetic alopecia is also known as common balding, male pattern balding, and female pattern balding. The onset of balding in females can be either at the time of menopause or in early adulthood. Most commonly the thinning of the hair is on the crown of the scalp.

On microscopy, the changes are similar in male and female pattern alopecia regardless of the time of onset. Progressive miniaturization is a characteristic feature. There is great variation in the diameter of the follicles. Streamers are seen below the miniaturized follicles. The normal terminal:vellus ratio of 2:1 is reduced. The inflammatory response in androgenetic alopecia is minimal, and mild perifollicular lymphohistiocytic inflammation may be seen.

ALOPECIA DUE TO NEVUS SEBACEOUS

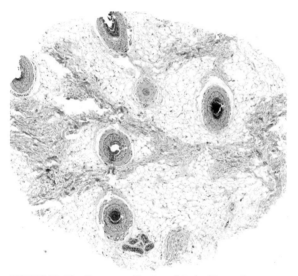

FIGURE 13.43   Transverse Section of Scalp Skin-Androgenetic Alopecia

Scarring alopecia is a recognized complication of nevus sebaceous. Clinically the lesions may present as alopecia.

On microscopy, the epidermis shows attachment of rudimentary hair follicles and sebaceous glands. The dermis shows scarring with abnormally positioned eccrine glands and immature sebaceous glands. Inflammation is not a feature in this condition.

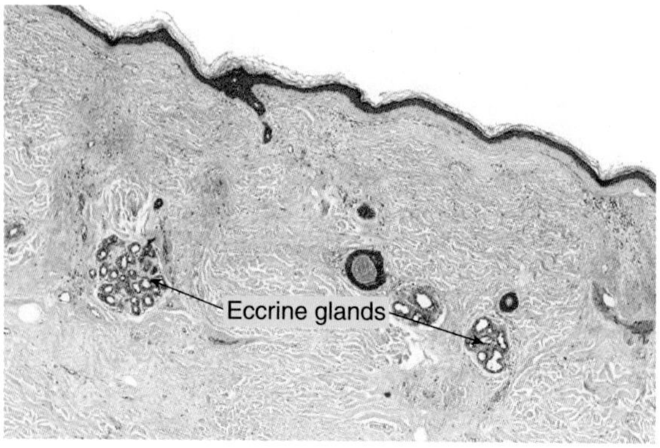

Eccrine glands

FIGURE 13.44   Alopecia Due to Nevus Sebaceous-Low Power

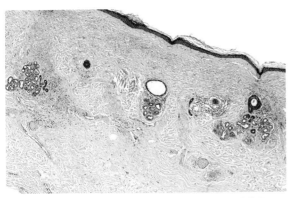

FIGURE 13.45   Alopecia Due to Nevus Sebaceous-High Power

TRICHOTILLOMANIA

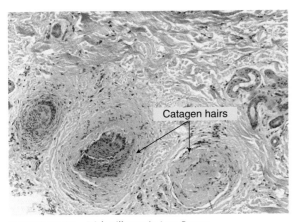

FIGURE 13.46   Trichotillomania-Low Power

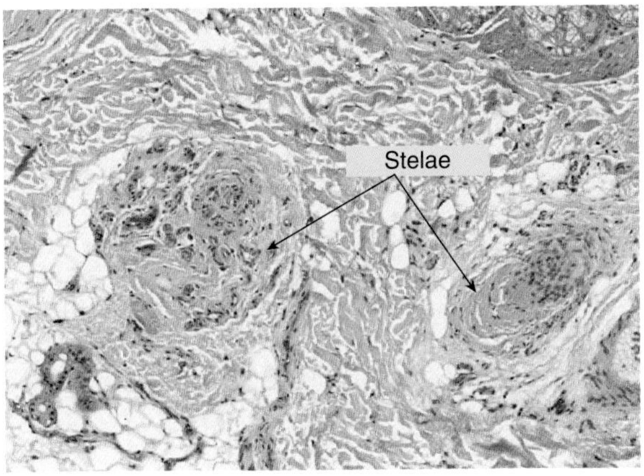

Trichotillomania is a form of alopecia resulting from deliberate avulsion of hairs by patients who may be under psychological stress. The crown and occipital scalp are commonly affected, but eyebrows trunk and pubic areas may be affected.

On microscopy, the characteristic features are the presence of numerous catagen hairs and the presence pigment casts within the dilated follicular infundibulum. This is the result of sudden termination of anagen phase. The interfollicular dermis may show some degree of scarring.

FIGURE 13.47   Stelae or Streamers in Trichotillomania

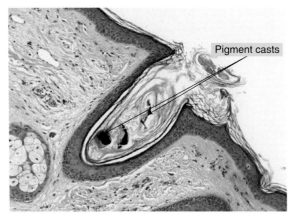

FIGURE 13.48 Pigment Casts in Trichotillomania-High Power

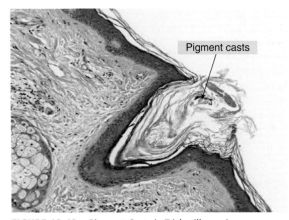

FIGURE 13.49 Pigment Casts in Trichotillomania

Nail Unit Biopsy Specimens

Biopsy of the nail unit and its individual structures requires a good working knowledge of the nail unit terminology and anatomy.

NAIL UNIT

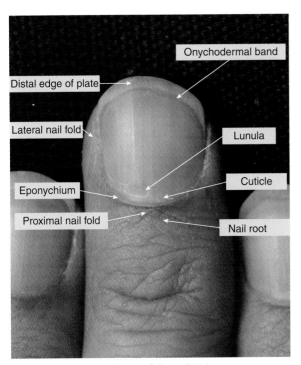

FIGURE 13.50   Dorsal View of the Nail Unit

The nail unit is composed of nail plate and the epithelial structures such as the proximal nail fold, the matrix, the nail bed, and the hyponychium. The nail plate is the translucent structure that overlies the distal digits of the hands and the feet. The proximal aspect of the nail plate has white semicircular areas called the lunulae. The dorsal surface of the nail bed is pink due to the extensive vasculature. The proximal nail fold has a dorsal and ventral epithelial surface, where the dorsal surface folds on itself to form the ventral surface. In between the two surfaces lies the eponychium, which is also known as the cuticle. The cuticle covers the potential space between the proximal nail fold and the nail plate. The nail matrix forms the entire length of the nail bed, which is the area beneath the nail plate, and lies in between the lunula and the hyponychium.

The hyponychium is located underneath the free edge of the nail plate. It indicates the transition from the nail bed to the normal epidermis of the fingers and toes. The part of the hyponychium that reflects on to the ventral surface of the nail plate is called the onychodermal band.

On microscopy, the nail plate is formed of squamous epithelium. The firm nature of the nail plate is due to the abundant calcium, sulfur protein, and other minerals such as iron and magnesium within it. The dorsal proximal nail fold does not contain hair follicles and sebaceous glands. The nail bed and the matrix are also formed of squamous epithelial cells. Unlike normal epidermal cells, the cells of proximal nail, and lateral nail folds, the cells of the matrix and the nail bed keratinize without forming a granular layer.

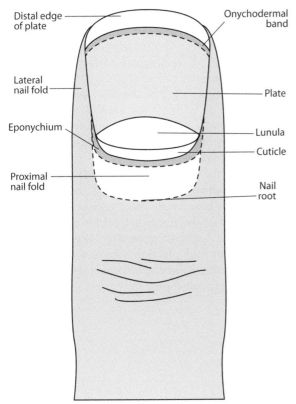

FIGURE 13.51   Dorsal View of the Nail Unit-Schematic Diagram

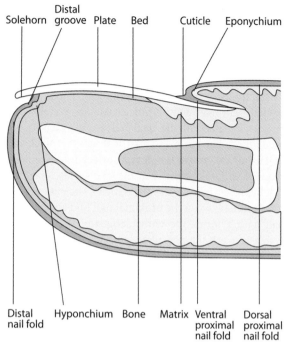

Solehorn   Distal groove   Plate   Bed   Cuticle   Eponychium

Distal nail fold   Hyponchium   Bone   Matrix   Ventral proximal nail fold   Dorsal proximal nail fold

FIGURE 13.52   Sagittal View of the Nail Unit-Schematic Diagram

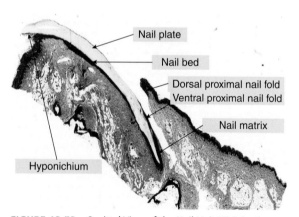

Nail plate

Nail bed

Dorsal proximal nail fold
Ventral proximal nail fold

Nail matrix

Hyponichium

FIGURE 13.53   Sagittal View of the Nail Unit-H&E Section

Biopsies of the Nail Unit

All nail surgeries are undertaken under anesthesia, with a digital nerve (or "ring") block or alternatively, utilizing a distal "wing" block using a 50:50 mixture of plain (i.e., containing no adrenaline), short-acting local anesthetic (e.g., lignocaine, prilocaine), and long-acting anesthetic (e.g., bupivacaine). In procedures such as nail bed surgery or removal of the nail matrix, a bloodless field is essential. This is usually achieved by use of a tourniquet (various different techniques can be used to accomplish this) intraoperatively (maximum tourniquet time approximately 15 minutes or less if there is a history of peripheral vascular disease).

Diagrams or clinical images accompanying the pathology request form indicating the site of the biopsy and with marking of orientation of longitudinal specimens of (e.g., fusiform incisions of the nail bed, en bloc longitudinal excision and lateral longitudinal biopsies) are particularly helpful for correct interpretation of nail biopsies. A specific request for longitudinal sectioning (rather than standard practice transverse "breadloaf" sectioning) of all longitudinally orientated specimens should be made on the pathology request form.

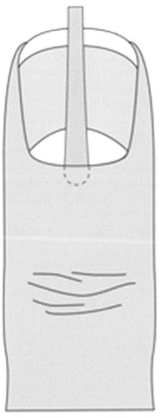

FIGURE 13.54   Schematic Diagram of Wedge Biopsy of
Proximal Nail Using an Elevator to Protect the Nail Matrix (a)

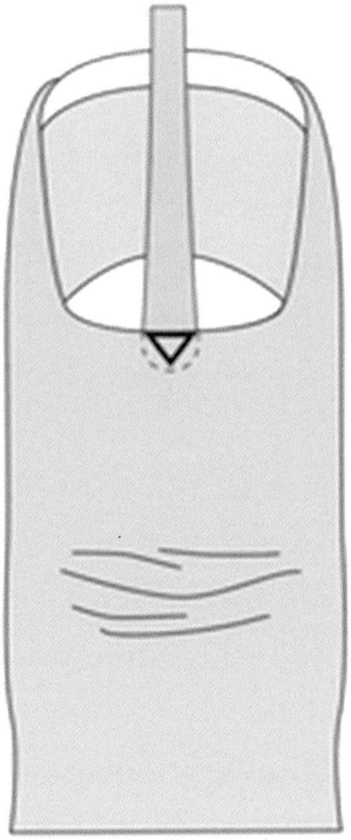

Schematic of Wedge Biopsy Proximal Nail Using an Elevator to Protect the Nail Matrix

Proximal nail fold biopsy are undertaken to diagnose disorders of the proximal nail fold such as neoplasms (melanoma, squamous cell carcinoma), precancerous conditions (squamous cell carcinoma in situ), and chronic refractory inflammatory dermatoses. Under local anesthetic, a Freer septal nail elevator is inserted under the proximal nail fold to protect the distal nail matrix immediately from inadvertent damage of the matrix. A wedge of proximal nail fold is then incised with a scalpel to the level of the nail elevator to include the ventral surface of the proximal nail fold. An alternative method is to take a 3-mm punch biopsy from the proximal nail fold without severing the ventral surface of the proximal nail fold.

FIGURE 13.55   Schematic Diagram of Wedge Biopsy of
Proximal Nail Using an Elevator to Protect the Nail Matrix (b)

NAIL MILD DYSPLASIA

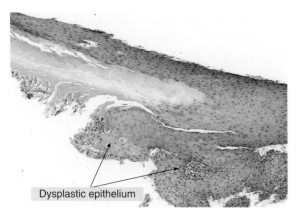

FIGURE 13.56   Nail-mild Dysplasia-Low Power

In situ and invasive squamous cell carcinoma of the nail is very rare.

Clinically, it most commonly presents as a nonhealing ulcer or discharging sinus.

On microscopy, the changes are seen as in other sites. The earliest change is in situ carcinoma. As the disease progresses, the neoplastic cells invade into the underlying stroma as islands and single cells. The grading of squamous cell carcinoma is done similar to other sites. The prognosis of ungual squamous cell carcinoma is worse compared with other cutaneous sites. They tend to metastasize earlier to regional lymph nodes.

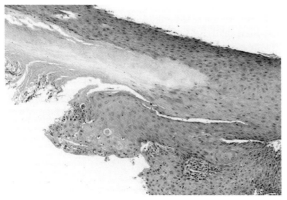

FIGURE 13.57   Nail-mild Dysplasia-Medium Power

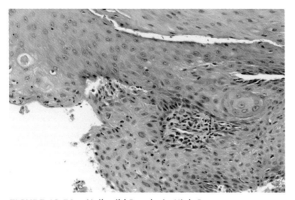

FIGURE 13.58   Nail-mild Dysplasia-High Power

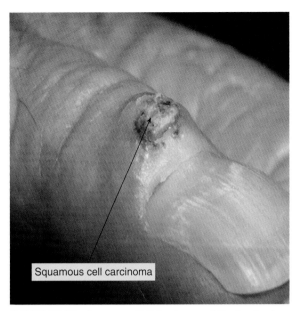

FIGURE 13.59 Squamous Cell Carcinoma of the Proximal Nail Fold

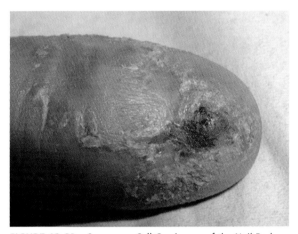

FIGURE 13.60 Squamous Cell Carcinoma of the Nail Bed

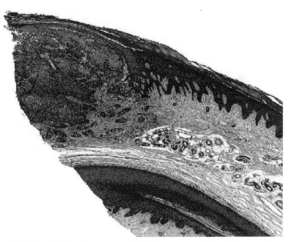

FIGURE 13.61 Squamous Cell Carcinoma of the Proximal Nail Fold-H&E Stain-Scanning View

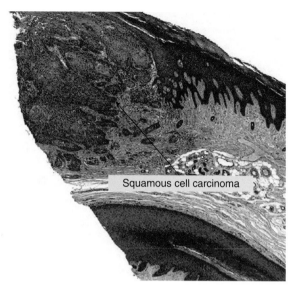

FIGURE 13.62   Squamous Cell Carcinoma of the Proximal Nail Fold-H&E Stain-Medium Power

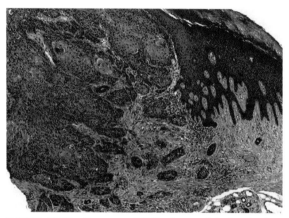

FIGURE 13.63   Squamous Cell Carcinoma of the Proximal Nail Fold-High Power

PROXIMAL ONYCHOMYCOSIS

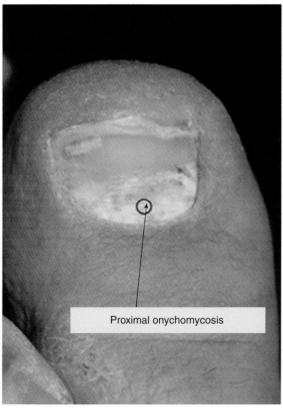

FIGURE 13.64   Proximal Onychomycosis and Planning for Proximal Nail Plate Biopsy by Punch Biopsy Method

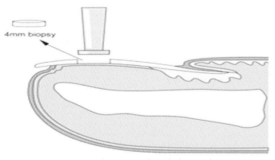

FIGURE 13.65   Punch Biopsy of Nail Plate-Schematic Diagram

Nail plate biopsy may be used for the diagnosis of proximal nail plate onychomycosis in cases where simple scrapings for mycological investigations have been unhelpful in confirming a diagnosis. This biopsy can be undertaken without local anesthetic. The nail is soaked in warm water for 10 minutes (or more) to soften the nail. The nail surface is scored with punch biopsy. The punch is twisted until the patient can feel the punch biopsy, indicating the ventral side of nail plate has been reached. The sample of nail can then removed for microbiological examination and histological examination with PAS (periodic acid-Schiff) staining.

Onychomycosis is the term used to denote fungal infections of the nail. This is caused by a variety of fungi, and they are seen in toe nails more commonly than finger nails. Peripheral vascular diseases and immunocompromised states are predisposing factors. The clinical presentation is classified on the basis of the location of the lesion as distal, proximal, lateral, subungual, and superficial. The causative organisms vary from *Candida albicans* to *Aspergillus* sp.

On microscopy, the fungal elements are seen in the deep portions of the biopsy and so a scraping may not yield a positive result. Additional changes such as hyperkeratosis, parakeratosis, and spongiosis of the epidermis with spongiotic vesicle formation are seen. The fungal elements may also be seen sandwiched in between the two layers of keratin surrounded by neutrophils. Very rarely, a granulomatous inflammation may be seen.

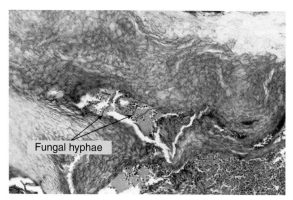

FIGURE 13.66   Fungal Hyphae in Proximal Nail Fold Biopsy-
H&E Section

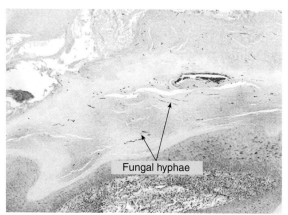

FIGURE 13.67   Fungal Hyphae in Proximal Nail Fold Biopsy-
PAS Stain-Low Power

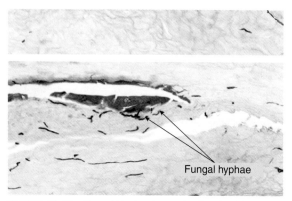

FIGURE 13.68   Fungal Hyphae in Proximal Nail Fold Biopsy-
PAS Stain-High Power

AVULSION TECHNIQUE, PUNCH BIOPSY, FUSIFORM BIOPSY

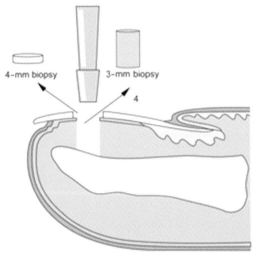

FIGURE 13.69   Nail Bed-Double Nail Plate Avulsion Technique of Nail Bed Biopsy Without Nail Avulsion-Schematic Diagram

Biopsies of the nail bed requires either complete or partial nail plate avulsion to expose the hyponychium, nail bed, distal nail matrix. If the proximal nail matrix needs to be visualized, retraction of the proximal nail fold to expose the proximal nail matrix is required.

Biopsies of the lesions of the nail bed and matrix can be undertaken either with punch biopsy or fusiform incisions down to the level of the bone.

For smaller localized pathology, the "window nail plate avulsion" or "double punch" nail plate avulsion technique may be utilized to expose the underlying nail bed to explore well-demarcated localized lesions, draining subungual hematomas, and acute paronychia and removing foreign bodies from the nail bed.

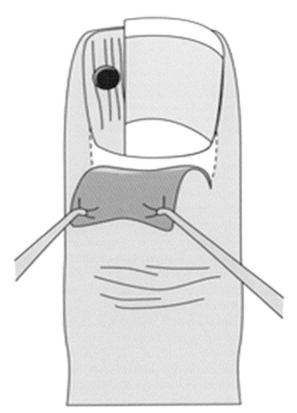

FIGURE 13.70   Nail Bed-Punch Biopsy After Partial Nail Avulsion-Schematic Diagram

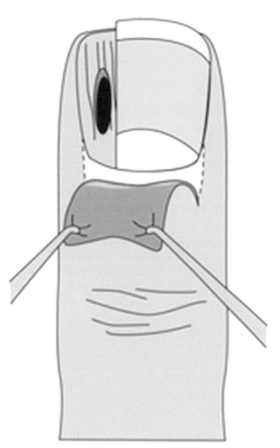

FIGURE 13.71   Fusiform Nail Biopsy After Partial Nail
Avulsion-Schematic Diagram

SUBUNGUAL MELANOMA

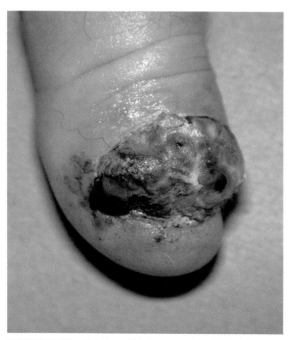

FIGURE 13.72   Sububgual Melanoma of the Nail Bed

Nail matrix biopsies are most commonly used for assessment and treatment of longitudinal melanonychia and for assessment of suspected malignant lesions affecting proximal nail fold, nail matrix, and nail bed (subungual lesions). Dermatoscopic assessment of the distal nail plate free margin in longitudinal melanonychia can useful to determine whether the proximal nail plate is involved (pigment confined to dorsal aspect of the nail plate) or distal nail plate (pigment confines to the ventral aspect of the nail plate). Biopsies larger than 3 mm in width or diameter are likely to leave permanent nail dystrophy. Biopsies 3 mm or less width are preferred where possible to reduce risk of nail dystrophy. If only the distal matrix is involved, a punch biopsy encompassing the whole area will suffice. The surface of the matrix is scored with a punch biopsy (then checked to assess if the correct area is identified). The punch biopsy is then twisted down to the level of the bone and sample gently removed with fine-tipped scissors. If the proximal matrix is affected, a longitudinal 3-mm fusiform ellipse of the affected matrix can be removed before suturing the wound defect with rapidly dissolving suture material. A small punch biopsy or narrow longitudinally orientated fusiform

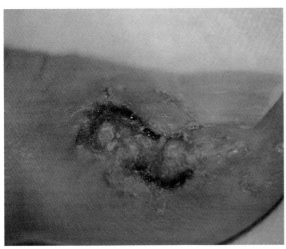

FIGURE 13.73   Amelanotic Melanoma with Ulceration of the Proximal and Lateral Nail Fold

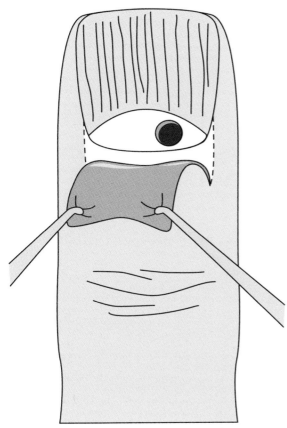

FIGURE 13.74   Nail Matrix-Punch Biopsy-Schematic Diagram

incisional biopsy is usually adequate to sample conditions that arise solely on the lateral nail fold without nail involvement.

Subungual melanoma may present in the intertriginous area or as longitudinal melanonychia. Amelanotic variants have also been described. In cases of longitudinal melanonychia where Hutchinson sign is present (i.e., the extension of melanocytic pigmentation to involve the proximal and/or lateral nail fold), a presumptive diagnosis of subungual melanoma is made, and further careful assessment and investigation is always required to differentiate it from benign causes of Hutchinson sign.

Causes of Hutchinson sign are as follows:

1. Subungual melanoma
2. Subungual hematoma
3. Congenital melanocytic nevus
4. Ethnic pigmentation
5. Posttraumatic (including post–nail biopsy)
6. Postradiation
7. Drugs (minocycline, zidovudine)
8. AIDS
9. Malnutrition
10. Peutz-Jegher syndrome
11. Laugier-Hunziker syndrome.

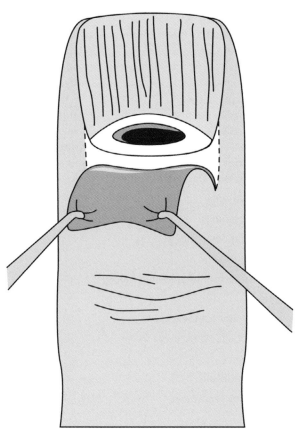

FIGURE 13.75   Nail Matrix-Punch Biopsy-Schematic Diagram

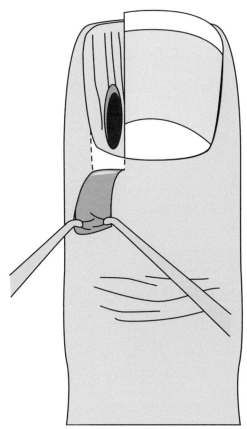

FIGURE 13.76   Proximal Nail Matrix-Longitudinal
Fusiform Biopsy

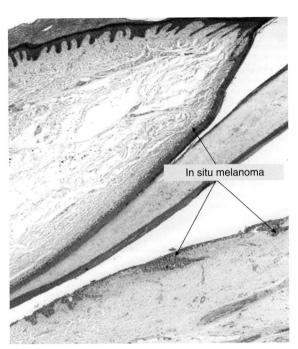

FIGURE 13.77   Subungual Melanoma in Situ-Low Power

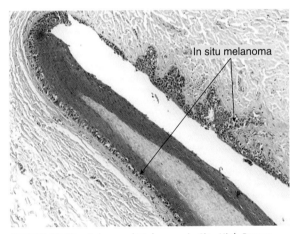

FIGURE 13.78   Subungual Melanoma in Situ-High Power

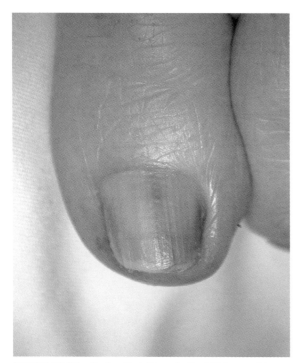

FIGURE 13.79   Benign Racial Longitudinal Melanonychia

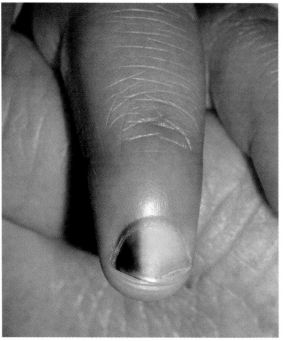

FIGURE 13.80   Congenital Melanocytic Naevus-Longitudinal Melanonychia

NAIL BIOPSY

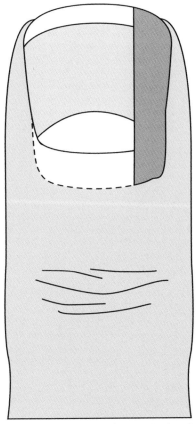

FIGURE 13.81   Lateral Longitudinal Nail Biopsy

If the nail lesion is large, an en bloc biopsy/excision of the matrix (whole matrix, nail plate, nail bed and hyponychium, and distal nail fold skin also removed) in the center or lateral portion of the nail unit (or lateral longitudinal biopsy), depending on the site of the lesion, is required.

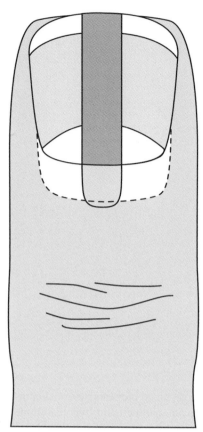

FIGURE 13.82   Planning of Central en bloc Longitudinal Nail Biopsy

BIBLIOGRAPHY

Baran R, Kechijian P. Hutchinson's sign: a reappraisal. J Am Acad Dermatol 1996;34(1):87–90.

Collins SC, Cordova K, Jellinek NJ. Alternatives to complete nail plate avulsion. J Am Acad Dermatol 2008;59(4):619–626.

Eedy D, Breathnach SM, Walker NPJ. Surgical Dermatology, 1st Ed. Oxford: Blackwell Science, 1996.

George R, Clarke S, Ioffreda M, Billingsley E. Marking of nail matrix biopsies with ink aids in proper specimen orientation for more accurate histologic evaluation. Dermatol Surg 2008;34(12):1705–1706.

Jellinek N. Nail matrix biopsy of longitudinal melanonychia: diagnostic algorithm including the matrix shave biopsy. J Am Acad Dermatol 2007;56(5):803–810.

Jellinek NJ. Nail surgery: practical tips and treatment options. Dermatol Ther 2007;20(1):68–74.

Elder D et al. Lever's Histopathology of Skin, 10th Ed. Philadelphia, PA: Lippincott Williams, 2010.

Richert B. Basic nail surgery. Dermatol Clin 2006;24(3):313–322.

Solomon AR. The transversely sectioned scalp biopsy specimen: the technique and algorithm for its use in the diagnosis of alopecia. Adv Dermatol 1994;9:127–157.

Sperling LC. An Atlas of Hair Pathology with Clinical Correlations. New York: Parthenon Publishing, 2003.

Templeton SF, Santa Cruz DJ, Solomon AR. Alopecia: histologic diagnosis by transverse sections. Semin Diagn Pathol 1996;13(1):2–18.

Thomas L, Dalle S. Dermoscopy provides useful information for the management of melanonychia striata. Dermatol Ther 2007;20(1):3–10.

Cutaneous Infiltrates

INTRODUCTION

The dermis and subcutaneous fat can be home to infiltration by several different types of cells. Many of these cells are normal constituents of the dermis. Excessive numbers of them are seen in inflammatory and neoplastic conditions explained in this chapter.

SWEET SYNDROME

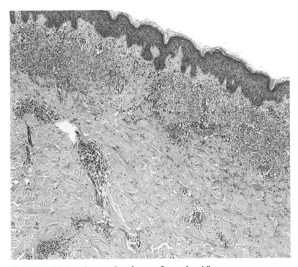

FIGURE 14.1   Sweet Syndrome-Scanning View

Sweet syndrome is also known as acute febrile neutrophilic dermatoses. It is a rare inflammatory disease in which sudden onset of painful nodules and plaques occur on the face and upper extremities associated with fever and peripheral blood leucocytosis. There is distinct association with myelomonocytic leukemia in 10 to 15% of cases. Leukemia may develop after the development of Sweet syndrome.

On microscopy, there is dense infiltration of neutrophils in the dermis and the subcutaneous fat. Leukocytoclasis with nuclear dust is seen. Focally, there is collection of neutrophils to form abscesses. Dermal edema is a feature that may sometimes lead to the formation of subepidermal vesicles. The vessels show endothelial swelling, but features of vasculitis are not seen.

Recently, there has been report of histiocytoid variant of Sweet syndrome. In this particular variant, there is infiltration of histiocytoid immature myelocytes in addition to neutrophils. This histological appearance also reinforces the association of Sweet syndrome with myelomonocytic leukemia and the fact that the possibility of histiocytoid Sweet syndrome should be considered when a diagnosis of leukemia cutis is made.

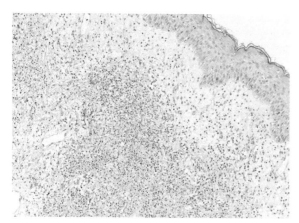

FIGURE 14.2   Sweet Syndrome-Low Power

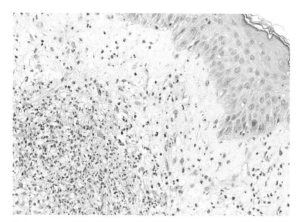

FIGURE 14.3   Sweet Syndrome-High Power

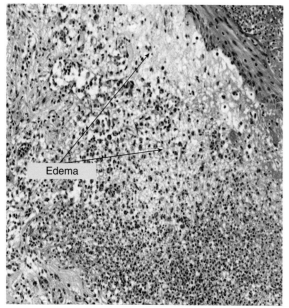

FIGURE 14.4   Sweet Syndrome—Dermal Edema

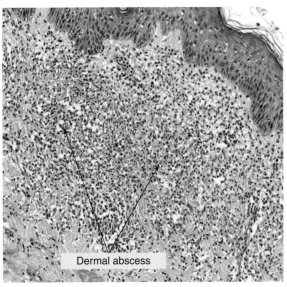

FIGURE 14.5   Sweet Syndrome—Dermal Abscess

NEUTROPHILIC URTICARIA

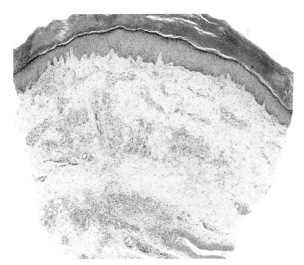

FIGURE 14.6   Neutrophilic Urticaria-Scanning View

Urticaria is a reaction pattern. This is clinically seen as transient erythematous papules or wheals, which may show central clearing. Acute urticaria can be triggered by viral illnesses and the use of antibiotics. On the other hand, chronic urticaria, which is defined as urticaria lasting for more than 6 weeks, is idiopathic in most cases. There may be triggering factors in chronic urticaria.

On microscopy, the basic pathological changes of urticaria are the result of vasodilatation and increased vascular permeability, which results in extravasation of protein and fluid into the dermis. Generally, the cell type involved in urticaria depends on the stage of the disease.

In neutrophilic urticaria, in early stages, there is perivascular infiltration and scattering of neutrophils in the interstitial dermal collagen. Very rarely, nuclear dusting may be present. Fibrinoid necrosis and other features of vasculitis are not seen. When the histological appearances are those of leukocytoclastic vasculitis and the clinical picture is that of urticaria, the term urticarial vasculitis is used.

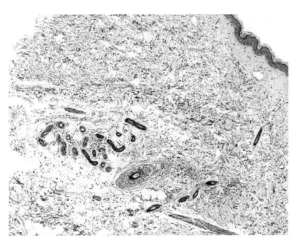

FIGURE 14.7   Neutrophilic Urticaria-Low Power

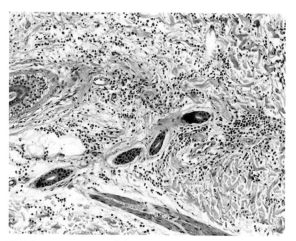

FIGURE 14.8   Neutrophilic Urticaria Periadnexal Infiltration

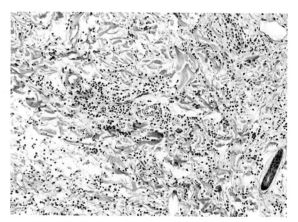

FIGURE 14.9   Neutrophilic Urticaria Interstitial Infiltration

NEUTROPHILIC ECCRINE HIDRADENITIS

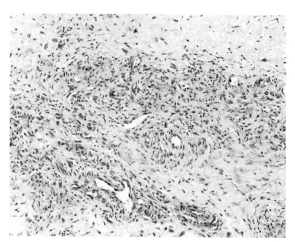

FIGURE 14.10   Neutrophilic Eccrine Hidradenitis

Neutrophilic eccrine hidradenitis is a rare disorder resulting from treatment for underlying malignancy. It is usually associated with treatment for leukemias but has been reported with other chemotherapeutic agents that contain a granulocyte-stimulating factor.

On microscopy, the main features are seen around the eccrine secretory ducts and glands. There is infiltration of neutrophils with vacuolar degeneration of the eccrine epithelium.

EOSINOPHILIC INFILTRATION

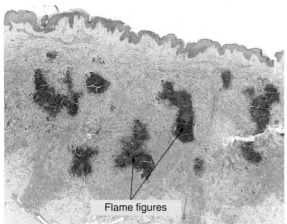

FIGURE 14.11 Eosinophilic Infiltration and Flame Figures in Eosinophilic Cellulitis

Eosinophilic cellulitis is also known as Well's syndrome. This is a tissue reaction pattern that occurs in a variety of conditions where there is infiltration of eosinophils. Many of the cases are idiopathic, but a number of other causes such as drug allergy, parasitic infections, and arthropod bite reaction are implicated as the etiological factors.

On microscopy, there is extensive infiltration of eosinophils in the dermis. Long-standing papillary dermal edema leads to subepidermal blister formation. The characteristic flame figures are formed by the major basic proteins released by eosinophilic degranulation, which get deposited in the normal collagen.

Eosinophilic infiltration of the dermis is also seen in eosinophilic folliculitis, which is a manifestation of HIV infection drug reaction and hypereosinophilic syndrome. Hypereosinophilic syndrome is an idiopathic disorder with systemic symptoms and persistent high blood eosinophilia. No identifiable cause is found.

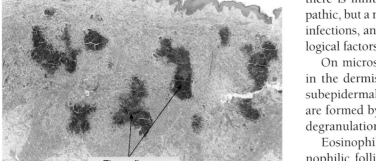

FIGURE 14.12 Flame Figure-High Power

EOSINOPHILS IN JUVENILE XANTHOGRANULOMA

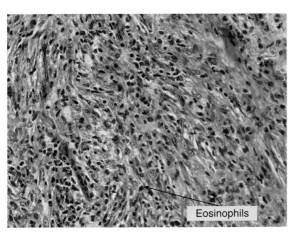

FIGURE 14.13 Eosinophils in Juvenile Xanthogranuloma

Eosinophils are an integral part of many histiocytic tumors of which juvenile xanthogranuloma is the commonest. Other tumors are reticulohistiocytoma and Langerhans cell histiocytosis.

PLASMA CELL INFILTRATION

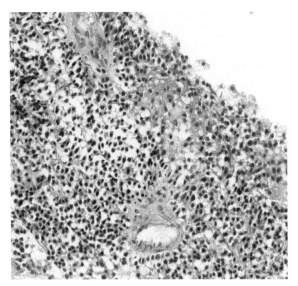

FIGURE 14.14   Plasma Cell Infiltration-Low Power

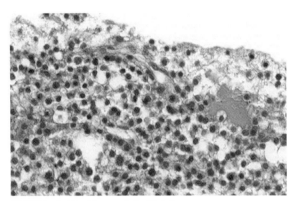

FIGURE 14.15   Plasma Cells-High Power

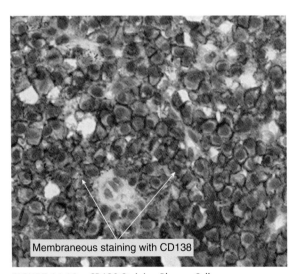

Membraneous staining with CD138

FIGURE 14.16   CD138 Staining Plasma Cells

Plasma cells are not normal constituents of the peripheral blood or skin. Plasma cells are commonly seen in biopsies of the lip and the mucous membranes. Increased numbers of plasma cells are seen in inflammatory and neoplastic conditions of the skin. Plasma cells are an important constituent of inflammatory diseases such as syphilis, rhinoscleroma, erythema nodosum leprosum, nodular amyloidosis, lupus erythematosus, morphea, and sometimes drug reactions. Plasma cells are also a prominent constituent of Castleman's disease.

Neoplastic monoclonal proliferation of plasma cells in the skin is termed cutaneous plasmacytoma. Multiple myeloma, extramedullary plasmacytoma in soft tissues, and very rarely plasma cell leukemias are the underlying malignancies associated with plasmacytomas. They usually arise as a metastatic deposit through bloodstream or lymphatics or by direct extension from the soft tissues and bone. Extremely rarely, primary cutaneous plasmacytomas arise without preexisting bone marrow or soft tissue disease.

On microscopy, these are located in the reticular dermis but may also extend into the subcutaneous fat. The tumor deposit is unencapsulated but generally circumscribed. The maturation seen within the plasma cells are variable, ranging from very mature cells to immature immunoblasts. Russell bodies, nuclear pleomorphism, binucleate forms, and mitotic activity are seen. Very rarely, plasmacytomas are polyclonal.

On immunohistochemical staining, plasmacytomas stain with epithelial membrane antigen (EMA), CD138, CD79a, and PC1. They may occasionally stain with cytokeratins.

MAST CELL INFILTRATION

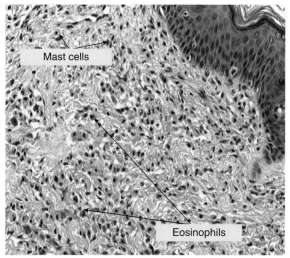

FIGURE 14.17   Mast Cell Infiltration

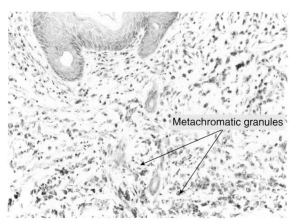

FIGURE 14.18   Toluidine Blue Staining Metachromatic Granules in Mast Cells

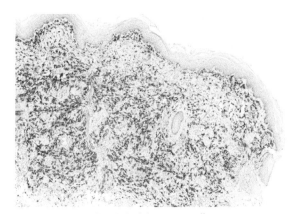

FIGURE 14.19   CD117 Staining Mast Cells

Mast cells are normally found in the skin in the superficial dermis and sometimes around blood vessels. Abnormally high numbers of mast cells are seen in inflammatory and neoplastic conditions, and this condition is called mastocytosis. Mast cells are formed in the bone marrow and produce a number of pharmacologically active substances when they degranulate. These substances include histamine, leukotrienes, and prostaglandin D2. The syncope, flushing, and pruritus, which are symptoms of mast cells, could be due to these substances. Increased numbers of mast cells have been associated with a number of inflammatory conditions such as wound healing, chronic inflammation, urticaria, atopic conditions, and psoriasis. Mastocytosis refers to the increase in mast cells in the skin or other organs. They are generally categorized as cutaneous mastocytosis, systemic mastocytosis, and malignant mast cell disease. Cutaneous mastocytosis is best represented by urticaria pigmentosa. Solitary mastocytoma and diffuse cutaneous mastocytosis are the other rare variants of mastocytosis occurring in childhood. Clinically, it presents as red-brown macules or plaques and are pruritic in less than 50% of cases. The lesions produce a wheal and flare when rubbed, called the Darier sign. Telangiectasia macularis eruptiva perstans is a rare form of mastocytosis in adults. Systemic involvement is commonly reported in this disease. Bone marrow is the most common tissue affected by mastocytosis. Malignant mast cell disease is extremely rare. Atypical mast cells are seen, and in addition to cutaneous sites, there is involvement of other organs leading to its enlargement.

On microscopy, the mast cell infiltrate is seen in the superficial dermis. It may be seen as an interstitial infiltrate or in a perivascular pattern. More than 15 mast cells per high power fields are considered pathological. Morphologically, mast cells in the infiltrate are the same as normal mast cells. Toludine blue and Giemsa stains the granules in mast cells pink and the process is called metachromatic staining.

LANGERHANS CELL HISTIOCYTOSIS

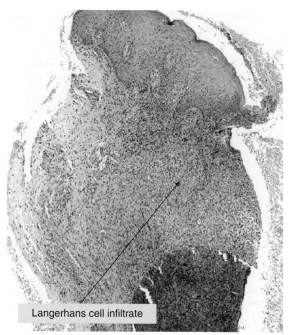

Langerhans cells belong to the group of dendritic cells, which may be of hemopoietic or mesenchymal in origin. They are nonphagocytic antigen-presenting cells. Only 2% of the cells are Langerhans cells in the epidermis. Clinically, Langerhans cell histiocytosis is a collective term for a spectrum of diseases affecting different organs of the body. They present in children younger than 2 years in most cases as cutaneous ulceration and as an erythematous rash. Systemic involvement has been reported in a large number of cases.

On microscopy, the Langerhans cells are seen in the subepidermal location. They are arranged as sheets and as small groups. The cells have eosinophilic cytoplasm and rounded or reniform nuclei. A mixture of other inflammatory cells such as lymphocytes and eosinophils may be seen within this histiocytic infiltrate.

Immunohistochemical stains positive in Langerhans cells histiocytosis are CD1a, S100 protein, and HLA-DR.

Langerhans cell infiltrate

FIGURE 14.20 Langerhans Cell Histiocytosis-Scanning View

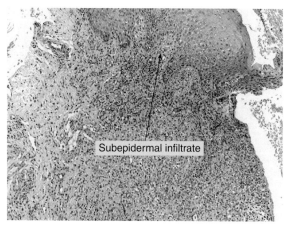

Subepidermal infiltrate

FIGURE 14.21 Langerhans Cell Histiocytosis-Low Power

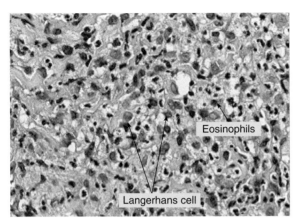

FIGURE 14.22   Langerhans Cell Histiocytosis-High Power

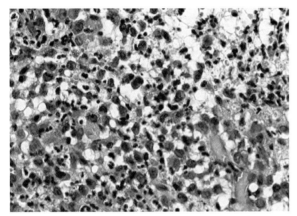

FIGURE 14.23   Langerhans Cell Histiocytosis—Another View

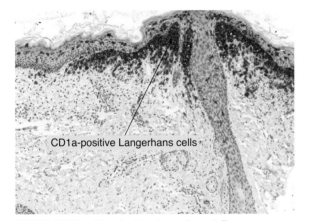

FIGURE 14.24   CD1a Positive Langerhans Cells

JUVENILE XANTHOGRANULOMA

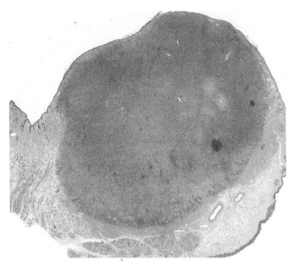

FIGURE 14.25 Juvenile Xanthogranuloma-Scanning View

Juvenile xanthogranuloma is a histiocytic tumor arising from non–Langerhans cell histiocytes. The non–Langerhans cell histiocytes originate from the monocyte lineage of cells. Clinically, the presentation is that of solitary or multiple papules and nodules on the upper part of the trunk. Most cases arise in children in the head and neck area and the upper extremities. Small numbers of cases of adult-onset juvenile xanthogranuloma have been reported.

On microscopy, the tumor is circumscribed but unencapsulated. It occupies the dermis and subcutaneous fat and may extend into the skeletal muscle. The cells are small histiocytes with ill-defined cytoplasmic borders. Mitotic activity and necrosis are rare. Areas of spindle cell xanthogranuloma may be seen, especially in the adult variant. Foam cells, which are lipidized histiocytes, are a characteristic feature in most cases. Touton giant cells are also a notable feature of juvenile xanthogranuloma.

The tumor cells are positive for CD68, CD163, Ham-56, and CD4. The cells are negative for S100 protein and CD1a.

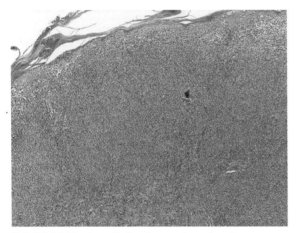

FIGURE 14.26 Juvenile Xanthogranuloma-Low Power

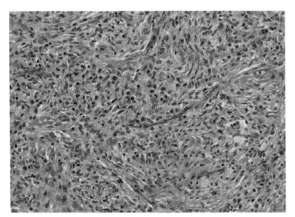

FIGURE 14.27 Juvenile Xanthogranuloma-High Power

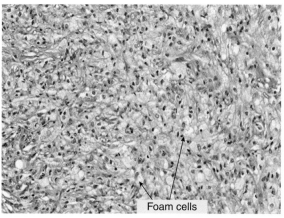

FIGURE 14.28   Juvenile Spindle and Foamy Cells

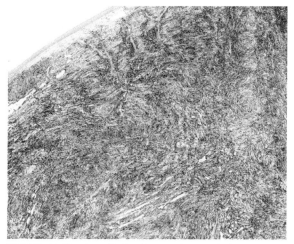

FIGURE 14.29   Juvenile Xanthogranuloma—CD68

RETICULOHISTIOCYTOMA

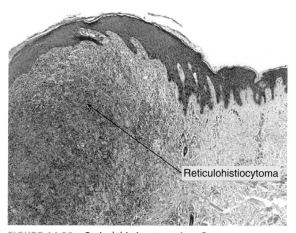

FIGURE 14.30   Reticulohistiocytoma-Low Power

Reticulohistiocytoma clinically presents as solitary or multiple small nodules in the head and neck area and upper trunk.

On microscopy, they are seen as poorly circumscribed dermal infiltrates. The cell population comprises histiocytes, multinucleate giant cells with glassy cytoplasm, and an admixture of other inflammatory cells, which may include eosinophils and neutrophils. Touton type giant cells are also seen.

Immunohistochemically, the cells are positive for CD68, CD163, and Ham-56. The cells are negative for CD1a and S100 protein.

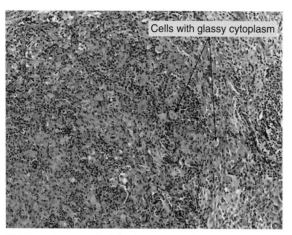

FIGURE 14.31   Reticulohistiocytoma-High Power

TENDINOUS XANTHOMA

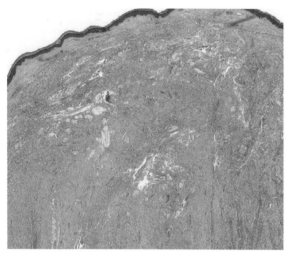

FIGURE 14.32   Tendinous Xanthoma-Scanning View

Xanthomas are neoplasms where there is infiltration of lipid-rich histiocytes. Clinically, they are present as nodules or plaques, which are yellow. They are further classified as eruptive, tendinous, tuberous, verruciform, planar, and plantar. Many of these entities are associated with abnormalities of fat metabolism. They may also arise in normolipemic states. This may be due to altered lipoprotein content and structure or an underlying lymphoproliferative disorder.

Tendinous xanthomas develop in ligaments and tendons. Clinically, they present as firm to hard nodules on hands and feet and on Achilles tendon. Tendinous xanthoma is most commonly associated with familial hypercholesterolemia.

On microscopy, the infiltrate is seen mainly in the dermis and subcutaneous tissue. There are aggregates of foam cells, which are lipidized cells. Inflammatory cells or Touton type of giant cells are not seen.

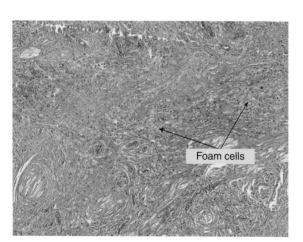

FIGURE 14.33   Tendinous Xanthoma-Medium Power

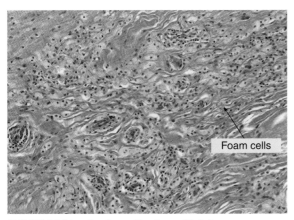

FIGURE 14.34   Tendinous Xanthoma-High Power

LYMPHOMATOID ARTHROPOD BITE REACTION

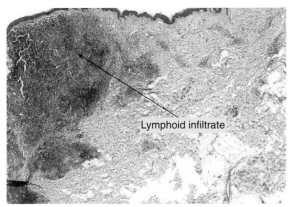

FIGURE 14.35   Lymphomatoid Arthropod Bite Reaction-Low Power

Lymphomatoid arthropod bite reaction is a reaction pattern resulting from the bites of insects notably scabies. Clinically, the lesions present as rounded reddish papules and nodules at the site of the bite. The remnants of the organism are very rarely identified from the nodule of a long-standing nature.

On microscopy, there is dense infiltration of lymphocytes in the dermis and subcutaneous tissue. This is sometimes seen in a multilobular pattern. The infiltrate is composed of lymphocytes, plasma cells, and eosinophils. There may be a scattering of eosinophils in the dermal collagen. The vessels may show endothelial cell thickening.

Immunohistochemically, the cells are positive for T-cell marker CD3. Some CD30-positive cells may be seen.

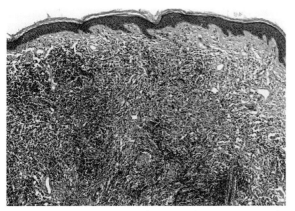

FIGURE 14.36   Lymphomatoid Arthropod Bite Reaction-High Power

CUTANEOUS LYMPHOID HYPERPLASIA

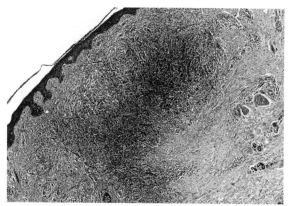

FIGURE 14.37   Cutaneous Lymphoid Hyperplasia-Low Power

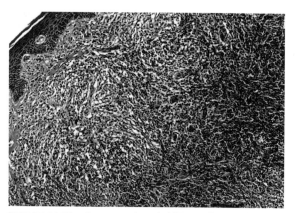

FIGURE 14.38   Cutaneous Lymphoid Hyperplasia-High Power

Cutaneous lymphoid hyperplasia is also known as pseudolymphoma or lymphocytoma cutis. A number of triggering factors have been postulated in the development of these lesions. They include the spirochete *Borrelia burgdorferi*, drugs, vaccinations, gold ear piercings, and medicinal leech therapy. Clinically, they present as solitary or multiple nodules on different parts of the body. The lesions developing following *B. burgdorferi* infection tend to localize on the ear lobe, nipple, and scrotum.

On microscopy, there is diffuse and nodular infiltration of lymphocytes in the dermis, which may extend into the subcutaneous fat. The germinal centers are not known to show the mantle zone, and they tend to coalesce with each other. The cell population comprises lymphocytes, plasma cells, and eosinophils.

Immunohistochemical stains show the cells to stain with CD20, CD10, and Bcl6, in a germinal-center cell pattern. The cells are negative for Bcl6. Many dendritic cells staining for CD21 and CD35 and a reactive population of cells staining for CD3 are also present.

Molecular analyses show a polyclonal pattern of arrangement of cells. Evidence for *B. burgdorferi* infection can be obtained by identifying *Borrelia* DNA by polymerase chain reaction, immunoblotting, or ELISA (enzyme-linked immunosorbent assay).

PRIMARY CD30-POSITIVE LYMPHOPROLIFERATIVE DISORDER

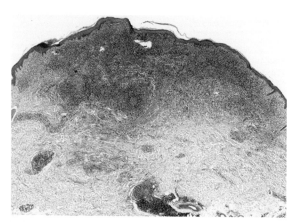

FIGURE 14.39   Primary CD30 Positive Lymphoproliferative Disorder-Low Power

Primary CD30-positive lymphoproliferative disorders belong to a spectrum of disorders of T-cell derivation. They range from purely benign conditions such as insect bite reaction, pityriasis lichenoides chronica, and pityriasis lichenoides et varioliformis acuta, to lymphomatoid papulosis and anaplastic large cell lymphoma at the malignant end of the spectrum. Clinically, the lesions present as nodules and papules in different parts of the body.

On microscopy, the overlying epidermis is unremarkable. The dermis shows diffuse and nodular infiltration of predominantly lymphocytes admixed with eosinophils as the case may be. Scattered CD30-positive cells are seen in the infiltrate.

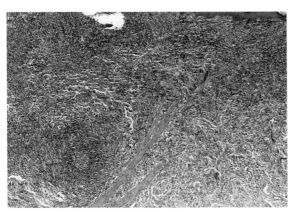

FIGURE 14.40 Primary CD30 Positive Lymphoproliferative Disorder-Medium Power

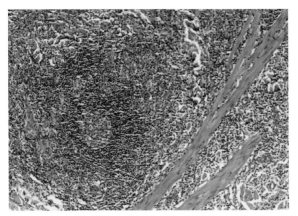

FIGURE 14.41 Primary CD30 Positive Lymphoproliferative Disorder-High Power

LYMPHOMATOID PAPULOSIS

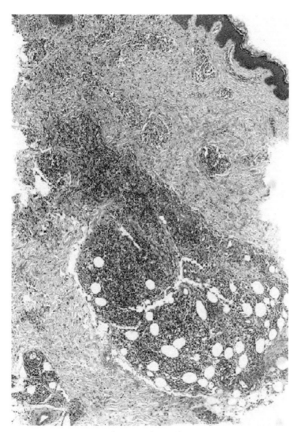

FIGURE 14.42   Lymphomatoid Papulosis-Scanning View

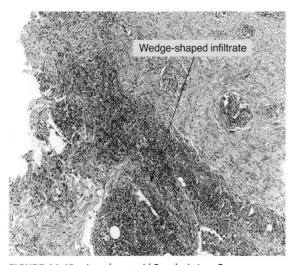

Wedge-shaped infiltrate

FIGURE 14.43   Lymphomatoid Papulosis-Low Power

In the recent WHO-EORTC (World Health Organization-European Organization for the Research and Treatment of Cancer) classification, lymphomatoid papulosis comes under cutaneous T-cell and NK-cell lymphomas as a subset of Primary Cutaneous CD30-positive lymphoproliferative disorder. Clinically, lymphomatoid papulosis presents as recurrent papules and nodules with a chronic course. Small reddish-brown papules and nodules are mainly seen in the upper extremities and trunk. These lesions are known to resolve spontaneously, and the interval between different episodes may vary. Ulceration is a common feature seen in many of the lesions.

On microscopy, three different patterns are described on the basis of the cell types.

Type A (histiocytic type) is the most common type of lymphomatoid papulosis where the classical wedge-shaped pattern of infiltration is described. There is variable epidermotropism. The cells are combination of large cells admixed with neutrophils and eosinophils.

Type B (mycosis fungoides type) is a rare variant where the predominant cells are the small cerebriform lymphocytes, although large CD30+ cells are also seen. There is prominent epidermotropism and a wedge-shaped infiltrate of small lymphocytes. The diagnosis of this type of lymphomatoid papulosis has to be made very carefully after clinicopathological correlation. This is to be sure that a possibility of mycosis fungoides is excluded.

Type C (anaplastic large cell lymphoma–like) is another unusual variant of lymphomatoid papulosis. The pattern of infiltration is that of nodules of large cells with nuclear pleomorphism similar to anaplastic large cell lymphoma. Mature lymphocytes and neutrophils are very few.

The diagnosis of lymphomatoid papulosis should be made only after close clinicopathological correlation.

Immunohistochemically, the neoplastic cells are of T-cell derivation. They express CD3 and CD4. CD30 expression is predominantly seen. The CD30-positive cells are arranged as small nodules and in sheets in lymphomatoid papulosis as opposed to scattered CD30-positive cells in CD30-positive inflammatory conditions. CD30-positive papular variant of mycosis fungoides should be carefully excluded in this context.

ALK-1 (anaplastic lymphoma kinase-1) is not expressed in lymphomatoid papulosis. JunB and c-Jun are expressed in a large number of cases of lymphomatoid papulosis.

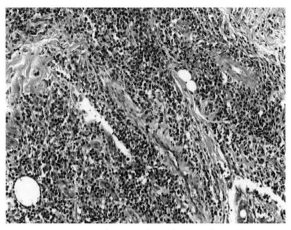

FIGURE 14.44   Lymphomatoid Papulosis-High Power

MYCOSIS FUNGOIDES

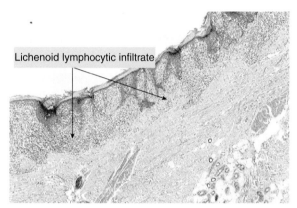

Lichenoid lymphocytic infiltrate

FIGURE 14.45   Mycosis Fungoides-Scanning View

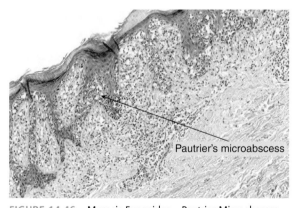

Pautrier's microabscess

FIGURE 14.46   Mycosis Fungoides—Pautrier Microabscess

Mycosis fungoides is the commonest type of cutaneous T-cell lymphoma. It is known to coexist with Hodgkin's lymphoma and lymphomatoid papulosis. Clinically, the disease presents as patch, plaque, and tumor. The patch stage is the earliest stage of the disease. It is usually seen in sun-protected sites, such as hip and buttock. The loss of elastic fibers in the skin in these patches gives the appearance of parchment paper–like appearance. The plaque stage is characterized by scaly lesions. The tumor stage is characterized by nodules and plaques, which may be solitary or extensive. The disease affects other organs such as lymph nodes, lung, liver, and spleen.

On microscopy, the appearances depend on the stage of the disease. In the earliest patch stage, there is a lichenoid infiltrate of lymphocytes in the papillary dermis and expanded reticular dermis. The dermal collagen is seen to be vertically orientated in the papillary dermis. Epidermotropism is readily seen, but collections of lymphocytes within the epidermis, called Pautrier microabscesses, are not that commonly seen. The epidermotropic lymphocytes have nuclei larger than the lymphocytes in the papillary dermis. They are usually seen in areas where there is hardly any spongiosis. The lymphocytes are also seen to align along the dermoepidermal junction. The latter two features are useful clues in the diagnosis of patch stage of mycosis fungoides.

The plaque stage of mycosis fungoides shows a dense lichenoid infiltrate of lymphocytes in the papillary dermis. Pautrier microabscesses is a notable feature in this stage. The lymphocytes show cerebriform nuclei and exhibit mild nuclear pleomorphism. Reactive germinal centers may be seen.

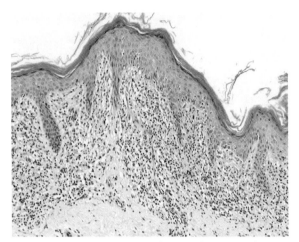

FIGURE 14.47   Mycosis Fungoides—Patch Stage-Medium Power

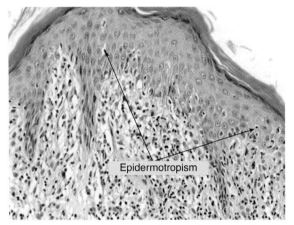

FIGURE 14.48   Mycosis Fungoides—Patch Stage-High Power

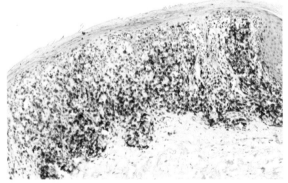

FIGURE 14.49   Mycosis Fungoides—CD4 Stain

In the tumor stage, the infiltrate is intense and is composed of lymphocytes arranged in nodules and sheets. The infiltrate fills the entire dermis and may even involve the subcutaneous fat.

Large cell transformation is a feature well-recognized in mycosis fungoides. The cells are larger than the usual and exhibit marked nuclear pleomorphism. With the expression of CD30, it may resemble anaplastic large cell lymphoma.

Immunophenotypically, most lymphocytes in mycosis fungoides express the helper cell profile. They stain positive for CD3, CD4, CD5, CD45Ro, and betaF1. Most cells are negative for CD8. A small number of cases may express the cytotoxic phenotype where the cells express CD8 positivity and show negative staining for CD4. CD20-staining B cells may be seen within the tumor.

A variety of clinical and histological variants of mycosis fungoides are described, which can be found on cutaneous lymphomas.

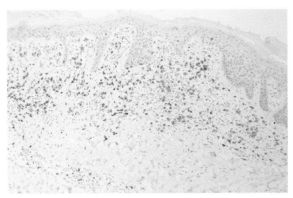

FIGURE 14.50   Mycosis Fungoides—CD8 Stain

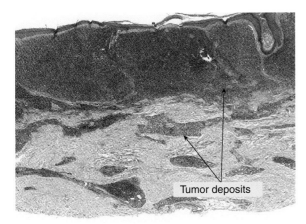

FIGURE 14.51   Mycosis Fungoides—Tumor Stage-Scanning View

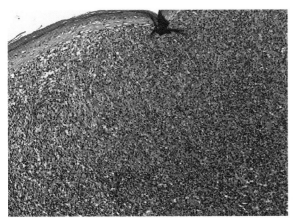

FIGURE 14.52   Mycosis Fungoides—Tumor Stage-Low Power

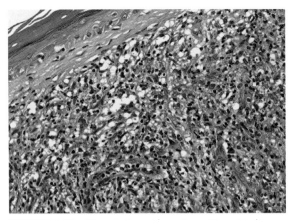

FIGURE 14.53   Mycosis Fungoides—Tumor Stage-Medium Power

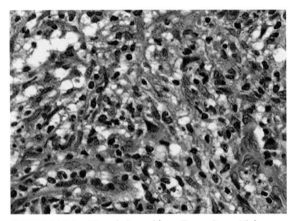

FIGURE 14.54   Mycosis Fungoides—Tumor Stage-High Power

PAGETOID RETICULOSIS

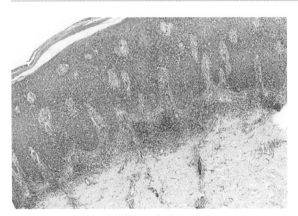

FIGURE 14.55   Pagetoid Reticulosis-Low Power

Pagetoid reticulosis is the term used to describe the solitary localized variant of mycosis fungoides. This variant is also known as Woringer-Kollop type. Clinically, it presents as scaly erythematous patch.

On microscopy, the epidermis is markedly hyperplastic and at times psoriasiform. There is marked epidermotropism. The intraepidermal infiltrate is composed of pleomorphic lymphocytes. These are of helper and cytotoxic types. CD30-positive cells may also be seen among the epidermotropic cells, which raise the possibility of variant of lymphomatoid papulosis.

The diagnosis of pagetoid reticulosis should be made very carefully after clinicopathological correlation and immunophenotypic studies. A solitary variant of the ordinary mycosis fungoides has been documented, which needs to be excluded with careful clinical history.

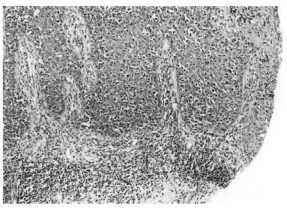

FIGURE 14.56   Pagetoid Reticulosis-High Power

ANAPLASTIC LARGE CELL LYMPHOMA

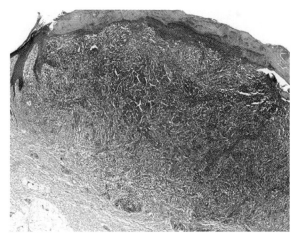

FIGURE 14.57   Anaplastic Large Cell Lymphoma-Low Power

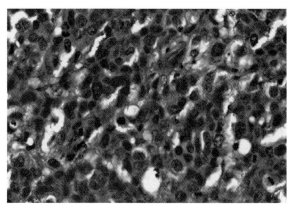

FIGURE 14.58   Anaplastic Large Cell Lymphoma-High Power

Cutaneous anaplastic large cell lymphoma presents primarily in the skin. Secondary involvement from an extranodal site should be excluded by complete investigations. This is a tumor of adults. The tumors are solitary or localized reddish-brown papules.

On microscopy, the overlying epidermis is usually ulcerated and shows pseudoepitheliomatous hyperplasia. The lesion is seen filling the entire dermis and subcutaneous fat. The tumor itself is composed of sheets of large cells with scanty cytoplasm and markedly pleomorphic nuclei with prominent nucleoli. Multinucleated forms may be seen.

Immunohistochemically, the cells are of the T-helper cell type, positive for CD3 and CD4 and negative for CD8. EMA and CD15 are negative. They also stain strongly and diffusely for CD30. Distinction from lymphomatoid papulosis can be difficult. The absence of staining of ALK-1 in purely cutaneous forms helps to differentiate from secondary anaplastic large cell lymphoma.

CUTANEOUS FOLLICLE CENTER LYMPHOMA

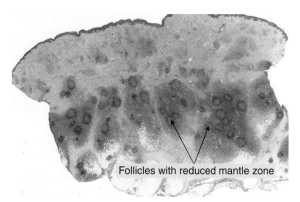

FIGURE 14.59   Cutaneous Follicle Center Lymphoma-Scanning View

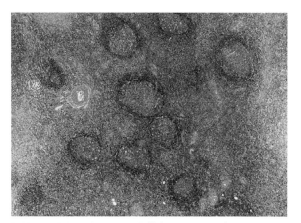

FIGURE 14.60   Cutaneous Follicle Center Lymphoma-Low Power—Absent or Reduced Mantle Zone

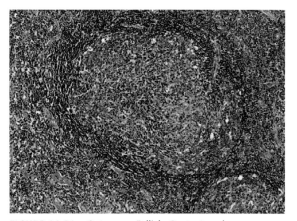

FIGURE 14.61   Cutaneous Follicle Center Lymphoma-Medium Power

Primary cutaneous follicle center lymphoma is diagnosed in the absence of extracutaneous manifestation after complete staging. Clinically, the lesions present in adult life. It presents as erythematous papules, plaques, and tumors. Ulceration is rare. The lesions may be diffuse or localized to one site.

On microscopy, the features vary with the type of lymphoma. In the follicular type, the follicles are a prominent feature and the entire lesion is seen as a nodule extending into the subcutaneous fat. The follicles show reduced or absent mantle zone. There is marked reduction in the number of tingible body macrophages. The neoplastic follicles comprise of centroblasts, centrocytes, and many reactive lymphocytes. In the diffuse type, the presence of follicles is not a prominent feature. The cells are seen diffusely as sheets and extend into the subcutaneous fat. The infiltrate is composed of mature lymphocytes, centrocytes, and centroblasts. The neoplastic cells are positive for B-cell markers such as CD20 and CD79a. This is seen in the follicular and diffuse type. Other markers such as paired box gene (PAX)-5 and interferon regulatory factor (IRF)-8 can be used to confirm the germinal center nature of the cells.

Genetically, the cells show monoclonal rearrangement of the J_H gene.

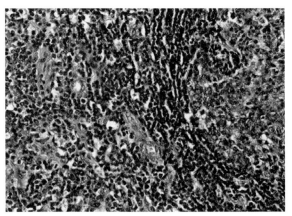

FIGURE 14.62   Cutaneous Follicle Center Lymphoma-High Power

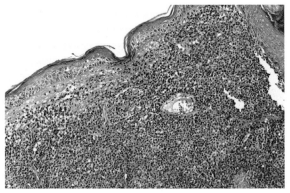

FIGURE 14.63   Primary Cutaneous Follicle Center Cell Lymphoma—Diffuse Type-Low Power

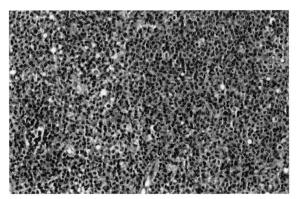

FIGURE 14.64   Primary Cutaneous Follicle Center Cell Lymphoma—Diffuse Type-High Power—Another View

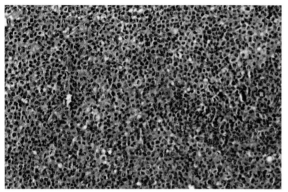

FIGURE 14.65 Primary Cutaneous Follicle Center Cell Lymphoma—Diffuse Type-High Power

LEUKEMIC INFILTRATE

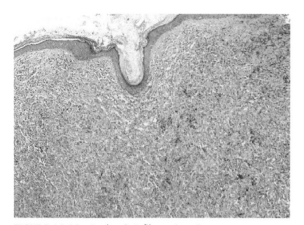

FIGURE 14.66 Leukemic Infiltrate-Low Power

Cutaneous leukemic infiltration is not uncommon. Chronic lymphocytic leukemia of the B-cell type is the most common type to infiltrate into the skin. Other subtypes, such as myelogenous leukemia, are also seen. Cutaneous deposits are referred to as myeloid sarcomas. Clinically, they present as papules and plaques and have characteristic reddish and violaceous color. Mucous membrane involvement is commonly seen.

On microscopy, the infiltrate involves the dermis and may extend into the subcutaneous fat. The cells are of moderate size and have scanty cytoplasm and rounded nuclei. Nuclear pleomorphism and mitotic activity are common. Immature myeloid precursors are also seen.

Immunophenotypically, the cells stain strongly for CD45, CD68, CD13, CD14, CD15, and myeloperoxidase.

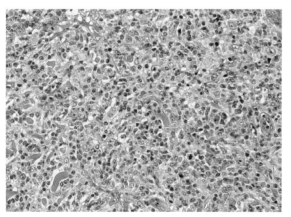

FIGURE 14.67 Leukemic Infiltrate-High Power

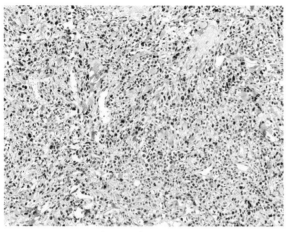

FIGURE 14.68   Myeloperoxidase Stain

METASTATIC HODGKIN DISEASE

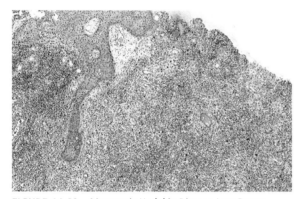

FIGURE 14.69   Metastatic Hodgkin Disease-Low Power

Cutaneous metastasis of Hodgkin disease is rare. Clinically, they present as papules, plaques, and nodules. Ulceration is commonly seen.

On microscopy, typical features of Hodgkin disease with the characteristic Reed-Sternberg cells are seen.

Immunohistochemically, the tumor cells satin positive for CD15 and CD30.

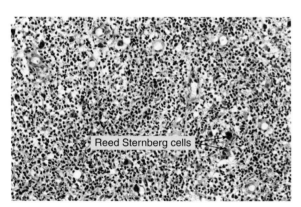

Reed Sternberg cells

FIGURE 14.70   Metastatic Hodgkin Disease-High Power

METASTATIC LOBULAR CARCINOMA OF BREAST

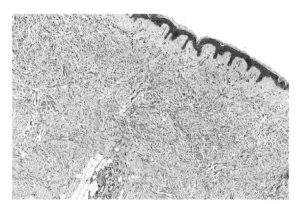

FIGURE 14.71   Metastatic Lobular Carcinoma of Breast-Low Power

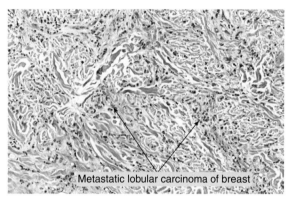

Metastatic lobular carcinoma of breast

FIGURE 14.72   Metastatic Lobular Carcinoma of Breast-High Power

Cutaneous metastasis is defined as deposition of tumor in the skin from a distant location. It represents approximately 2% of all cases. Scalp is considered the most common site of metastasis because of its rich vascularity. The metastasis could be the cutaneous manifestation of an underlying disorder, when it is termed precocious metastasis. When the metastasis occurs at the same time of development of the primary disease, it is called synchronous metastasis, and when it develops months or years after the development of the primary malignancy, it is called metachronous metastasis.

Clinically, most metastases are seen as nodules or plaques. Most often the metastasis is seen adjacent to the primary site. Melanoma appears to be the most frequent primary tumor to metastasize. Other primary sites of carcinomas such as lung, breast, gastrointestinal tract, thyroid, and genitourinary tract are also well known to metastasize to the skin. Leiomyosarcoma and mesothelioma very rarely metastasize to the skin. Sister Mary Joseph nodule was first described by Sister Joseph, a nursing superintendent at the Mayo Clinic in Rochester, Minnesota. The lesion is characteristically seen on the umbilicus as an ulcerated nodule. The primary tumor has been identified to be carcinoma from the breast, ovary, endometrium, gastrointestinal tract, or urological tract. Renal cell carcinoma is a tumor well known to metastasize to the skin. Renal cell carcinoma metastasis raises the differential diagnosis of all clear cell tumors of the skin, either primary or secondary. Metastatic gastrointestinal stromal tumor and metastatic adenocarcinoma of the rete testis are exceedingly rare. In all cases of cutaneous metastasis, the history is helpful in confirming the diagnosis.

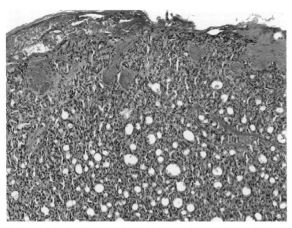

FIGURE 14.73 Metastatic Follicular Carcinoma of Thyroid-Low Power

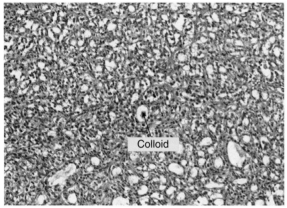

FIGURE 14.74 Metastatic Follicular Carcinoma of Thyroid-Medium Power

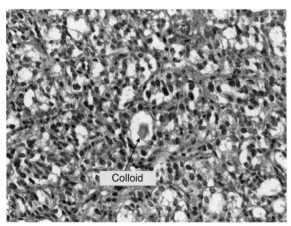

FIGURE 14.75 Metastatic Follicular Carcinoma of Thyroid-High Power

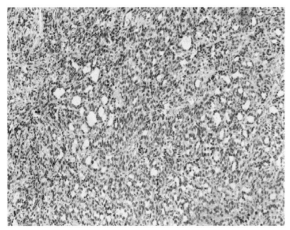

FIGURE 14.76 Metastatic Follicular Carcinoma of Thyroid—
TTF1 Stain

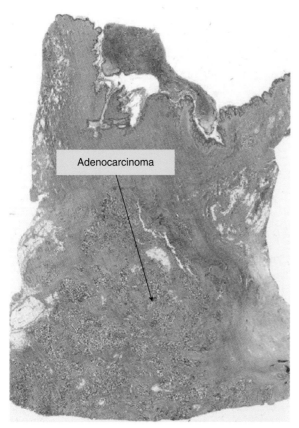

FIGURE 14.77 Sister Mary Joseph Nodule-Scanning View

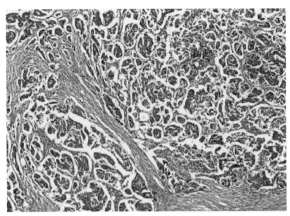

FIGURE 14.78   Sister Mary Joseph Nodule-Low Power

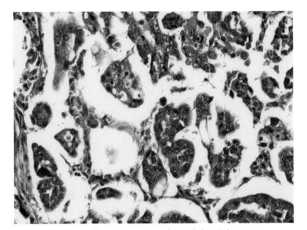

FIGURE 14.79   Sister Mary Joseph Nodule-High Power

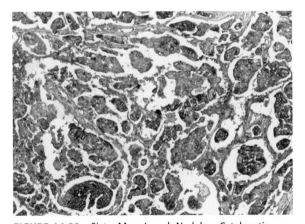

FIGURE 14.80   Sister Mary Joseph Nodule—Cytokeratin

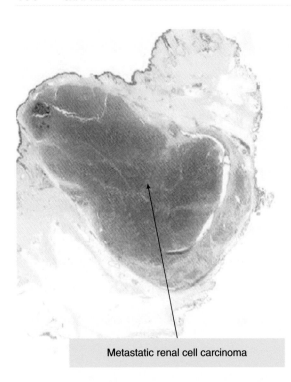

Metastatic renal cell carcinoma

FIGURE 14.81   Metastatic Renal Cell Carcinoma-Scanning
View

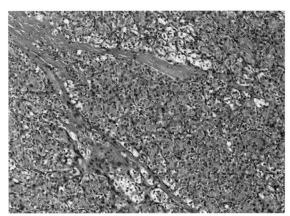

FIGURE 14.82   Metastatic Renal Cell Carcinoma-Low Power

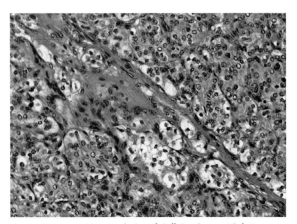

FIGURE 14.83   Metastatic Renal Cell Carcinoma-High Power

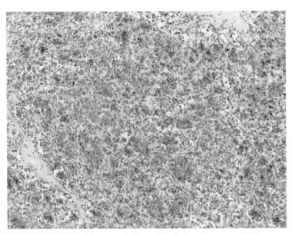

FIGURE 14.84   Metastatic Renal Cell Carcinoma—RCC Antigen

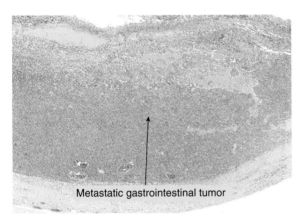

Metastatic gastrointestinal tumor

FIGURE 14.85   Metastatic Gastrointestinal Stromal Tumor-Low Power

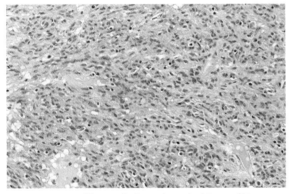

FIGURE 14.86   Metastatic Gastrointestinal Stromal Tumor-High Power

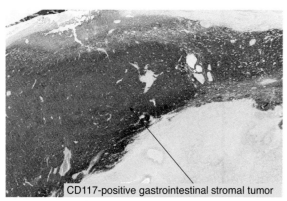

FIGURE 14.87 Metastatic Gastrointestinal Stromal Tumor—CD117

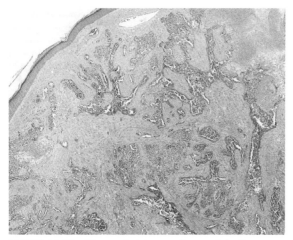

FIGURE 14.88 Metastatic Adenocarcinoma of the Rete Testis-Low Power

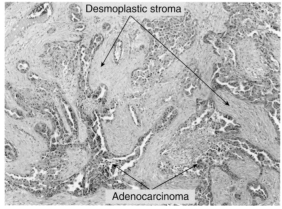

FIGURE 14.89 Metastatic Adenocarcinoma of the Rete Testis-High Power

BIBLIOGRAPHY

Cerroni L, Gatter K and Kerl H. Skin Lymphoma—The Illustrate Guide, 3rd Ed. Blackwell Wiley, 2009.
Elder D et al. Lever's Histopathology of Skin, 10th Ed. Philadelphia, PA: Lippincott Williams, 2010.
Weedon D. Skin Pathology, 3rd Ed. Churchill Livingstone, 2009.

Soft Tissue Tumors of the Skin

INTRODUCTION

Soft tissue tumors are a group of benign and malignant neoplasms seen within the dermis and subcutaneous tissue, with the cell of origin from the mesenchyme. It includes tumors originating from fibroblasts, myofibroblasts, smooth muscle cells, neural cells, pericytes, endothelial cells, and adipocytes. The tumors arising from the adipocytes are located in the subcutaneous fat and are analyzed in Chapter 11.

ACRAL FIBROKERATOMA

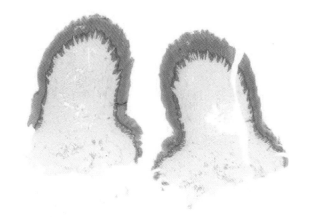

Acral fibrokeratomas are group of benign tumors originating in the dermal connective tissue. They encompass acquired digital fibrokeratoma, acquired periungual fibrokeratoma. Occasional lesions may be seen in sites other than digits. Clinically, they appear as solitary dome-shaped papules occurring on the digits. Multiple acral fibromas with a myxoid background are reported in patients with retinoblastomas.

On microscopy, the overlying epidermis is markedly acanthotic and hyperkeratotic. The dermis shows vertically orientated bundles of collagen. Scattered fibroblasts are also seen. There may be few inflammatory cells of chronic nature.

FIGURE 15.1   Acral Fibrokeratoma-Scanning View

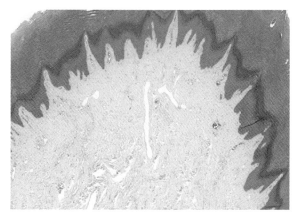

FIGURE 15.2   Acral Fibrokeratoma-Low Power

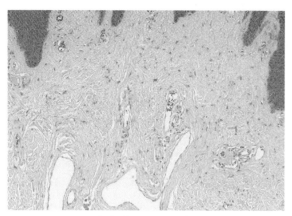

FIGURE 15.3   Acral Fibrokeratoma-High Power

SUBUNGUAL FIBROMA

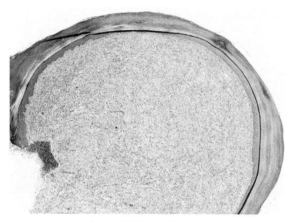

FIGURE 15.4   Subungual Fibroma-Low Power

Subungual and periungual fibrokeratomas are benign tumors associated with tuberous sclerosis. Clinically, they are usually multiple and may be located under the nail fold.

On microscopy, the overlying epidermis is hyperkeratotic and acanthotic. There is dermal proliferation of bland-looking cells admixed with stellate fibroblasts. Nuclear pleomorphism and mitotic activity are not seen.

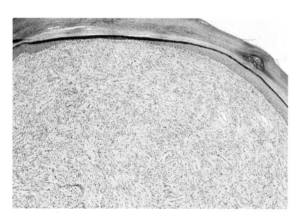

FIGURE 15.5   Subungual Fibroma-Medium Power

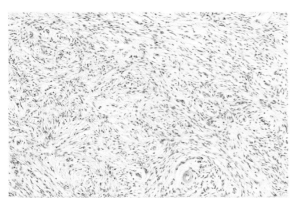

FIGURE 15.6   Subungual Fibroma-High Power

SUPERFICIAL ACRAL FIBROMYXOMA

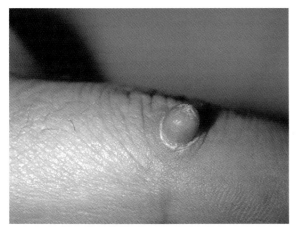

FIGURE 15.7   Superficial Acral Fibromyxoma

Superficial acral fibromyxoma as the name implies has a predilection for hands and feet. Clinically, they present as slowly enlarging mass.

On microscopy, the tumor is entirely dermal and is composed of spindle-shaped and oval cells set in a myxocollagenous matrix. There is no nuclear pleomorphism. Occasional mitotic figures may be seen. No atypical mitoses are seen. Multinucleated giant cells may be seen.

The cells stain strongly and diffusely for CD34.

Superficial acral fibromyxomas are benign tumors but can pose diagnostic difficulties histologically with other CD34 positive myxoid tumors.

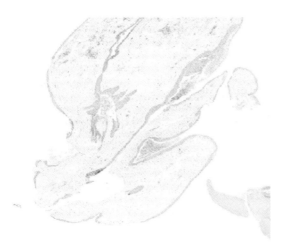

FIGURE 15.8   Superficial Acral Fibromyxoma-Scanning View

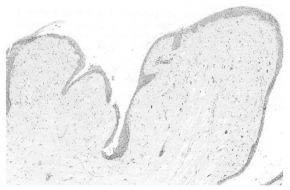

FIGURE 15.9   Superficial Acral Fibromyxoma-Low Power

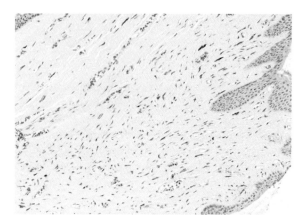

FIGURE 15.10   Superficial Acral Fibromyxoma-High Power

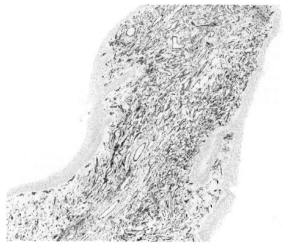

FIGURE 15.11   Acral Fibromyxoma—CD34 Stain

FIBROUS STROMAL POLYP

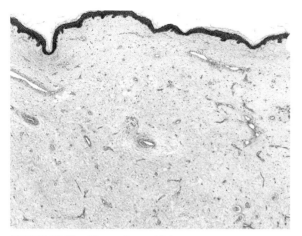

FIGURE 15.12   Fibrous Stromal Polyp

Fibrous stromal polyp is also known as "pseudosarcomatous stromal polyp." Clinically, this presents as a skin tag, slightly larger than the usual fibroepithelial polyps.

On microscopy, the overlying epidermis is unremarkable. The stroma of the polyp is formed of loose connective tissue and shows scattered blood vessels and bizarre stromal cells. The stromal cells are in fact fibroblasts. There is no mitotic activity.

FIGURE 15.13   Fibrous Stromal Polyp-High Power

SCLEROTIC FIBROMA

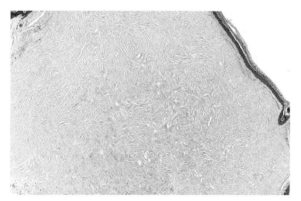

FIGURE 15.14   Sclerotic Fibroma-Low Power

Sclerotic fibroma is a rare benign tumor that occurs in Cowden's syndrome. It is known by different names such as circumscribed storiform collagenoma, plywood fibroma, and hypocellular fibroma. Clinically, it is seen as solitary or multiple flesh-colored papules. The entire lesion is thought to be formed of type 1 collagen.

On microscopy, the overlying epidermis is thinned out. The tumor is located in the dermis and is unencapsulated and circumscribed. It is formed of laminated pattern of collagen arranged in a storiform pattern. The cellularity is very sparse and the cells appear to be fibroblasts. There is no mitotic activity. Occasional cells stain for CD34.

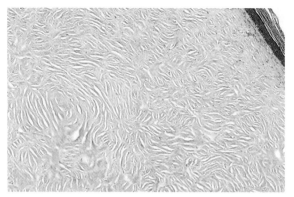

FIGURE 15.15   Sclerotic Fibroma-High Power

FIBROMATOSIS

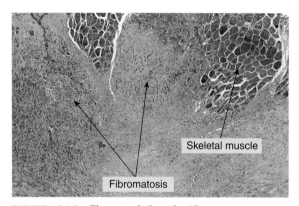

FIGURE 15.16   Fibromatosis-Scanning View

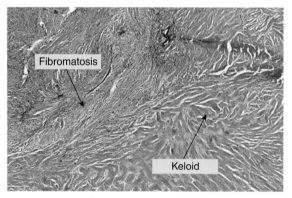

FIGURE 15.17   Fibromatosis-Low Power with Keloid
Formation

Fibromatosis is a broad term used to describe the proliferation of fibroblasts and rarely myofibroblasts. This is a well-defined entity and should not be used for benign reactive proliferation of fibroblasts. Fibromatosis can be broadly classified into superficial and deep types. The superficial type rarely involves the skeletal muscle. The superficial type of fibromatosis is known by different names depending on the location of the tumor. They are palmar fibromatosis also known as "Dupuytren's disease," plantar fibromatosis also known as "Ledderhose's disease," and penile fibromatosis also known as "Peyronie's disease".

On microscopy, all subtypes show similar appearances. The early lesions are very cellular. They form nodules of cells with ill-defined borders. Sweeping fascicles of cells are also seen. The cells are seen to infiltrate the underlying skeletal muscle and they chew up the muscle. The cells have spindle-shaped nuclei with tapering ends and scanty eosinophilic cytoplasm. Nuclear pleomorphism and mitotic activity are not seen.

Immunohistochemically the cells stain characteristically with beta-catenin. The cells are also positive for smooth muscle actin (SMA) that stains the myofibroblasts in a typical tram tack appearance, staining the membrane and the cytoplasm.

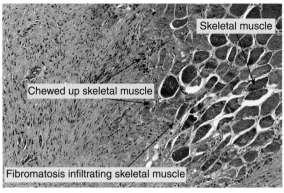

FIGURE 15.18   Fibromatosis-High Power

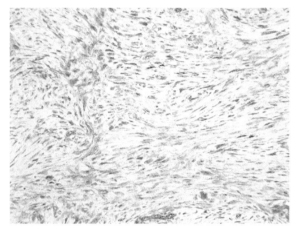

FIGURE 15.19   Nuclear Beta Catenin in Fibromatosis

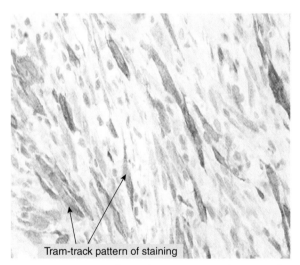

FIGURE 15.20   Smooth Muscle Actin–Tram Track Pattern of Staining

NODULAR FASCIITIS

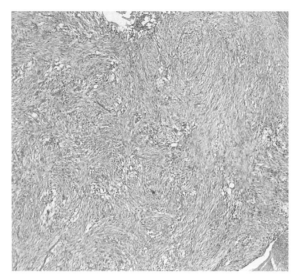

FIGURE 15.21 Nodular Fasciitis-Low Power

Nodular fasciitis is the most common benign mesenchymal lesion misdiagnosed as sarcoma. It was originally described as subcutaneous pseudosarcomatous fibromatosis in 1955 by Kornwaler et al. Clinically the lesion classically appears on the shoulder and the upper extremities. Head and neck is also a common site. Nodular fasciitis is also known to give history of rapid growth.

On microscopy, nodular fasciitis is known to occur in a subcutaneous, intramuscular, and deep fascial location. The subcutaneous type is the most common. The lesion is ill defined and is composed of immature fibroblasts and myofibroblasts arranged in bundles and fascicles. There is abundant myxoid ground substance in the background. Areas of edema and extravasated red blood cells are characteristically seen. Mitotic figures are readily seen, but atypical mitoses are never found. Multinucleated giant cells, hemosiderin deposition, and foamy macrophages may be seen. The earlier lesions tend to show myxoid change, but the more mature lesions may show hyalinized and fibrotic areas.

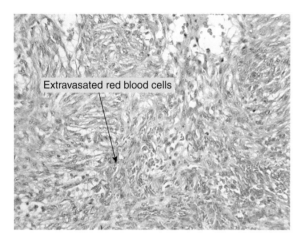

Extravasated red blood cells

FIGURE 15.22 Nodular Fasciitis-High Power

DERMATOFIBROMA

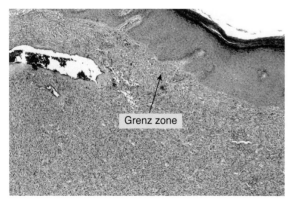

Grenz zone

FIGURE 15.23 Dermatofibroma-Low Power. Grenz Zone

Dermatofibroma is a fibrohistiocytic lesion and is the most common benign mesenchymal tumor found in the skin. The term "dermatofibroma" is used when the lesion is located in the dermis and the subcutaneous fat. In a deeper location, the term "fibrous histiocytoma" is more aptly used. Some authors are of the view that this may be a reactive condition secondary to insect bite. The most frequent location is the lower extremities although the lesion may occur in other sites. Clinically they present as small nodules with a central dimple in certain cases. The overlying skin may have a reddish hue. Involvement of the skeletal muscle is extremely rare.

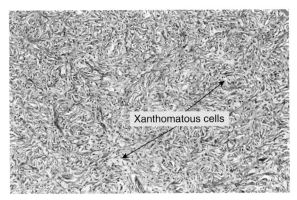

FIGURE 15.24   Dermatofibroma—Xanthomatous Cells

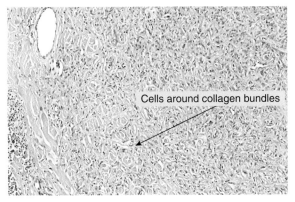

FIGURE 15.25   Dermatofibroma—Cells Wrapping Round Collagen

On microscopy, the tumor is seen in the dermis and very rarely involves the subcutaneous tissue, in a focal manner, as tonguelike projections. The characteristic grenz zone separating the tumor from the overlying epidermis is a common feature. The epidermis shows hyperplastic changes in large majority of cases. Folliculosebaceous induction is a rare feature but recorded. Here the epidermis shows proliferation of basaloid cells in an architecture resembling early buds of a basal cell carcinoma. Occasionally, primitive follicular buds and lobules of sebaceous glands may also be seen. This change is thought to be due to the cytokines released by the tumor stimulating the epidermis and the follicular epithelium. The tumor is very ill-defined at the peripheral and the deep edges. It is composed of short spindly or stellate cells arranged in a vague storiform pattern and single cells intersecting collagen bundles. Xanthomatous cells containing lipid in their cytoplasm may also be seen. Touton giant cells with wreath-like arrangement of cells around the periphery are a notable feature. The cells also show the characteristic wrapping round collagen bundles. Nuclear pleomorphism and mitotic activity are not seen. Hemosiderin pigment may be a conspicuous feature in the pigmented variant of dermatofibroma. Scattered lymphocytes in varying numbers are also seen. Rarely granular cell change, clear cell change, and marked hyalinization are also noted.

Immunohistochemical stains show positive staining with SMA. CD34 stains in a characteristic edge pattern, where the staining is seen only at the periphery of the lesion.

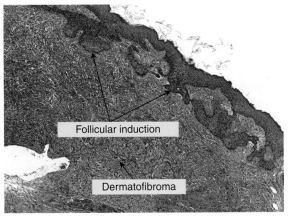

FIGURE 15.26   Dermatofibroma with Folliculosebaceous Induction

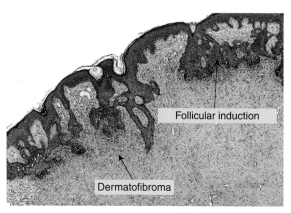

FIGURE 15.27   Follicular Induction Overlying
Dermatofibroma Almost Resembling Basal Cell Carcinoma

DEEP FIBROUS HISTIOCYTOMA

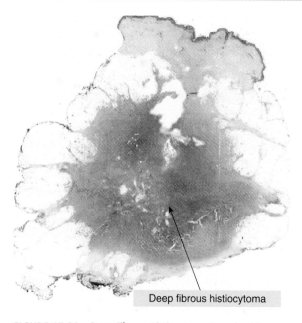

FIGURE 15.28   Deep Fibrous Histiocytoma-Scanning View

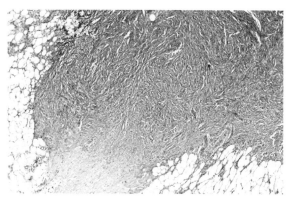

FIGURE 15.29   Deep Fibrous Histiocytoma—Base

Deep fibrous histiocytoma is an uncommon variant of dermatofibroma. Fibrous histiocytoma occurs in the deep dermis and the subcutaneous tissue. It has also been documented in the deep soft tissue. Similar to dermatofibroma, the commonest site is the lower extremities. Less commonly other deep soft tissue locations and visceral sites have also been documented. Clinically the tumor presents as small papules and nodules.

On microscopy, the tumor is located in the soft tissue with minor involvement of the dermis. The morphological appearances are similar to the usual dermatofibroma. The cells are arranged in a vague storiform pattern and intersect in between collagen bundles. The cellularity of the tumor is very variable. The commonest pattern is that seen in a cellular fibrous histiocytoma. The cells are closely packed with formation of multinucleated giant cells and the occasional mitotic figure. Very rarely, more than 10 mitoses have been reported. Necrosis and lymphovascular space permeation are exceptionally rare, although they have been documented in deep benign fibrous histiocytoma.

Immunohistochemically, CD34 stains the cells at the periphery. SMA stains the cells uniformly throughout the lesion. Deep fibrous histiocytoma is known to recur in 20% of cases and it very rarely metastasizes. Malignant change in a fibrous histiocytoma is easily identified by marked nuclear pleomorphism and increased mitotic activity with many atypical forms.

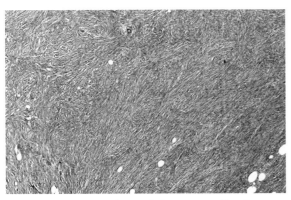

FIGURE 15.30   Deep Fibrous Histiocytoma-Medium Power

ATROPHIC DERMATOFIBROMA

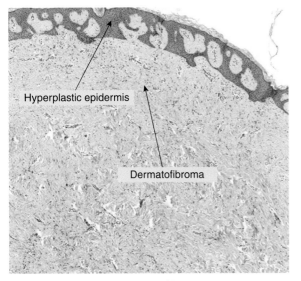

Hyperplastic epidermis

Dermatofibroma

FIGURE 15.31   Atrophic Dermatofibroma

Atrophic dermatofibroma is not an uncommon variant of dermatofibroma. Clinically, it presents as areas of thickening or small plaques on the extremities.

On microscopy, the overlying epidermis is hyperplastic. The tumor is located in the dermis. The cellularity is sparse and the cells infiltrate in between the collagen bundles. Wrapping round collagen is also seen. Atrophic dermatofibroma can be easily missed histologically because of the very poor cellularity of the tumor.

EPITHELIOID DERMATOFIBROMA

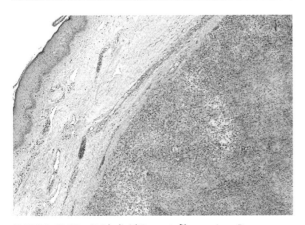

FIGURE 15.32   Epithelioid Dermatofibroma-Low Power

Epithelioid dermatofibroma is a histological variant of dermatofibroma. The clinical presentation is similar to ordinary dermatofibroma.

On microscopy, the overlying epidermis is hyperplastic. The dermis shows features of typical dermatofibroma, but with more than 50% of the cells showing epithelioid morphology. Epithelioid cells have ample eosinophilic cytoplasm and rounded vesicular nuclei. Because of the presence of epithelioid cells, this variant of dermatofibroma may be mistaken for a Spitz naevus. The S100 protein decorating the cells of the Spitz naevus should be useful in differentiating the two tumors.

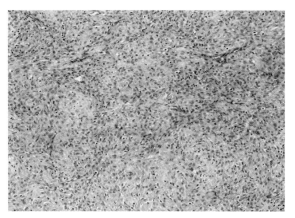

FIGURE 15.33   Epithelioid Dermatofibroma-High Power

ANEURYSMAL DERMATOFIBROMA

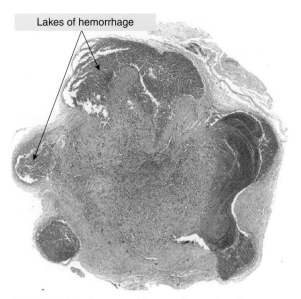

Lakes of hemorrhage

FIGURE 15.34   Aneurysmal Dermatofibroma-Low Power

Aneurysmal dermatofibroma is a variant of dermatofibroma with a history of rapid growth. This is thought to be due to the spontaneous hemorrhage that occurs in these tumors. Clinically, they appear as blue-black nodules resulting from the hemorrhage within the tumor.

On microscopy, the tumor shows large blood-filled spaces in the periphery lined by tumor cells. The adjacent areas show features of ordinary dermatofibroma. Hemosiderin pigment and brisk mitotic activity are seen within the tumor. There is a 20% chance of recurrence in aneurysmal dermatofibroma.

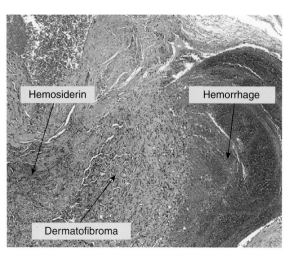

Hemosiderin   Hemorrhage

Dermatofibroma

FIGURE 15.35   Aneurysmal Dermatofibroma-High Power

DERMATOFIBROSARCOMA PROTUBERANS

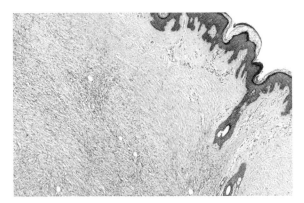

FIGURE 15.36   Dermatofibrosarcoma Protuberans-Low Power

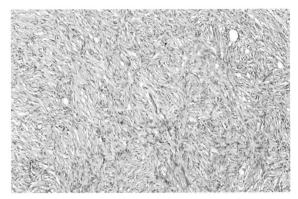

FIGURE 15.37   Dermatofibrosarcoma—Storiform Pattern Protuberans-Low Power

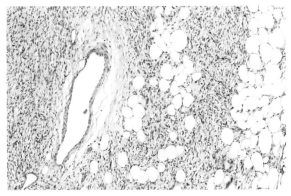

FIGURE 15.38   Dermatofibrosarcoma Protuberans— Sieve-Like Pattern

Dermatofibrosarcoma protuberans is a tumor related to the fibroblasts and is of intermediate malignant potential. They have a high chance of recurrence but very rarely metastasize. Clinically, the tumor presents as solitary or multiple nodular masses. The most frequent sites affected are the upper extremities and the trunk. Dermatofibrosarcoma protuberans is well known for its indolent growth. The initial manifestation may be that of flattened plaque which may remain stationary for over many years. Multiple nodules may develop over the years. It can rarely occur in children.

On microscopy, the tumor has a diffuse pattern of infiltration. The tumor is located in the dermis and the subcutaneous fat. The overlying epidermis is thinned out or normal. The major bulk of the tumor shows a classical storiform pattern of arrangement of cells. Toward the periphery the tumor is seen to grow around adnexal structures and in the deep subcutaneous fat it has the classical infiltrative lacelike pattern. The tumor cells are fibroblastic and have scanty cytoplasm and slender nuclei with tapering ends. Mitotic activity, fewer than 5 per 10 high power fields, is seen. Nuclear pleomorphism is not seen. Inflammatory cells and xanthoma cells are not a feature seen in this tumor. Myoid nodule which is condensation of myofibroblasts around blood vessels is a feature noted in dermatofibrosarcoma protuberans.

Sarcomatous transformation of dermatofibrosarcoma protuberans is very rare. The sarcomatous change is seen in fascicular growth pattern as opposed to storiform growth seen in dermatofibrosarcoma protuberans and should constitute at least 5–10% of the tumor, with increase in mitotic activity and diminished CD34 staining. The chances of distant metastasis after sarcomatous transformation are remote if the tumor is adequately excised.

Immunohistochemically, dermatofibrosarcoma protuberans stains diffusely and strongly with CD34.

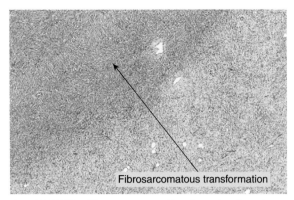

FIGURE 15.39   Fibrosarcomatous Transformation-Scanning View

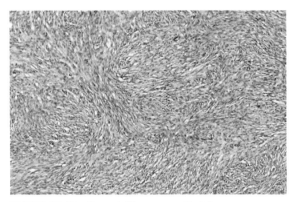

FIGURE 15.40   Dermatofibrosarcoma Protuberans—Fibrosarcomatous Areas-High Power

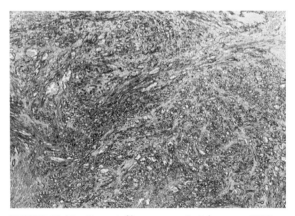

FIGURE 15.41   Dermatofibrosarcoma Protuberans—CD34

MYXOID DERMATOFIBROSARCOMA PROTUBERANS

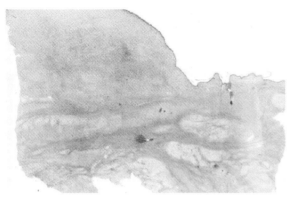

FIGURE 15.42   Myxoid Dermatofibrosarcoma Protuberans-Scanning View

Myxoid change in dermatofibrosarcoma protuberans is not very uncommon. The myxoid areas could be focal or extensive. In the latter situation, the cellularity is markedly reduced. Myxoid change in neurofibroma and myxoid liposarcoma enters the differential diagnosis. Strong and diffuse staining for CD34 is helpful in confirming the diagnosis.

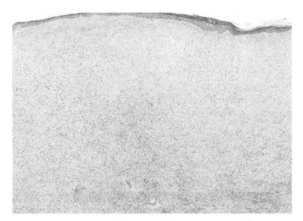

FIGURE 15.43   Myxoid Dermatofibrosarcoma Protuberans-Low Power

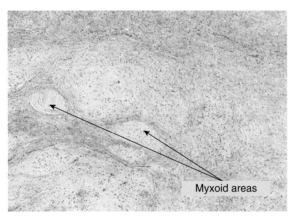

FIGURE 15.44   Myxoid Dermatofibrosarcoma Protuberans—Myxoid Areas

FIGURE 15.45   Myxoid Dermatofibrosarcoma Protuberans—
Storiform Areas

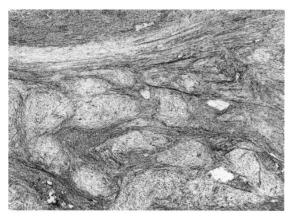

FIGURE 15.46   Myxoid Dermatofibrosarcoma Protuberans—
CD34

ACRAL MYXOINFLAMMATORY FIBROBLASTIC SARCOMA

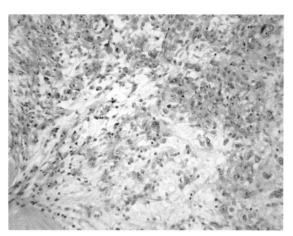

FIGURE 15.47   Acral Myxoinflammatory Fibroblastic
Sarcoma—Myxoid Areas

As the name implies, acral myxoinflammatory fibroblastic sarcoma is a tumor affecting the acral sites predominantly. The upper extremities are much more commonly affected than the lower extremities. Clinically, most often they present as small cysts or tenosynovitis.

On microscopy, in majority of cases the tumor occupies the subcutaneous tissue as multinodular masses. Myxoid change within the tumor is conspicuous. In addition, a pronounced inflammatory infiltrate is also seen. This is formed of variable mixtures of eosinophils, lymphocytes, plasma cells, and sometimes neutrophils. Lymphoid follicle with germinal centers may also be seen. The cellular component includes spindle cells with atypical nuclei and larger cells with eosinophilic cytoplasm and vesicular nuclei and prominent nucleoli. The latter cells show resemblance to Reed-Sternberg cells or virocytes. Mitotic activity is very low and necrosis is not a feature in this tumor. Very rarely, ganglion-like cells are also noted.

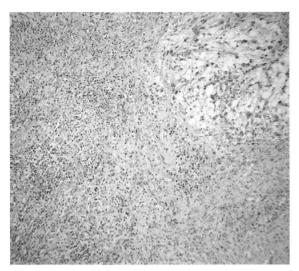

FIGURE 15.48   Acral Myxoinflammatory Fibroblastic Sarcoma

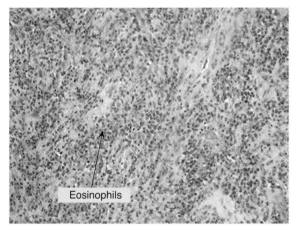

FIGURE 15.49   Acral Myxoinflammatory Fibroblastic Sarcoma—Inflammatory Areas

EPITHELIOID CELL SARCOMA

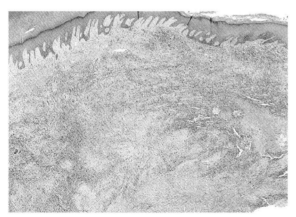

FIGURE 15.50   Epithelioid Cell Sarcoma-Scanning View

Immunohistochemically, the tumor cells stain with CD34, CD68, and SMA. There is negative staining with S100, HMB-45, Melan A, and EMA.

No specific cytogenetic abnormality has been identified. Acral myxoinflammatory fibroblastic sarcoma is a tumor with a high propensity for local recurrence. There has been a single case of histologically documented metastasis in a regional lymph node.

Epithelioid cell sarcoma is an uncommon tumor affecting young adults. The tumor involves the extremities and is known to arise from the flexor aspect of the fingers and hands. Less common sites include the lower extremities and the shoulder. Clinically the presentation is very variable. The superficial tumors that are invariably dermal, present as woody lumps and are very slow-growing and painless. They eventually ulcerate and present as a nonhealing ulcer.

On microscopy, the classic type of epithelioid cell sarcoma is the most common. The classic type is a dermal tumor exhibiting granulomatous appearance. The proximal type which is uncommon and is usually located within the muscle. Epithelioid cell sarcoma has a characteristic multinodular arrangement of cells with areas of geographic necrosis. The cells forming the tumor are either spindle-shaped or epithelioid. Nuclear pleomorphism and mitotic activity are not very conspicuous.

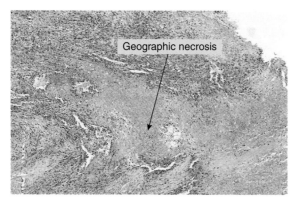
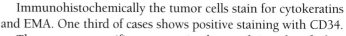

FIGURE 15.51   Epithelioid Cell Sarcoma-Low Power—
Geographic Necrosis

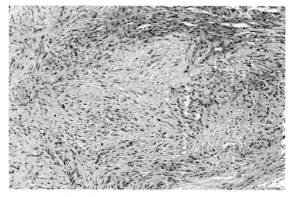

FIGURE 15.52   Epithelioid Cell Sarcoma-Low Power—
Spindle and Epithelioid Cell Infiltration

ATYPICAL FIBROXANTHOMA

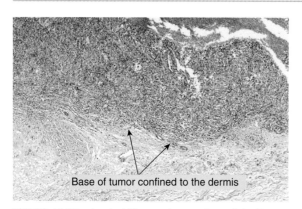

FIGURE 15.53   Atypical Fibroxanthoma—Base of the Tumor

Immunohistochemically the tumor cells stain for cytokeratins and EMA. One third of cases shows positive staining with CD34.

There are no specific cytogenetic abnormalities identified in epithelioid cell sarcoma. Several dermal and deep granulomatous conditions such as granuloma annulare, necrotizing infections, and rheumatoid nodule enter the differential diagnosis histologically. Malignant tumors with a prominent epithelioid cell component should also be considered in the differential diagnosis.

Atypical fibroxanthoma presents as nodule or plaque on the sun-exposed site of the elderly individuals. Scalp is the most common location.

On microscopy, the overlying epidermis may or may not be ulcerated. The tumor is entirely dermal and is well circumscribed. In most cases, it is seen in close apposition with the overlying epidermis, although not arising from it. The tumor cells are usually closely packed and exhibit marked nuclear pleomorphism with many bizarre cell forms. The majority of the cells are spindle-shaped, although cells with foamy cytoplasm are also seen. Necrosis is not a feature although occasional mitotic figures may be seen. Several histological subtypes are described, which include clear cell, granular cell, pigmented cell, and the commonest spindle-cell variant. A variable mixture of inflammatory cell infiltration is also seen. The features of aggressive behavior include infiltration into subcutaneous fat, vascular invasion, and presence of necrosis. Tumors that show any of these features are designated pleomorphic sarcomas.

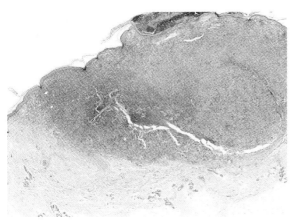

FIGURE 15.54   Atypical Fibroxanthoma-Low Power

Immunohistochemically, the tumor cells are known to stain with CD68 and CD10.

The histological features of atypical fibroxanthoma can also be confused with a poorly differentiated squamous cell carcinoma, melanoma, and leiomyosarcoma. The absence of staining of cytokeratins (MNF116, AE1/AE3, CK14, CK5/6) and p63 excludes a squamous cell carcinoma. Negative staining of S100, Melan A, and HMB45 excludes the possibility of a melanoma and negative staining SMA, Desmin, and h-caldesmon exclude a leiomyosarcoma.

There has been reports of atypical fibroxanthoma recurring because of incomplete removal. Recently, a case of atypical fibroxanthoma that metastasized to the lymph nodes has been reported.

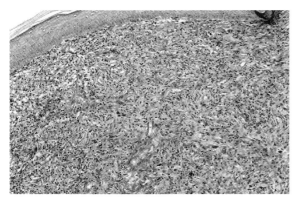

FIGURE 15.55   Atypical Fibroxanthoma-High Power

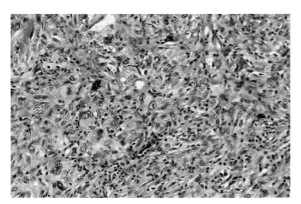

FIGURE 15.56   Atypical Fibroxanthoma-High Power—Another View

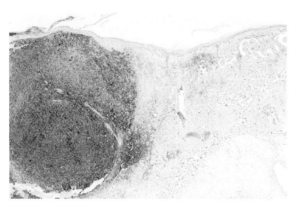

FIGURE 15.57   Atypical Fibroxanthoma—CD10

MYXOFIBROSARCOMA

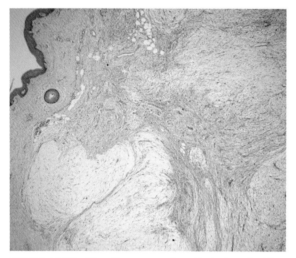

FIGURE 15.58   Myxofibrosarcoma-Low Grade-Scanning View

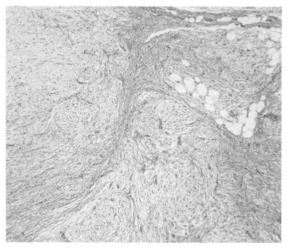

FIGURE 15.59   Myxofibrosarcoma-High Power

Myxofibrosarcoma is a rare tumor clinically presenting as painless masses in elderly individuals. The tumor is known to be common in the upper extremities.

On microscopy, myxofibrosarcoma is located in the dermis and the subcutaneous fat. The characteristic scanning view is that of multiple large lobules of myxoid areas separated by broad fibrous bands containing tumor cells. Because of the marked myxoid appearance of the tumor, hypo and hypercellular areas are commonly seen. The hypocellular areas are seen in the myxoid areas and the hypercellular areas are seen within the solid fibrous bands. The term "myxofibrosarcoma" is used when more than 50% of the tumor is occupied by the myxoid areas. The tumor cells have scanty cytoplasm and spindle-shaped slender nuclei reminiscent of myofibroblasts. The tumor is graded into low and high grade categories based on the nuclear pleomorphism, mitotic activity and necrosis. The low-grade areas show mild nuclear pleomorphism and scanty mitotic activity. In the high-grade areas the cells are markedly pleomorphic with bizarre cell forms. Brisk mitotic activity is noted in this area.

Immunohistochemically, the cells stain with SMA and focally with CD34. Low-grade myxofibrosarcomas recur if incompletely excised, but very rarely metastasize. The high-grade tumors tend to metastasize more frequently.

FIBRO-OSSEOUS PSEUDOTUMOR

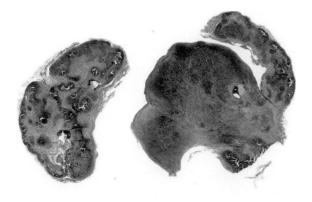

FIGURE 15.60   Fibro-Osseous Pseudotumor of Digits

Fibro-osseous pseudotumor of the digits is a rare tumor. It is usually seen in the subcutaneous tissue of the digits in young individuals.

On microscopy, the tumor has a multinodular growth pattern and is composed of an intermixture of cartilage, bone, and fibrous tissue. Calcification could be a notable feature. Features of malignancy such as nuclear pleomorphism and mitotic activity are not seen in this tumor and the behavior is entirely benign.

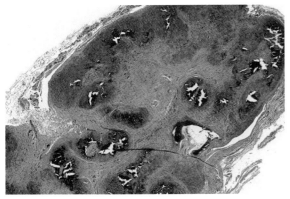

FIGURE 15.61   Fibro-Osseous Pseudotumor of Digits-Medium Power

CUTANEOUS LEIOMYOMA

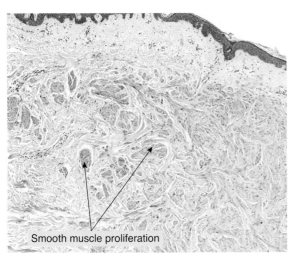

Smooth muscle proliferation

FIGURE 15.62   Cutaneous Leiomyoma-Low Power

Benign smooth muscle tumors of skin are called "leiomyomas." They arise in several clinical settings. They are broadly classified into five groups: (a) solitary leiomyomas, (b) multiple leiomyomas, (c) angioleiomyomas, (d) genital leiomyomas, and (e) leiomyomas with additional mesenchymal components.

Solitary and multiple leiomyomas arise from the arrector pili muscle. The numbers of the lesion vary from being solitary to many crops of lesions. Pain is a common symptom. Genital leiomyomas are located in the vulva and the scrotum and rarely in the nipples. Cutaneous angiolipoleiomyomas are very rare lesions and may develop following trauma.

On microscopy, leiomyomas are poorly circumscribed dermal tumors. They arise from the arrector pili muscles and are seen as a haphazard proliferation of smooth muscle cells in between dermal collagen. The cells have eosinophilic cytoplasm and blunt-ended or "cigar-shaped" nuclei. Nuclear pleomorphism and mitotic activity are absent.

The tumor cells stain strongly with SMA, Desmin, and h-caldesmon. Genital leiomyomas stain with oestrogen and progesterone receptors.

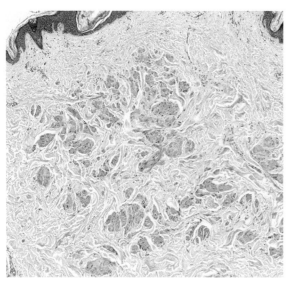

FIGURE 15.63 Cutaneous Leiomyoma-Medium Power

ANGIOLEIOMYOMA

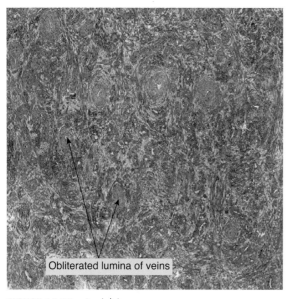

Obliterated lumina of veins

FIGURE 15.64 Angioleiomyoma

Angioleiomyoma also known as "vascular leiomyoma" is a variant of cutaneous leiomyoma. Clinically, they arise as painful nodules on the lower extremities predominantly. They are less frequently seen on other parts of the body.

On microscopy, angioleiomyomas are circumscribed tumors unlike cutaneous leiomyomas. They are thought to arise from the veins and so the smooth muscle proliferation is seen around small venous channels. Some of them have obliterated lumen due to the proliferation of smooth muscle around them.

The smooth muscle cells stain strongly for SMA, Desmin, and h-caldesmon.

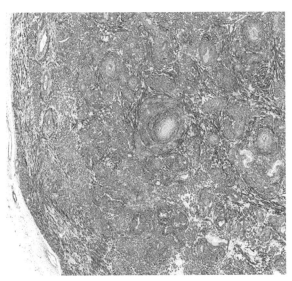

FIGURE 15.65   Angioleiomyoma—Smooth Muscle Actin

CUTANEOUS LEIOMYOSARCOMA

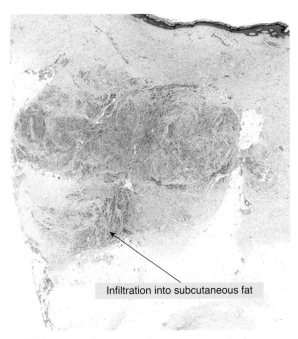

Infiltration into subcutaneous fat

FIGURE 15.66   Cutaneous Leiomyosarcoma—Grade 1-Scanning View

Cutaneous leiomyosarcomas are rare tumors. Clinically, they present as solitary skin-colored nodules. Occasionally they are painful. They are known to arise from the arrector pili muscles, the smooth muscle around the veins, and the smooth muscle around the eccrine glands. Very rarely, multiple nodules may be seen when the possibility of metastasis should be considered.

On microscopy, the tumor is not encapsulated and may be partly circumscribed. The base of the tumor and the periphery show the infiltrative appearance. The tumor itself is cellular and is composed of cells with eosinophilic cytoplasm and spindle-shaped nuclei with blunt ends. Nuclear pleomorphism can vary from mild to severe depending on the grade of the tumor. Bizarre cell forms may also be seen. Mitotic activity also is variable. Any tumor with a mitotic activity of more than 3 per high power fields is considered leiomyosarcoma. Infiltration into the deep subcutaneous tissue is another important diagnostic feature apart from nuclear pleomorphism and mitotic activity.

Immunohistochemically, the tumor cells stain for SMA, Desmin, and h-caldesmon. The SMA stains the nucleus and cytoplasm of the cells, characteristic of its nature. A small percentage of leiomyosarcomas may also stain with cytokeratins.

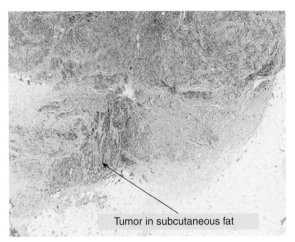

Tumor in subcutaneous fat

FIGURE 15.67   Leiomyosarcoma—Base

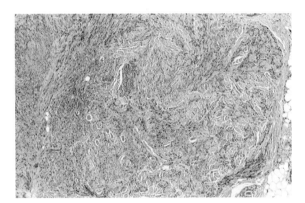

FIGURE 15.68   Cutaneous Leiomyosarcoma-High Power

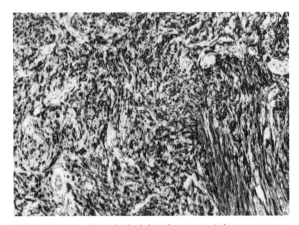

FIGURE 15.69   Desmin Staining Cutaneous Leiomyosarcoma

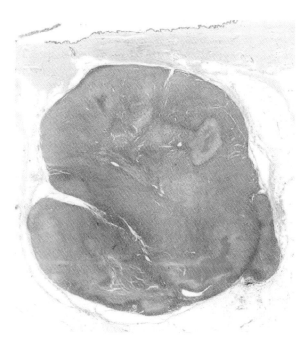

FIGURE 15.70   Cutaneous Leiomyosarcoma—High Grade

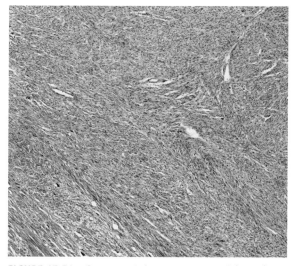

FIGURE 15.71   Cutaneous Leiomyosarcoma—High Grade-
High Power

CAPILLARY HEMANGIOMA

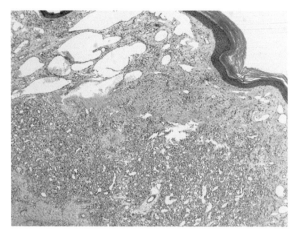

FIGURE 15.72   Capillary Hemangioma-Scanning View

Capillary hemangioma is one of the most common vascular tumors and can arise in any age and site. Clinically, they present as bright red or bluish lobulated lesions.

On microscopy, the tumor is located in the dermis and has the characteristic lobular architecture. There is proliferation of capillaries and in places the vessels are dilated similar to cavernous hemangioma. The lining cells are large and mitotically active in early lesions. In mature lesions there may be fibrosis. The main differential diagnosis is with a vascular malformation. Human erythrocyte glucose transporter (GLUT-1) stains the hemangioma but not the vascular malformation.

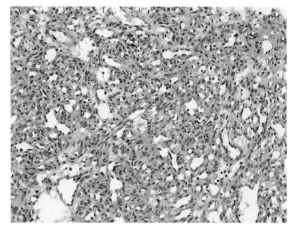

FIGURE 15.73   Capillary Hemangioma-Medium Power

PYOGENIC GRANULOMA

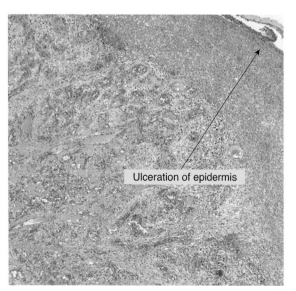

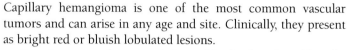

Ulceration of epidermis

FIGURE 15.74   Pyogenic Granuloma-Low Power

Pyogenic granuloma is a common vascular tumor seen in children and young adults. The clinical presentation is usually that of an ulcerated nodule. It arises in a wide variety of anatomical sites including the oral cavity.

On microscopy, the tumor is polypoid and is covered by ulcerated epidermis. The dermis shows proliferation of capillaries of variable sizes. The lining endothelial cells may be swollen in the superficial part of the tumor due to the secondary changes of overlying ulceration. There is usually an infiltrate of neutrophils from the ulcerated epidermis. The deeper part of the tumor shows features exactly similar to that of capillary hemangioma.

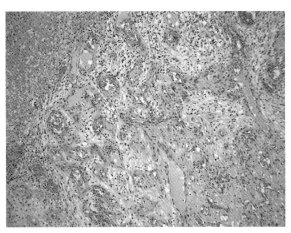

FIGURE 15.75   Pyogenic Granuloma-High Power

CAVERNOUS HEMANGIOMA

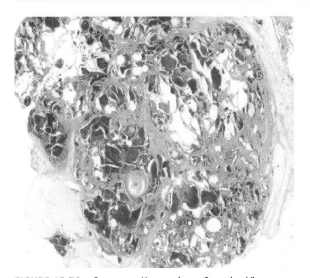

FIGURE 15.76   Cavernous Hemangioma-Scanning View

Cavernous hemangioma has similar incidence as that of capillary hemangioma. Clinically, they tend to be larger bright red lesions and can occur in any anatomical sites. Cavernous hemangiomas are associated with multiple enchondromas in Maffucci's syndrome and cavernous hemangioma can coexist with hemangiomas of the gastrointestinal tract in Blue rubber bleb syndrome.

On microscopy, cavernous hemangiomas show dilated congested vessels lined by flattened endothelial cells. The lobular architecture is absent. The vessels may vary in thickness. Inflammatory cell infiltration is also rarely seen.

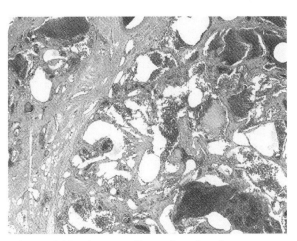

FIGURE 15.77   Cavernous Hemangioma-Low Power

MICROVENULAR HEMANGIOMA

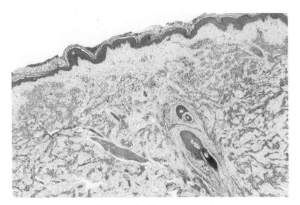

FIGURE 15.78 Microvenular Hemangioma-Low Power

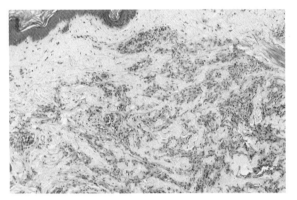

FIGURE 15.79 Microvenular Hemangioma-High Power

Microvenular hemangioma is a vascular lesion that has predilection for the extremities and trunk. Clinically, they present as small reddish nodules.

On microscopy, the tumor shows proliferation of thin-walled vascular channels with compressed lumina intersecting collagen bundles. The endothelial cells lining the vessels do not exhibit any atypia. The histological appearances raise the differential diagnosis of patch stage of Kaposi's sarcoma. CD34 staining of the spindle cells of Kaposi's sarcoma should be a useful diagnostic clue.

EPITHELIOID HEMANGIOMA

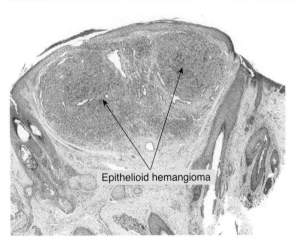

Epithelioid hemangioma

FIGURE 15.80 Epithelioid Hemangioma-Scanning View

Epithelioid hemangioma is a vascular lesion which is uncommon. There is still controversy as to whether this is a neoplastic or reactive lesion secondary to trauma. Clinically, epithelioid hemangioma has a predilection for the head and neck region. They present as dark-brown or reddish nodules. They rarely ulcerate secondary to trauma. They are also reported in deep visceral sites such as ovary, testis, and also breast and lymph nodes.

On microscopy, the lesion is dermal in a large majority of cases. It may involve the subcutaneous fat. The lesion is seen as lobulated nodules composed of vascular channels with a moderate infiltrate of inflammatory cells. The blood vessels can be of varying luminal sizes and are characteristically lined by epithelioid endothelial cells. The endothelial cells are enlarged with ample cytoplasm and prominent nuclei and sometimes vacuolated cytoplasm. Nuclear pleomorphism and mitotic activity are not seen in the endothelial cells. The inflammatory infiltrate has a conspicuous eosinophilic component but also has variable numbers of lymphocytes, histiocytes, and plasma cells. Lymphoid aggregates with prominent germinal centers may be seen.

Epithelioid hemangioma is a benign lesion and has no associations with other vascular tumors.

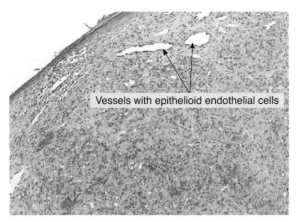

FIGURE 15.81   Epithelioid Hemangioma-Low Power

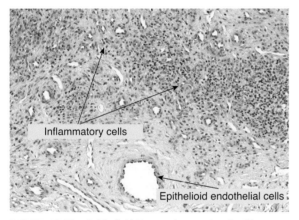

FIGURE 15.82   Epithelioid Hemangioma—Another View

ACQUIRED TUFTED HEMANGIOMA

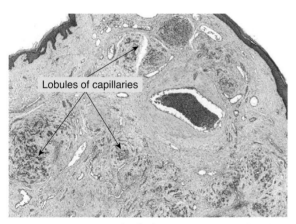

FIGURE 15.83   Acquired Tufted Hemangioma-Scanning View

Acquired tufted hemangioma is a benign vascular tumor. It is commonly seen in the older age group as reddish nodules over various anatomical sites.

On microscopy, the tumor is dermal and is composed of lobules of small-sized capillaries arranged randomly in the dermis in a cannon ball appearance. The capillaries may be not be canalized completely. The periphery of the tumor shows dilated and sometimes slit-like vascular spaces. The tumor behaves in a benign fashion.

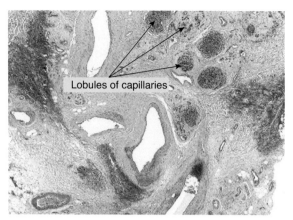

FIGURE 15.84   Acquired Tufted Hemangioma—Scanning Another View

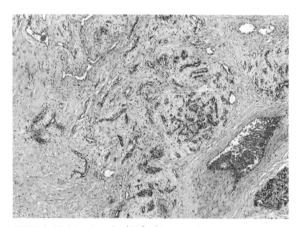

FIGURE 15.85   Acquired Tufted Hemangioma—Scanning-High Power

ANGIOKERATOMA

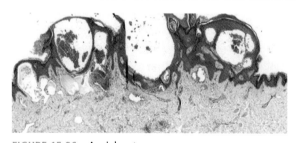

FIGURE 15.86   Angiokeratoma

Angiokeratomas is the broad term used to describe five different variants. They are angiokeratoma of Fordyce, angiokeratoma of Mibelli, angiokeratoma circumscriptum corporis diffusum, and solitary and multiple angiokeratomas.

On microscopy, all the clinical variants show similar appearances. There are dilated blood vessels in the papillary dermis which impinge on to the epidermis. The reticular dermis is usually not involved.

GLOMUS TUMOR

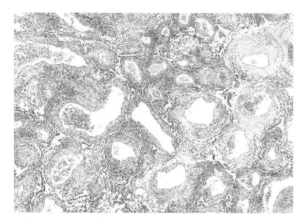

FIGURE 15.87   Glomus Tumor-Scanning View

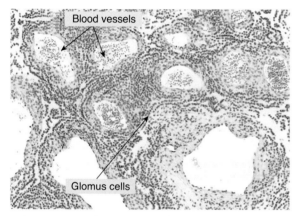

Blood vessels

Glomus cells

FIGURE 15.88   Glomus Tumor-High Power

Glomus tumors are neoplasms arising from the glomus bodies. They are specialized arteriovenous anastomoses and are thought to be involved in thermoregulatory mechanisms. Glomus tumors are common and have a predilection for fingers and toes. Clinically they present as painful bluish-red nodules. Rarely they present as multiple nodules. They are reported to arise in rare sites such as ovary and retroperitoneum.

On microscopy, glomus tumors are circumscribed but not encapsulated. The tumor is composed of blood vessels of varying sizes lined by flattened endothelial cells. The vessels are lined by proliferation of glomus cells. Glomus cells have scanty cytoplasm and rounded bland nuclei. Mitotic figures and nuclear pleomorphism are rare. The histological variants of glomus tumors described are glomangiomas and glomangiomyomas. Glomangiomas exhibit dilated vascular spaces lined by glomus cells in the periphery. Glomangiomas contain smooth muscle cells in their walls. Benign glomus tumors rarely recur if incompletely excised.

Malignant change in a glomus tumor is very rarely reported. The features of malignancy are deep location of the tumor and size more than 2 cm or more than 5 mitoses/50 high power fields or atypical mitoses. Glomus tumor of uncertain malignant potential is used when the criteria of malignancy are not entirely satisfied, but the tumor is either more than 2 cm or in a deep location and has high mitotic activity. About a third of the cases of malignant glomus tumor is known to metastasize.

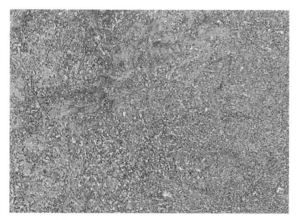

FIGURE 15.89   Glomus Tumor of Uncertain Malignant Potential-Low Power

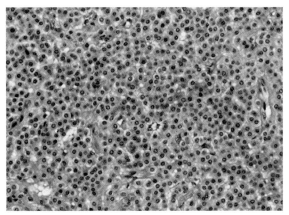

FIGURE 15.90   Glomus Tumor of Uncertain Malignant Potential-High Power

INTRAVASCULAR FASCIITIS

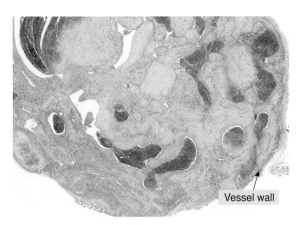

Vessel wall

FIGURE 15.91   Intravascular Fasciitis-Scanning View

Intravascular fasciitis occurs in children and young adults. The lesion commonly presents as flesh-colored plaques and nodules on the shoulder and back. Less commonly, it occurs on other sites.

On microscopy, the features are essentially those of nodular fasciitis. The spindle-cell proliferation is contained within a markedly dilated vascular lumen. Features of congestion may also be seen. The lesion is not known to recur and has no malignant potential.

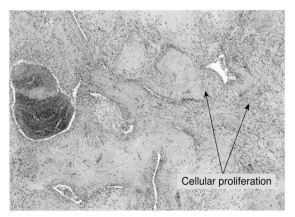

Cellular proliferation

FIGURE 15.92   Intravascular Fasciitis-High Power

INTRAVASCULAR PAPILLARY ENDOTHELIAL HYPERPLASIA

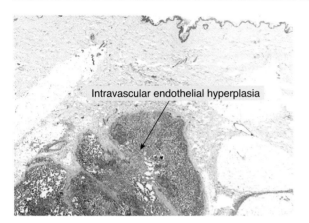

FIGURE 15.93   Intravascular Papillary Endothelial Hyperplasia-Scanning View

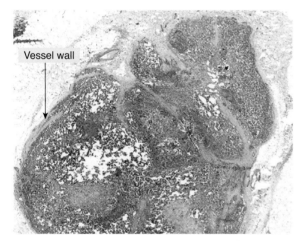

FIGURE 15.94   Intravascular Papillary Endothelial Hyperplasia in Subcutis

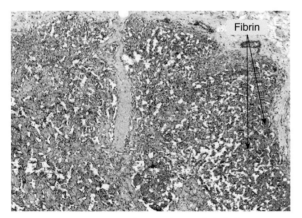

FIGURE 15.95   Intravascular Papillary Endothelial Hyperplasia-High Power

Intravascular papillary endothelial hyperplasia is also known as "Masson's tumor." This is considered a reactive lesion. A history of trauma is not elicited most of the time. Clinically the lesion is most commonly seen in the head and neck area and the upper extremities as reddish blue papules and nodules. Occasionally it may be cystic.

On microscopy, the vessel lumen is almost completely obliterated by several papillae lined by endothelial cells. The endothelial cells do not exhibit any nuclear atypia, hobnailing, or mitotic figures. The vessel wall is massively thickened and fibrotic. Elsewhere in the lumen there may be features of an organized thrombus and hemosiderin deposition. Very rarely subsequent to the rupture of the vessels, the papillary growth may be seen in an extravascular location. This appearance, particularly, can be confused with an angiosarcoma. However, the absence of nuclear pleomorphism and the intravascular location of the papillary proliferation together with features of rupture of the vessel should aid in confirming the diagnosis of intravascular papillary endothelial hyperplasia, which is a benign condition with no features of malignancy.

BACILLARY ANGIOMATOSIS

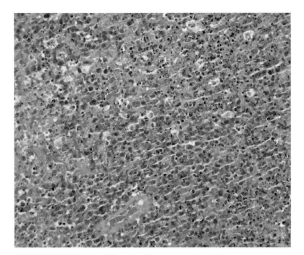

FIGURE 15.96   Bacillary Angiomatosis-Low Power

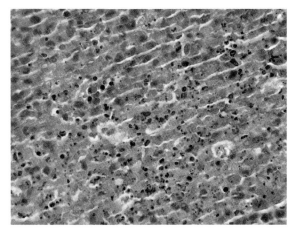

FIGURE 15.97   Bacillary Angiomatosis-High Power

Bacillary angiomatosis is a tumorlike lesion seen predominantly in a cutaneous location. It is accompanied by systemic symptoms and the lesions may be seen in other sites such as lymph nodes, spleen, soft tissue, and bone. Immunocompromised individuals are most susceptible to acquire this disease. The causative agent is thought to be *Bartonella henselae* or *Bartonella quintana*. Clinically the cutaneous lesions are multiple and are seen on the head and neck and extremities. They appear as dark red or brownish small papules.

On microscopy, the epidermis is ulcerated in most of the cases. The dermis shows proliferation of vascular spaces which are closely packed and lined by swollen endothelial cells. Many neutrophils with neutrophilic dust are seen. Histiocytes and plasma cells also form a major component of the inflammatory infiltrate. Mitotic activity and nuclear atypia may be noted. As the lesions progress the vascular spaces may be difficult to identify and the inflammatory infiltrate predominates. There are several reports of bacillary angiomatosis coexisting with Kaposi's sarcoma. Detection of human herpes virus-8 (HHV-8) by immunohisto-chemistry or by polymerase chain reaction (PCR) will be useful in excluding the latter.

The organisms can be demonstrated by Warthin-Starry stain or by PCR to identify the *Bartonella* species.

CUTANEOUS ANGIOMYXOMA

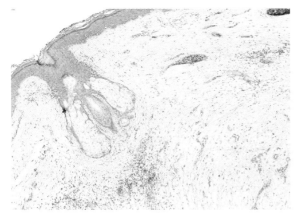

FIGURE 15.98   Cutaneous Angiomyxoma

Cutaneous myxoma is a benign neoplasm described as occurring in the setting of Carney's complex. Carney's complex includes cardiac myxomas, spotty pigmentation (multiple lentigines), and endocrine overactivity. It is an autosomal dominant familial disorder. Cutaneous myxomas associated with Carney's complex are seen around the eyelids. On other occasions, tumor is seen mainly on the trunk and the head and neck area. It may also be seen on the extremities. Clinically, they appear as soft flesh-colored nodules of varying sizes.

On microscopy, the tumor is predominantly dermal and may extend to the subcutaneous fat. The overlying epidermis may be mildly acanthotic. It is a poorly circumscribed lobular or multinodular tumor that is extensively myxoid. The cellularity is very sparse with scattered cells arranged in no definite pattern. Mitotic figures and nuclear atypia are rare. A conspicuous feature of this tumor is the presence of many thin-walled vascular channels set in the myxoid background. An inflammatory infiltrate predominantly of neutrophils is a notable feature of this tumor.

Immunohistochemically the tumor cells stain with CD34. Cutaneous myxomas recur if they are incompletely excised. There is no malignant potential.

KAPOSI'S SARCOMA

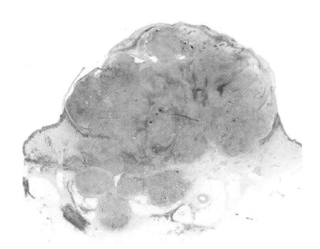

FIGURE 15.99   Kaposi's Sarcoma-Scanning View

Kaposi's sarcoma is a chronic disease induced by HHV-8. Whether Kaposi's sarcoma is a neoplasm or a reactive condition is still controversial. Several studies have been carried out on this aspect and the lesion has been shown to be monoclonal and polyclonal.

Kaposi's sarcoma develops in four clinical settings.

1. Chronic Kaposi's sarcoma—it develops especially in men belonging to certain parts of the world such as Poland, Russia, and central parts of Africa. Majority of these patients go on to develop a second malignancy, either a lymphoid malignancy or a sarcoma. The lesions are mainly seen on the lower limbs. The disease tends to have a prolonged course.

2. Lymphadenopathic Kaposi's sarcoma—this type is most commonly seen in African children and primarily affects the lymph nodes. Skin lesions are rare. The course of the disease is fulminant and in most of the cases there is involvement of the internal organs.

3. Transplantation-associated Kaposi's sarcoma—it develops in patients who already had a renal transplant. The clinical course of the disease depends on the stage of the disease and the immunosuppressive state of the person.

4. AIDS-related Kaposi's sarcoma—this is a well-established association with about 40% of patients with AIDS developing Kaposi's sarcoma. The profound immunosuppression caused by the AIDS virus is thought to be the predisposing factor.

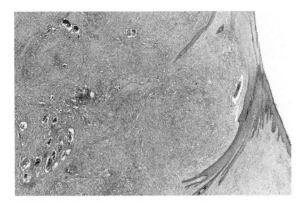

FIGURE 15.100   Kaposi's Sarcoma-Low Power

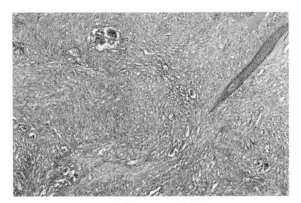

FIGURE 15.101   Kaposi's Sarcoma-High Power

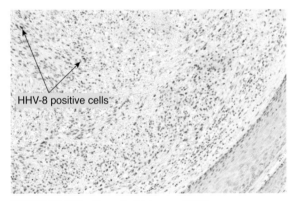

FIGURE 15.102   Kaposi's Sarcoma—HHV8

All the clinical variants of Kaposi's sarcoma manifest similar symptoms to a large extent. Clinically, Kaposi's sarcoma is seen as purplish or reddish papules and plaques in the early stages. The tumor stage could manifest as large ulcerated masses mainly in the lower extremities.

On microscopy, regardless of the clinical background, Kaposi's sarcoma shows features in three different stages.

1. Patch stage—the overlying epidermis is unremarkable. The lesion is centered on the papillary and reticular dermis. There is proliferation of thin-walled small blood vessels characteristically arranged parallel to the overlying epidermis. The endothelial cells lining the vessels show no evidence of cytological atypia or multilayering. The vascular proliferation is surrounded by inflammatory cells composed mainly of lymphocytes and plasma cells.

2. The plaque stage—it is more advanced. The epidermis is uninvolved. The dermal proliferation of blood vessels is much more pronounced and is seen in an ill-defined pattern parallel to the overlying epidermis. The endothelial cells are still flattened with no multilayering. The intervening dermis shows spindle cells with elongated tapering nuclei. Inflammatory cells composed of lymphocytes and plasma cells are present among the inflammatory cells.

3. Nodular or tumor stage—the epidermis is usually thinned out and ulcerated. The dermal tumor shows closely packed spindle-shaped cells with the vasculature closely intermingled with it. Extravasated red blood cells and inflammatory cells are seen. Hemosiderin pigment and small eosinophilic hyaline globules are seen. The hyaline globules are seen more commonly in AIDS-related Kaposi's sarcoma. In the later stages of the disease fibrosis may supervene.

The vasculature and spindle cells are positive for CD31 and CD34. The causative organism HHV-8 can be detected using immunohistochemical markers or PCR.

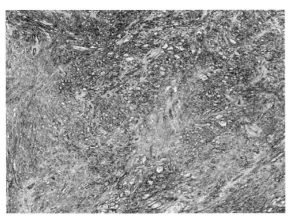

FIGURE 15.103   Kaposi's Sarcoma—CD34

CUTANEOUS ANGIOSARCOMA

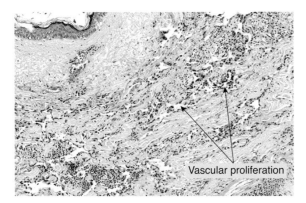

FIGURE 15.104   Cutaneous Angiosarcoma-Low Power

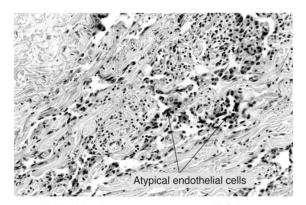

FIGURE 15.105   Cutaneous angiosarcoma-High Power

Angiosarcoma is the one of the rarest soft tissue tumors. They are known to arise in the older age group and the prognosis depends on the clinical setting in which they arise. The commonest type is the cutaneous angiosarcoma with and without association with lymphedema. Other types are angiosarcoma of the breast and postirradiation angiosarcoma. Angiosarcoma associated with lymphedema is extremely rare. The commonest types of cutaneous angiosarcoma are idiopathic cases that arise in the head and neck areas of elderly individuals. Clinically, in the earliest stage the tumor presents as an area of bruising. Large chronic lesions may be ulcerated.

On microscopy, the overlying epidermis may be intact or ulcerated depending on the stage of the disease. In the earliest lesions, there is proliferation of vascular spaces that are seen to intersect collagen bundles in a diffuse pattern. The tumor is extensive and very ill-defined. The endothelial lining of the vessels shows hobnailed appearance with nuclear atypia and mitotic activity. The cells also show multilayered appearance. In the later stage, the malignant endothelial cells show tumor aggregates and diffuse sheetlike arrangement. The tumor cells form vascular lumina. Mitotic activity and necrosis are prominent. The cells exhibit marked nuclear pleomorphism with prominent nucleoli. Other cell types such as epithelioid cells and spindle cells also form a dominant component in angiosarcoma. In such situations, other spindle-cell sarcomas, melanomas, and carcinomas enter the differential diagnosis. Careful use of the immunohistochemical markers should confirm the diagnosis.

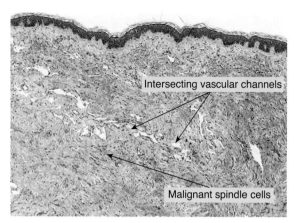

FIGURE 15.106   Postirradiation Angiosarcoma-Low Power

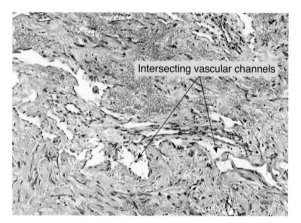

FIGURE 15.107   Postirradiation Angiosarcoma-High Power

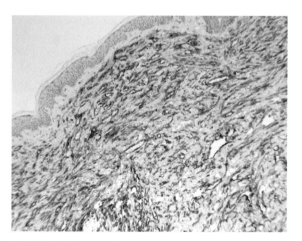

FIGURE 15.108   Angiosarcoma—CD31 Stain

Angiosarcomas stain strongly and diffusely with vascular markers CD31 and CD34.

Postirradiation angiosarcoma follows therapeutic radiation for several diseases. Most commonly it is seen following radiation for breast carcinoma, when the earliest changes can be difficult to diagnose histologically. Atypical vascular proliferation is the term used in such situations. Angiosarcoma in any setting is a very aggressive tumor with grave prognosis.

MORTON'S NEUROMA

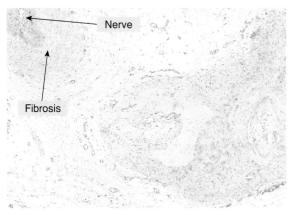

FIGURE 15.109   Morton's Neuroma-Low Power

Morton's neuroma is a reactive proliferation of fibrous tissue and is not a true neoplasm. It is seen almost exclusively in women because of ill-fitting shoes. Clinically, it presents as intermittent pain in the feet and toes.

On microscopy, there is extensive secondary fibrosis and chronic inflammation surrounding proliferated nerve fibers. Very rarely, hyalinization of the endoneurial vessels may be seen.

PALISADED ENCAPSULATED NEUROMA

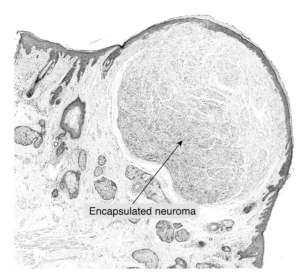

FIGURE 15.110   Palisaded Encapsulated Neuroma-Scanning View

Palisaded encapsulated neuroma is not an uncommon benign neural tumor and presents as solitary flesh-colored nodule on the face of elderly individuals.

On microscopy, the tumor is located in the dermis and may extend into the subcutaneous fat. It is circumscribed and encapsulated. The neuroma is formed of proliferated Schwann cells. Nuclear pleomorphism and mitotic figures are not seen. There are no additional stromal changes such as hyalinization and fibrosis.

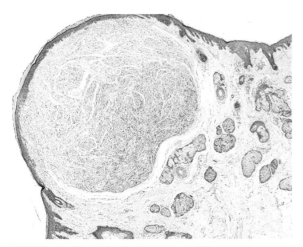

FIGURE 15.111   Palisaded Encapsulated Neuroma-Low Power

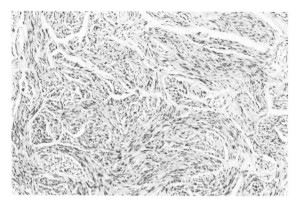

FIGURE 15.112   Encapsulated Neuroma-High Power

NEUROFIBROMA

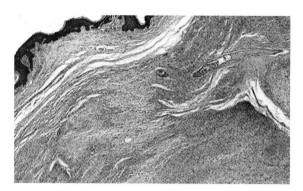

FIGURE 15.113   Neurofibroma-Low Power

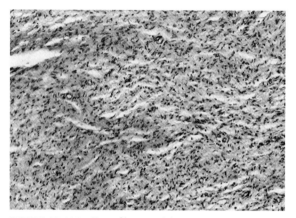

FIGURE 15.114   Neurofibroma-High Power

Neurofibromas are very common tumors. Clinically they are seen as localized or sporadic, diffuse, and plexiform neurofibromas. Localized neurofibromas are the most common types of neurofibromas. The diffuse and plexiform variants are associated with neurofibromatosis 1 (NF1). Localized neurofibromas present as painless skin-colored nodules on various anatomical sites. They may arise in connection with a nerve when they expand the nerve in a fusiform pattern.

On microscopy, neurofibromas are nonencapsulated and not circumscribed. They are seen in the dermis in a diffuse pattern. Occasionally, the cells are closely packed and may resemble a Schwannoma. The cells are short and spindly and they have nuclei with tapering ends. Scattered mast cells and lymphocytes are seen among the neural cells. Vascularity is not a prominent feature, a finding useful in excluding the possibility of a myxoma particularly when the neurofibroma shows myxoid change. Nuclear pleomorphism and mitotic activity are not features seen in sporadic or localized neurofibroma.

The S100 protein stains about 30–40% of the cells in a neurofibroma. There has been reports of positive staining of CD34 in neurofibromas. Malignant change in a neurofibroma is exceptionally rare.

Diffuse and plexiform neurofibromas occur in the setting of NF1. It is an autosomal dominant genetic disease affecting 1 in 2500–3000 live births. There are several criteria for the diagnosis of NF1. The reader is referred to more detailed text books for reference. Malignant change in a neurofibroma associated with NF1 occurs very rarely and that too in a deep-seated plexiform lesion. The genetic changes involve p16 and p19 and hence a useful test is immunohistochemical demonstration of p16 in neurofibroma which is absent in malignant peripheral nerve sheath tumor.

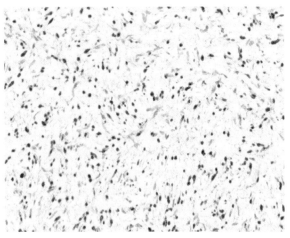

FIGURE 15.115   S100 in Neurofibroma

DENDRITIC CELL NEUROFIBROMA WITH PSEUDOROSETTES

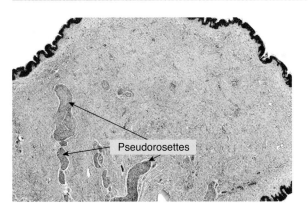

FIGURE 15.116   Dendritic Cell Neurofibroma with Pseudorosettes-Scanning View

Dendritic cell neurofibroma with pseudorosettes is a rare variant of neurofibroma. Clinically, they present as solitary nodules in different parts of the body.

On microscopy, the tumor is formed of two different types of cells. Type 1 cells are small and with dark-staining nuclei and scanty cytoplasm. Type 11 cells are larger with eosinophilic cytoplasm and vesicular nuclei. The aggregation of Type 1 cells around the Type 11 cells forms the pseudorosettes. Nuclear pleomorphism and mitotic activity are not features of this tumor.

Both cell types stain strongly for S100 and CD57. Dendritic cell neurofibroma is entirely benign and recurrences have not been reported.

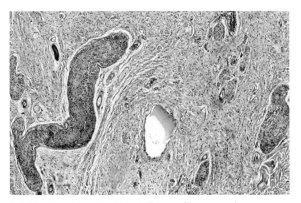

FIGURE 15.117   Dendritic Cell Neurofibroma with Pseudorosettes-Medium Power

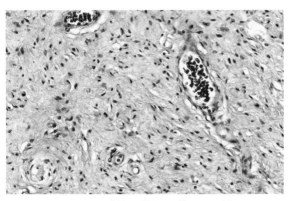

FIGURE 15.118   Dendritic Cell Neurofibroma with Pseudorosettes-High Power

SCHWANNOMA

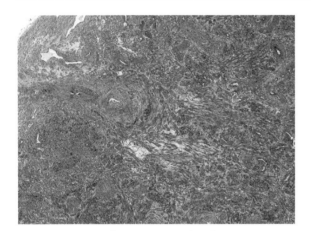

FIGURE 15.119   Schwannoma-Scanning View

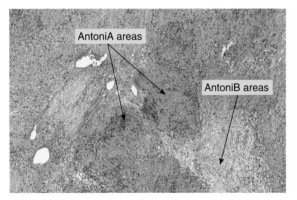

FIGURE 15.120   Schwannoma—AntoniA and AntoniB Areas

Schwannoma is also known as "neurilemmoma." This is a benign nerve sheath tumor. Clinically, they are seen in young to middle-aged individuals. They are most commonly seen in the head and neck area and the upper and lower extremities. The spinal nerve roots and ulnar nerve are most commonly affected. They are also seen in deeper locations such as mediastinum and retroperitoneum. Large majority of cases are sporadic. They are known to be slowly growing tumors.

On microscopy, schwannomas are encapsulated tumors surrounded by a fibrous capsule. The capsule contains the epineurium and the residual nerve fibers. The tumor is rarely dermal. Most often they are seen in the subcutaneous fat or deeper tissues. The classical schwannoma shows AntoniA and AntoniB areas. AntoniA areas show closely packed spindle cells. The cells have hyperchromatic nuclei and scanty cytoplasm. They are arranged in interlacing fascicles. The palisading of cells and arrangement of rows of cells with intervening fibrillary processes called "Verocay bodies" are also seen. AntoniB areas are less cellular. Spindle-shaped cells arranged in a haphazard pattern with edematous and microcystic changes are characteristically seen in AntoniB areas. Occasional mitotic figures and random nuclear atypia may be seen.

Schwannomas stain strongly and diffusely with S100.

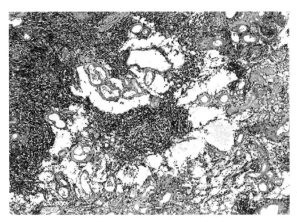

FIGURE 15.121   Schwannoma—Microcystic Changes

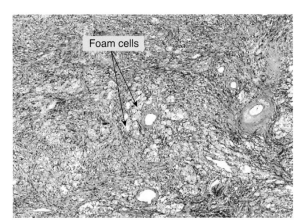

FIGURE 15.122   Schwannoma—Foam Cells

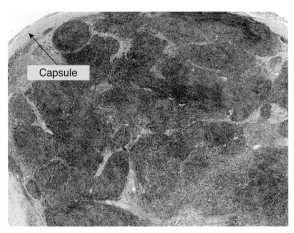

FIGURE 15.123   Schwannoma–S100

NEUROTHEKEOMA

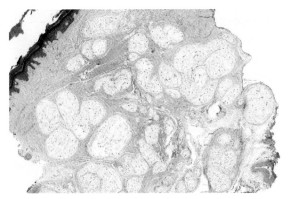

FIGURE 15.124   Neurothekeoma-Low Power

Neurothekeomas are also known as "nerve sheath myxomas." They are benign neural tumors. They are more commonly seen in children and young adults in the head and neck areas and upper extremities.

On microscopy, the tumor is formed of lobules of myxoid tissue separated by fibrous bands. The amount of myxoid substance (hyaluronic acid) can vary. In some cases, there is marked increase in cellularity with nuclear pleomorphism and mitotic activity. The cells are bland with scanty cytoplasm and oval or spindle-shaped nuclei.

Neurothekeomas stain with S100 and PGP9.5 and are not known to have any malignant potential.

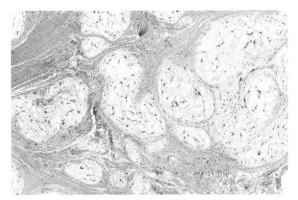

FIGURE 15.125   Neurothekeoma-Medium Power

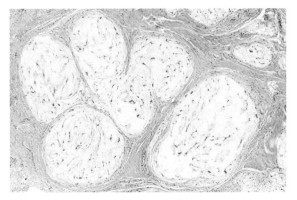

FIGURE 15.126   Neurothekeoma-High Power

CELLULAR NEUROTHEKEOMA

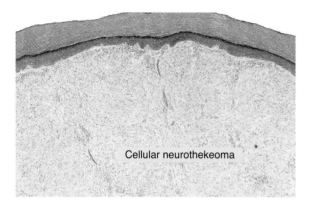

FIGURE 15.127   Cellular Neurothekeoma-Low Power

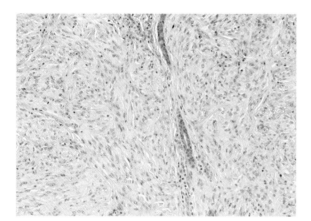

FIGURE 15.128   Cellular Neurothekeoma-High Power

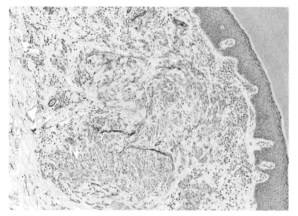

FIGURE 15.129   Cellular Neurothekeoma—CD163

Cellular neurothekeoma is a recently described benign tumor. It is commonly seen in children and young adults in the head and neck areas and upper extremities. Clinically, they are seen as small flesh-colored nodules.

On microscopy, they are poorly circumscribed tumors occupying the dermis. They may extend into the subcutaneous fat. The cells are arranged in sheets or small lobules separated by thin fibrovascular septae. The cell type is either epithelioid or spindle-shaped. Mitotic activity may be seen but atypical mitotic figures are not seen. Unlike the usual neurothekeoma, myxoid change is not seen.

Cellular neurothekeoma is a tumor of uncertain histogenesis. The tumor cells stain strongly with NKIC3 (CD63) (melanoma marker) and PGP9.5 and a small number of cases stain with SMA. The cells are consistently negative for S100. Because of the positive staining with NKIC3, the tumor is thought to belong to the family of Pecomas.

GRANULAR CELL TUMOR

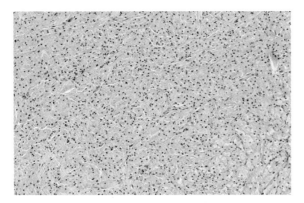

FIGURE 15.130   Granular Cell Tumor-Medium Power

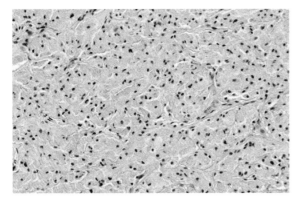

FIGURE 15.131   Granular Cell Tumor-High Power

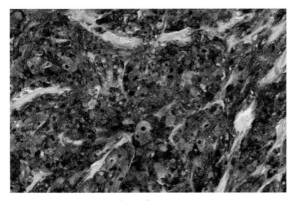

FIGURE 15.132   Granular Cell Tumor—S100 Stain

Granular cell tumor is a neoplasm of uncertain histogenesis. There are reports favoring a Schwann cell origin. Other studies have indicated an origin from "neural crest–derived peripheral nerve–related cell." Clinically, the tumors are seen as flesh-colored nodules. They are either solitary or multiple and are seen in a wide variety of sites including the oral cavity.

On microscopy, the tumor is composed of cells arranged in sheets. The cells are large with distinct cytoplasmic borders and characteristic granular cytoplasm. They have vesicular rounded nuclei. The overlying epidermis shows pseudoepitheliomatous hyperplasia.

Immunohistochemically, the tumor cells stain strongly with S100 protein, NKIC3, and PGP9.5.

Malignant change in a granular cell tumor is rare. Size greater than 5 cm, vascular invasion, nuclear pleomorphism, and mitotic activity are indicators of malignant behavior.

MERKEL CELL CARCINOMA

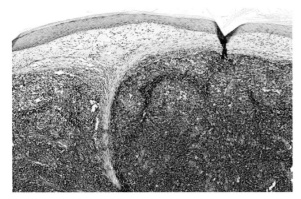

FIGURE 15.133   Merkel Cell Tumor-Low Power

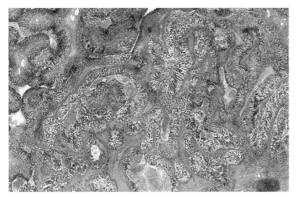

FIGURE 15.134   Merkel Cell Carcinoma-Low Power—Note the Glandular Pattern of Arrangement of Cells

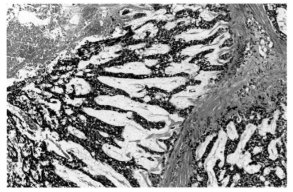

FIGURE 15.135   Merkel Cell Carcinoma-High Power—Note the Myxoid Change

Merkel cell carcinoma is a primary neuroendocrine carcinoma of skin. It is a tumor affecting sun-damaged skin of elderly individuals. Merkel cell carcinoma most commonly affects the head and neck areas but other sun-exposed sites are not exempted. Clinically, the tumor presents as painless skin-colored nodule. It can be of varying sizes, with giant types being described. The tumor is frequently ulcerated. There is a high incidence of Merkel cell carcinoma in patients who received organ transplants. The cell of origin of Merkel cell carcinoma is still controversial. The different options put forward are that they could be arising from the Merkel cells in the epidermis, the neuroendocrine cells of the dermis, or the pluripotential stem cells. The favored theory is that they arise from the Merkel cells in the epidermis.

On microscopy, Merkel cell carcinoma is centered in the dermis and may extend to the subcutaneous fat. In a small percentage of cases there is upward extension into the epidermis. The pattern of arrangements of the tumor is varied. It can be seen as solid sheets, nests separated by thin fibrovascular septae, and also as cords and ribbons of cells. Glandular differentiation has also been reported. Myxoid change is recorded in some cases. The cells have scanty cytoplasm and rounded or oval nuclei with irregular chromatin pattern described as salt and pepper appearance. Mitotic activity and apoptotic figures are frequently seen. Rarely the cells may exhibit a spindle-cell morphology. Amyloid deposition is seen as a secondary change. Lymphovascular invasion has been documented in some cases.

Immunohistochemically, Merkel cell carcinoma shows the characteristic features of neuroendocrine carcinoma. They stain with the neuroendocrine markers such as synaptophysin and chromogranin. The diagnostic staining pattern is that of paranuclear dot positivity with low-molecular-weight cytokeratin (Cam5.2) and CK20. TTF1 and CK 7 are negative, which is a useful feature to differentiate Merkel cell carcinoma from metastatic small cell carcinoma, particularly from primary sites such as lung. The cells also stain positively for EMA, CD117, and BerEp4. The cells are negative for S100 and CD45, which is again useful in excluding the possibilities of melanoma and lymphoma, respectively.

Merkel cell carcinoma is a very aggressive tumor with a recurrence rate of 40% and distant metastasis of 35%. The tumor spreads to the regional lymph nodes and also to visceral organs such as liver, skin, and lung.

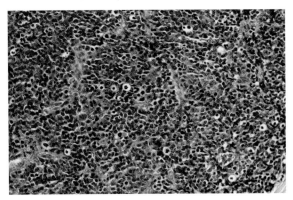

FIGURE 15.136   Merkel Cell Carcinoma-High Power—Note the Mitotic Activity and Apoptotic Figures

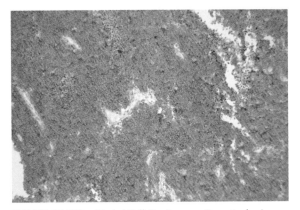

FIGURE 15.137   Merkel Cell Carcinoma—Synaptophysin Staining

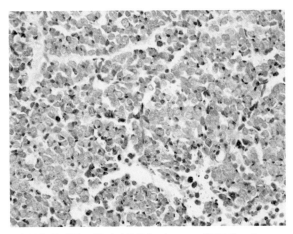

FIGURE 15.138   Merkel Cell Carcinoma—CK20 Showing Paranuclear Dot Positivity

CLEAR CELL SARCOMA OF TENDON SHEATH

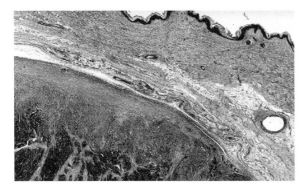

FIGURE 15.139   Clear Cell Sarcoma-Scanning View

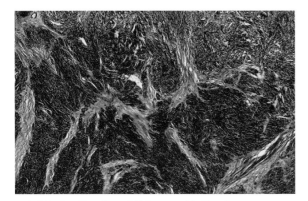

FIGURE 15.140   Clear Cell Sarcoma-Medium Power

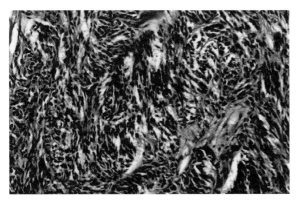

FIGURE 15.141   Clear Cell Sarcoma-High Power

Clear cell sarcoma of tendon sheaths is also known as "malignant melanoma of soft parts." The tumor is classically seen in the lower extremities in the region of the ankle. They are less frequently seen on the knee and the thigh. Clear cell sarcoma commonly affects the young adults. Clinically, they present as an enlarging mass.

On microscopy, the tumor does not involve the epidermis. Junctional activity is not a feature in this tumor. The cells are arranged as compact nests separated by thin fibrovascular septae. The cells have distinct cell borders with pale or clear cytoplasm. The nuclei are vesicular with prominent nucleoli. The nuclei exhibit varying degrees of pleomorphism and mitotic activity. The mitotic rate is generally not high. The clear cell appearance of the tumor is due to the presence of glycogen within the cytoplasm of the cells. Melanin pigment is absent in almost all the primary cases but can easily be identified in metastatic clear cell tumors.

Immunohistochemically, clear cell sarcoma stains strongly for S100, Melan A, and HMB45.

Clear cell sarcoma is considered to be a neuroectodermal tumor. It has a unique translocation t(12; 22) (q13; q12) which is not identified in melanoma. This feature is most useful in differentiating clear cell sarcoma from metastatic melanoma.

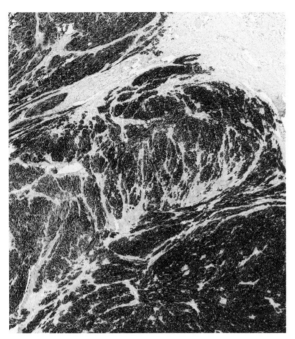

FIGURE 15.142   Clear Cell Sarcoma of Tendon Sheath—S100 Stain

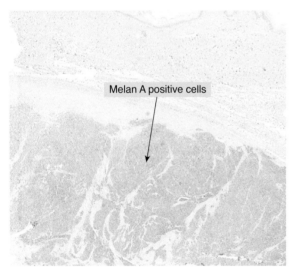

FIGURE 15.143   Clear Cell Sarcoma of Tendon Sheath— Melan A

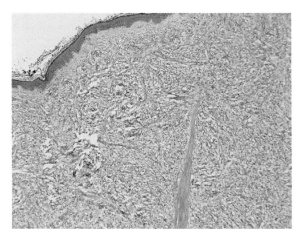

FIGURE 15.144   PEComa-Scanning View

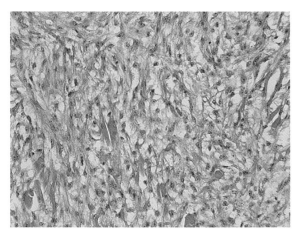

FIGURE 15.145   PEComa-Low Power

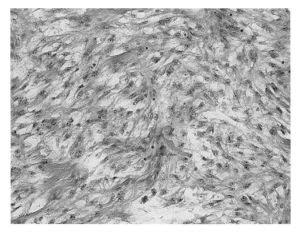

FIGURE 15.146   PEComa—Spindle Cell Appearance

PEComa also known as "perivascular epithelioid cell tumor" is a rare neoplasm occurring in the skin and the soft tissues. They belong to a spectrum of tumors that include the deep tumors such as angiomyolipoma, clear cell (sugar tumor) of lung, and clear cell myelomonocytic tumor of falciform ligament. Clinically, they present as nodules and plaques on the trunk and extremities.

On microscopy, the tumor is located in the dermis and extends to the subcutaneous fat. It is composed of cells arranged in sheets and no definite pattern. The cells characteristically have clear cytoplasm and rounded or spindle-shaped nuclei. Mitotic activity and nuclear pleomorphism are not seen. Very rarely, malignant changes have been reported.

Immunohistochemically, the cells stain with NKIC3, MelanA, HMB45, and SMA and focally with Desmin. The cells are negative for S100 and cytokeratins.

PEComas are considered as benign tumors and very rare reports of malignant variants have been documented.

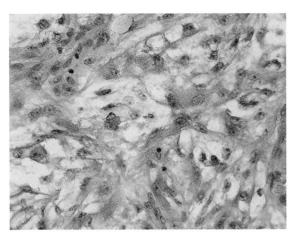

FIGURE 15.147   PEComa-High Power

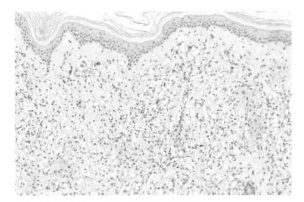

FIGURE 15.148   HMB45 Staining in PEComa

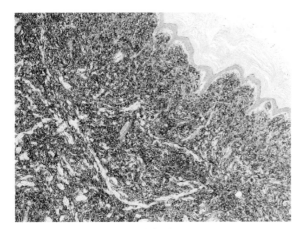

FIGURE 15.149   NK1C3 Staining in PEComa

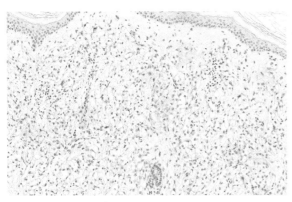

FIGURE 15.150   Melan A Staining in PEComa

BIBLIOGRAPHY

Elder D et al. Lever's Histopathology of Skin, 10th Ed. Philadelphia, PA: Lippincott Williams, 2010.

Luzar B, Calonje E. Superficial acral fibromyxoma: clinicopathological study of 14 cases with emphasis on a cellular variant. Histopathology 2009;54:374–393.

McKee PH. Pathology of the Skin, 3rd Ed. Mosby, Elsevier, 2005.

Michal M, Fanburg-Smith JC, Mentzel T, Kutzner H, Requena L, Zamecnik M, Miettinen M. Dendritic cell neurofibroma with pseudorosettes—a report of 18 cases of distinct and hitherto unrecognized neurofibroma variant. Am J Surg Pathol 2001;25(5):587–594.

New D, Bahrami S, Malone J, Callen JP. Atypical fibroxanthoma with regional lymph node metastasis. Report of a case and review of the literature. Arch Dermatol 2010;146(12):1399–1404.

Weiss SW, Goldblum JR. Enzinger and Weiss's Soft Tissue Tumors, 5th Ed. Mosby, 2007.

Note: Page locators followed by f and t indicates figure and table respectively.